The Quest for Quality in the NHS

A chartbook on quality of care in the UK

Sheila Leatherman
Kim Sutherland

Foreword by
Denis Pereira Gray

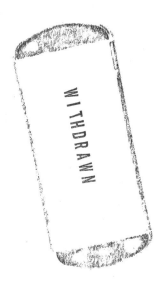

WITHDRAWN

Radcliffe Publishing
Oxford · Seattle

Radcliffe Publishing Ltd
18 Marcham Road
Abingdon
Oxon OX14 1AA
United Kingdom

www.radcliffe-oxford.com

Electronic catalogue and worldwide online ordering facility.

British Library Cataloguing in Publication Data

A catalogue record for this book is available from the British Library.

ISBN 1 85775 790 4

Typeset by Anne Joshua & Associates, Oxford
Printed and bound by Nuffield Press Ltd., Abingdon, Oxon

Contents

The Nuffield Trust

FOR RESEARCH AND POLICY
STUDIES IN HEALTH SERVICES

The Nuffield Trust is one of the leading independent health policy charitable trusts in the UK. It was established as the Nuffield Provincial Hospitals Trust in 1940 by Viscount Nuffield (William Morris), the founder of Morris Motors. In 1998 the Trustees agreed that the official name of the trust should more fully reflect the Trust's purposes and, in consultation with the Charity Commission, adopted the name The Nuffield Trust for Research and Policy Studies in Health Services, retaining 'The Nuffield Trust' as its working name.

The Nuffield Trust's mission is to promote independent analysis and informed debate on UK healthcare policy. The Nuffield Trust's purpose is to communicate evidence and encourage an exchange around developed or developing knowledge in order to illuminate recognised and emerging issues.

It achieves this through its principal activities:

- bringing together a wide national and international network of people involved in UK healthcare through a series of meetings, workshops and seminars
- commissioning research through its publications and grants programme to inform policy debate
- encouraging inter-disciplinary exchange between clinicians, legislators, academics, healthcare professionals and management, policy makers, industrialists and consumer groups
- supporting evidence-based health policy and practice
- sharing its knowledge in the home countries and internationally through partnerships and alliances.

To find out more, please refer to our website or contact:

The Nuffield Trust
59 New Cavendish St
London
W1G 7LP
Website: www.nuffieldtrust.org.uk
Email: mail@nuffieldtrust.org.uk
Tel: +44 (0)20 7631 8458
Fax: +44 (0)20 7631 8451

Charity number: 209201

Other Nuffield Trust publications

The Quest for Quality in the NHS: a mid-term evaluation of the ten-year quality agenda
Professor Sheila Leatherman and Dr Kim Sutherland

This report examines the return on the investment in quality of healthcare made in the NHS by the government since they came to power in 1997. This study presents a follow-on to a report published in 1998 at the outset of the Labour Government's reform: *Evolving Quality in the New NHS. Policy, process and pragmatic considerations*, which is also available from The Nuffield Trust. *Quest for Quality in the NHS* offers current analysis of progress made with improving the quality of healthcare in the NHS and, in Chapter nine, contains the most up-to-date analysis of the performance of the English NHS since the abolition of the internal market in 1997.
ISBN 0 11 703286 7   Price: £30.00
A4 Paperback: pp69   2003

Improving the Credibility of Information on Health Care Outcomes: the cardiac surgery demonstration project
Leon G Fine, Bruce E Keogh, Maria Orlando, Shan Cretin, Mairi M Gould, Edited by Caroline White

This report, based on a study carried out jointly with RAND and the Society of Cardiothoracic Surgeons of Great Britain and Ireland, is a contribution to the discussion on the need for systematic internal and external monitoring of the clinical performance of healthcare professionals and hospitals. It demonstrates the feasibility of producing and publishing risk-adjusted data on the outcome of cardiac artery bypass graft surgery (CABG) and should be essential reading for anyone concerned with how clinical outcome data should be produced and disseminated in the public domain.
ISBN 1-902089-90-1   Price: £10.50
A4 paperback: pp40   2003

Foreword

The Nuffield Trust has long been interested in the quality of healthcare. Its Trustees have continued to back a variety of approaches in clarifying issues and informing patients, professionals and policy makers.

Perhaps best known was the Trust's Rock Carling Lecture by Professor Archie Cochrane (1972) whose *Effectiveness and Efficiency* proved a world famous stimulus to the evidence-based movement and which has now spawned Cochrane centres around the world.

On the patient-centred approach, the Trust was fortunate to have John Fry as a Trustee for many years and he espoused the patient-centred generalist philosophy of care. More recently, the Trust has supported work on the analysis of individual performance by one group of surgeons (Fine *et al.*, 2003)

The third approach has been more recent. The Trust has been pleased to publish the work of Professor Sheila Leatherman. The book by Sheila Leatherman and Kim Sutherland (2003) provided fascinating comparisons between five English speaking nations – Australia, Canada, New Zealand, the UK and the USA. In effect, it benchmarked the NHS. This proved to be one of the major recent statements on the quality of care in the NHS.

Leatherman and Sutherland have continued to apply their techniques within the UK. This is particularly timely as the advent of devolution makes such benchmarking of great interest. Health is now a devolved function in Northern Ireland, Scotland and Wales and the UK seems to be developing four increasingly different health services. The Trust's interest in this is long established (most recently in *The New EU Health Policy and the NHS Systems* (Greer SL, 2005)).

This chart book is both a method and a result. It is a method in that it shows what can be done and offers a model of what ideally should be regular recurrent reporting by some organisation independent of Government and the Department of Health. It is a result in that it displays more clearly than is available elsewhere the present position in healthcare in four different parts of the UK.

The Trustees are most grateful to Sheila Leatherman and Kim Sutherland and are pleased to publish this chart book with Radcliffe Publishing.

Denis Pereira Gray
Chairman of the Trustees
The Nuffield Trust
May 2005

References

Cochrane A (1972) *Effectiveness and Efficiency*. Nuffield Trust, London.

Fine LG, *et al.* (2003) *Improving the Credibility of Information on Health Care Outcomes: the cardiac surgery demonstration project*. Nuffield Trust, London.

Greer SL (2005) *The New EU Health Policy and the NHS Systems*. Nuffield Trust, London.

Leatherman S and Sutherland K (2003) *The Quest for Quality in the NHS: a mid-term evaluation of the ten-year quality agenda*. TSO, Norwich.

This chartbook is a compendium of data, encapsulating the efforts of many analysts and researchers who study the healthcare systems in the United Kingdom and other countries. We are indebted to all those who have produced useful data and are involved in efforts to further the field of quality measurement and performance assessment.

We owe a special debt of gratitude to The Nuffield Trust, in particular to John Wyn Owen, who first invited us to evaluate the quality improvement efforts instigated in England in 1997. The Nuffield Trust supports health policy work, both ours and that of a much wider network of colleagues around the world, and makes a valuable contribution to many varied policy debates. This chartbook represents the sequel to our report published by The Nuffield Trust in 2003, *The Quest for Quality in the NHS: a mid-term evaluation of the ten-year quality agenda.*

For many years our work has benefited from excellent support in England, most notably from the Chief Medical Officer (CMO) Professor Sir Liam Donaldson, and experts from a range of organisations. For their help and advice in the production of this chartbook, we owe particular thanks to John Fox from the Health and Social Care Information Centre; Michael Fleming from the Department of Health; Veena Raleigh, Robert Irons, Paul Sims and Gerrard Abi-Aad from the Healthcare Commission; and Azim Lakhani, Daniel Eayres and Jim Coles from the National Centre for Health Outcomes Development (NCHOD).

We would like to acknowledge and thank the various individuals who have helped us through the maze of data and the complicated contextual issues in Scotland, Wales and Northern Ireland, in particular: Ruth Hall, Ken Alexander, Robin Jones and Wendy Chatham in Wales; and David Steel, Rod Muir and Graham Mitchell in Scotland. We also thank Northern Ireland's Deputy Chief Medical Officer Ian Carson for his interest in this endeavour and the stated ambition to work with us more closely on future related projects.

Douglas McCarthy, who is a co-author of three chartbooks published in the US, has been a source of invaluable help and advice in the conceptual and technical tasks of this project. Kathleen Lohr at RTI International in North Carolina has provided excellent review and editing. Sandra Dawson at the Judge Institute of Management, University of Cambridge, has over many years been an unstinting supporter of our work. Behind the scenes, but playing critical roles in administrative and research support and publishing assistance, are Sara Massie and Sue Tolleson-Rinehart at University of North Carolina, Kim Beazor and Helena Scott at The Nuffield Trust, Lindsey Clarke at the Health Foundation, and Paula Moran at Radcliffe Publishing.

Finally, we would like to express our appreciation to the people, too many to list here, who have encouraged us over the past seven years, tirelessly answering queries, providing policy context and forthright advice. We can honestly say that we have never been turned down in our many, many searches, whether it be for one more piece of data to fill a specific hole, or for perspectives and insights on 'the big questions'.

It continues to be our pleasure and privilege to work with the venerable institution of the National Health Service.

Sheila Leatherman
Kim Sutherland

Sheila Leatherman, an internationally recognised health expert, is Research Professor at the School of Public Health, The University of North Carolina at Chapel Hill, and a Senior Associate of The Judge Institute of Management and Distinguished Associate of Darwin College at the University of Cambridge, England. She conducts research and policy analysis in the United States and the United Kingdom, focusing on quality of care, health systems reform, performance measurement and improvement, and the economic implications of implementing quality enhancing interventions in healthcare delivery. Leatherman is an elected member of the Institute of Medicine of the US National Academy of Sciences (2002) and an elected member of the National Academy of Social Insurance (1997).

Professor Leatherman is widely published and is author of a series of chartbooks on quality of healthcare in the US, supported by the Commonwealth Fund; general (2002), child health (2004), Medicare (2005). In the UK, she was commissioned by The Nuffield Trust to assess the Government's proposed quality reforms for the National Health Service in 1997–98 and evaluated the mid-term impact of the 10-year quality agenda in the NHS, resulting in publication of the book, *Quest for Quality in the NHS*, in December 2003. This book is the sequel.

Appointed by President Clinton, she served on the President's Advisory Commission on Consumer Protection and Quality in the Health Care (1997–98), chairing the sub-committee to develop a national strategy for quality measurement and reporting, subsequently serving as Co-Chair of the Strategic Framework Board tasked to develop the blueprint for the newly developing National Quality Forum of the US (1999–2000). She has a broad background in healthcare management in State and Federal health agencies, as chief executive of a Health Maintenance Organisation (HMO), and as senior executive of the largest national managed care company in the US. She is a Trustee of the American Board of Internal Medicine Foundation, a Senior Advisor to The Nuffield Trust (UK) and to The Health Foundation (UK), and serves on the Board of Directors of the international organisation Freedom From Hunger.

Kim Sutherland BSc, MSc, MBA, PhD is a Senior Research Associate at the Judge Institute of Management, University of Cambridge. Her work concentrates on interactions between research evidence, policy and clinical practice within the NHS. Her current research interests focus on quality of healthcare, and organisational change. In 1997–98, together with Sheila Leatherman, she was funded by The Nuffield Trust to evaluate the Labour Government's 10-year quality agenda for the NHS. In 2002–03, the same team undertook a mid-term review of progress in implementing that agenda and improving performance.

She is currently working as co-Principal Investigator in a multi-disciplinary, multiyear project, funded by the Health Foundation, which seeks to monitor performance and inform efforts to improve quality and cost-effectiveness in the NHS. Her work has been published both in peer-reviewed journals, including *British Medical Journal, Quality and Safety in Health Care, International Studies of Management and Organisation* and *Journal of Health Services Research and Policy*, and in books – as co-author of *Organisational Change: a review for health care managers, professionals and researchers* (for which she was awarded the British Association of Medical Managers' Book of the Year Award 2002) and *The Quest for Quality in the NHS: a mid-term evaluation of the ten-year quality agenda* (2003) and as a contributing author in *The Encyclopaedic Dictionary of Organisational Behaviour* (2005).

Summary of charts

Chart	Level of Analysis	Data Source	Findings	Page
1 Effectiveness				
1.1 Mortality from causes considered amenable to healthcare	1.1a UK and four international comparators 1998 1.1b England, Wales 1993–2003	National statistics ONS	In 1998, the UK had the highest mortality rates of the five countries compared (87.4/100 000 and 173.1/100 000 including and excluding ischaemic heart disease, respectively). Mortality rates were consistently higher in Wales than in England. Both countries have seen a steady decline in rates, reflecting improvements in healthcare.	2
1.2 Cancer mortality rates: international comparison	UK and five international comparators	OECD	Mortality rates from cancer in the UK have been falling steadily, but in 1999 were still high relative to comparator countries. In 1999, 184.7 deaths per 100 000 were attributed to cancer in the UK, compared to 151.3 deaths per 100 000 in Sweden.	4
1.3 Mortality rates from common cancers (lung, colorectal, breast and prostate)	1.3a UK males 1990–2002 1.3b UK females 1990–2002	ONS	Mortality rates for the four most common cancers have declined since 1990. Particularly noteworthy is the marked decrease in the death rate for lung cancer among males, from 87.9 deaths per 100 000 in 1990 to 58.3 deaths per 100 000 in 2002. Mortality rates for lung cancer in women remained fairly static.	5
1.4 Premature deaths from cancer: progress against a target	England 1995–2002	ONS	Between 1995–97 and 2000–02, England achieved a 10% reduction in the cancer mortality rate.	6
1.5 Five-year relative survival rates for common cancers (lung, colon, breast, prostate)	England and Wales 1991–95 and 1996–99 Scotland 1992–96 and 1997–2001	ONS ISD Scotland	Five-year survival rates rose in all four common cancers over time. The greatest improvement was in prostate cancer survival rates, which increased by 9.4% in Scotland between 1992–96 and 1997–2001; and by 11.2% in England between 1991–95 and 1996–99. England and Wales differed little from Scotland in terms of survival rates.	7
1.6 Breast cancer mortality rates	England and four international comparators 1990 and 1999	Commonwealth Fund International Working Group on Quality Indicators	Despite a 21% reduction between 1990 and 1999, England continued to have the highest breast cancer mortality rates among these comparator countries: 28.9 deaths per 100 000 as compared to the lowest rate in Australia, with 21.9 per 100 000.	9

Chart	Level of Analysis	Data Source	Findings	Page
1.7 Breast cancer survival and screening rates	1.7a England and four international comparators ~1992–97, ~2000 1.7b Intra-UK 1999–2002	Commonwealth Fund International Working Group on Quality Indicators ONS	Of the five countries compared, the US had the highest survival rates from breast cancer, with 86% of women alive five years after diagnosis; and England had the lowest, with 75%. Within UK countries, screening rates ranged from 67% coverage in Wales to 75% coverage in Scotland.	10
1.8 Colorectal cancer mortality rates	1.8a England and four international comparators 1990 and 1999 1.8b Intra-UK 2002	Commonwealth Fund International Working Group on Quality Indicators ONS	Between 1990 and 1999, deaths from colorectal cancer fell significantly. In 1999, of the countries compared, New Zealand had the highest mortality rate (28.0 per 100 000 population) and the US the lowest (17.4 per 100 000). Within the UK, England had the lowest rate and Scotland the highest. UK colorectal cancer mortality rates differ between males and females. The difference in 2002 was at its widest in Scotland where the male mortality rate was 78% higher than the female rate.	12
1.9 Colorectal cancer survival rates	Scotland 1977–2001 (time of diagnosis)	Scottish Cancer Registry, ISD	Improvement in survival rates from colorectal cancer (in patients 15–74 years) has been sustained and substantial. More people survived for 10 years following a diagnosis in the early 1990s than survived for three years following a diagnosis in the late 1970s. Female survival for 1997–2001 was generally higher than male survival.	13
1.10 Childhood leukaemia survival rates	England and four international comparators ~1992–97	Commonwealth Fund International Working Group on Quality Indicators	Survival rates for childhood leukaemias are high. In England, three-quarters of children diagnosed with leukaemia were alive five years after initial diagnosis; a rate comparable with that in other countries.	15
1.11 Circulatory disease mortality rates	1.11a UK and five international comparators 1990–2001 1.11b UK 1971–2002	OECD ONS	UK mortality rates from circulatory disease have shown a marked decrease. UK rates were similar to the EU average rate in 1999 (data not shown) although they were among the highest of the comparator countries. In the UK the drop in mortality rates was 55% for both males and females in the 30 years between 1972 and 2002.	17
1.12 Premature deaths from circulatory disease: progress against a target	England 1995–2002	ONS	*Our Healthier Nation* (1999) set a target to reduce the death rate from circulatory disease among people under 75 years by at least 40% by 2010, using 1995–97 as a baseline. As of 2002, a 23% reduction in the rate of deaths had been achieved.	18

Chart	Level of Analysis	Data Source	Findings	Page
1.13 Mortality from coronary heart disease	UK and five international comparators 1999	WHO mortality database	In 1999, the UK had the highest mortality rate in people aged $\leq$ 75 years from CHD among the comparator countries. Compared to France, UK mortality rates were four times higher for females and around three times higher for males.	20
1.14 Coronary heart disease mortality rates	Intra-UK 1997–2002	ONS	For both males and females, Scotland had the highest mortality rate from CHD. In 2002, there were 246 male deaths and 96 female deaths per 100 000 population attributed to CHD in Scotland, compared to 192 male and 65 female deaths per 100 000 in England, which had the lowest rates.	21
1.15 Explaining the decline in CHD mortality	England and Wales 1981–2000	Unal et al., 2004	Smoking cessation was the largest contributor to the declining mortality rate from CHD; it was estimated to account for almost half of the rate of decline. Clinical processes and treatment contributed 42% of the overall deaths prevented or postponed; personal risk factors or behavioural factors contributed 58%.	22
1.16 Mortality from acute myocardial infarction	England and four international comparators 1990 and 1999	Commonwealth Fund International Working Group on Quality Indicators	Mortality rates from AMI have decreased significantly in recent years. England's mortality rate fell by 42% between 1990 and 1999. Despite this considerable progress, mortality rates in England remained high in comparison to those in comparator countries.	24
1.17 Managing acute myocardial infarcts	England, 2002–04; and Wales 2004	MINAP	The percentage of hospitals achieving the targets for DTN30 and secondary prevention of AMI improved greatly since 2002. In 2004, Welsh hospitals, although performing extremely well in secondary prevention measures, did less well in the thrombolysis measures; none achieved the CTN60 standard.	25
1.18 Thrombolysis rates after AMI	England 2002–04	MINAP	In March 2002, 59% of patients were treated within 30 minutes of arriving at hospital. By September 2004, this figure had increased to 84%. The proportion of people being thrombolysed within one hour of calling for professional help, which is clinically more meaningful, was 32% in March 2002 and 54% in September 2004.	26

Chart	Level of Analysis	Data Source	Findings	Page
1.19 Revascularisation rates and mortality from heart disease	UK and four international comparators 2000	OECD	The relationship between mortality rates from heart disease and the rate of revascularisation is weak. Most noteworthy are results from the UK, where uniquely among the countries compared, mortality rates exceed revascularisation rates, suggesting underuse of the procedure.	28
1.20 Appropriateness of revascularisation procedures	Case study of three London hospitals Patients tracked 1996–99 (treated 1996–97).	Hemingway et al., 2001	PTCA was substantially underused: only 36% of patients (327 of 908) who could have benefited from PTCA received it, whereas 6% of patients (34 of 568) for whom PTCA was not appropriate received it. CABG was underused: only 57% of patients (765 of 1353) who could have benefited from CABG received it, whereas 8% of patients (15 of 186) for whom CABG was not medically appropriate received it. Patients who did not receive the treatment recommended by the expert panel were more likely to suffer subsequent cardiac health problems.	29
1.21 Deaths within 30 days of coronary artery bypass graft (CABG)	England 1998–99 to 2002–03	NCHOD, using HES data	Between 1998–99 and 2002–03 a 26% decrease in the rate of deaths within 30 days of CABG was recorded.	30
1.22 Statin use in Europe	1.22a England and 13 international comparators 2000 1.22b Intra-UK 2003	1.22a Walley et al., 2004 1.22b DHSSPS, Northern Ireland	England in 2000 dispensed about 24 defined daily doses per 1000 population per day (DDD). Norway dispensed two and a half times that amount. Data for 2003 show prescribing rates for England more than double those for 2000. Among UK countries in 2003, Wales dispensed the most statins (86.2 DDDs) and England the least (50.9 DDDs).	32
1.23 Stroke mortality	1.23a England and three international comparators circa 2000 1.23b England, Wales and Scotland 1993–2003	1.23a Commonwealth Fund International Working Group on Quality Indicators 1.23b ONS, ISD Scotland	In 2001, England's mortality rate from stroke (38.8 per 100 000 population) was lower than that in Australia (47.1 per 100 000) but higher than that in the US (23.6 per 100 000) and New Zealand (10.1 per 100 000). Mortality rates in the countries of the UK have declined over the past 10 years, with Scotland showing the most rapid rate of improvement in outcomes.	34
1.24 Mortality from diabetes	England, Wales 1993–2003	DH Mortality Extracts	Mortality rates, both when diabetes is identified as the underlying cause of death and when diabetes is simply mentioned on the death certificate, remained fairly static from 1993 to 2003. Mortality rates in both categories were higher in Wales than in England.	36

Chart	Level of Analysis	Data Source	Findings	Page
1.25 Diabetic control in children	1.25a England, Wales and Northern Ireland 2002 1.25b Scotland 1993–2003	Diabetes UK; Paediatric Diabetes Audit Scottish Morbidity Records, ISD Scotland	Levels of control in diabetic children in England, Wales and Northern Ireland in 2002 were poor, with less than one in five diabetic children maintaining blood glucose readings within recommended levels. The rate of emergency admissions for diabetic children in Scotland increased by 16% between 1993 and 2003.	37
1.26 Measures indicating poor diabetic control	England 1998–99 to 2002–03	HES	The number of episodes of ketoacidosis rose 19% from 17.97 per 100 000 in 1998–99 to 21.43 in 2002–03. The rate of lower limb amputations in diabetics in England remained fairly static at about 8.5 per 100 000 between 1998–99 and 2002–03.	38
1.27 Influenza vaccinations (in people ≥ 65 years)	1.27a UK and four international comparators 2004 1.27b Intra-UK 2004	Commonwealth Fund International Health Policy Survey	Of UK respondents ≥ 65 years of age, 74% indicated that they had been vaccinated, the second highest rate of the countries compared. Within the UK, reported vaccination rates differed greatly, ranging from 62% in Wales to 82% in Scotland.	40
1.28 Childhood vaccinations by age 2	1.28a Intra-UK 2000–04 1.28b Intra-UK 1993–2004	Health Protection Agency (and country agencies)	Across the UK, the level of coverage in childhood vaccinations has generally been high (around 95%). However, MMR vaccination rates have fallen in all countries of the UK over the past 10 years; most dramatically in England from a high of 91.5% in 1996 to 79.9% in 2003.	41
1.29 Antibiotic prescribing patterns	1.29a Scotland 1996–2003 1.29b England and Wales 1998	QIS, Scotland Wrigley *et al.*, 2002	Children are normally prescribed antibiotics in liquid form (and few other patients are) so the amount of liquid antibiotics dispensed can be used as a proxy for prescribing rates in children. Between 1996 and 2003, liquid antibiotic prescribing rates fell by one-third. In 1998, prescribing rates for antibiotics among general practices in England and Wales varied more than five-fold, ranging from 300 to nearly 1597 prescriptions per 1000 patients; with a median of 660 per 1000 patients.	42
1.30 Suicide rates	England and Wales and four international comparators Circa 2000	Commonwealth Fund International Working Group on Quality Indicators	The suicide rate in England and Wales in 2000 (6.0 per 100 000 people) was low compared to rates in comparator nations. New Zealand had the highest rate with 13.2 per 100 000 overall and had an even higher rate, 29.3 per 100 000 for persons aged 20–29.	45

Chart	Level of Analysis	Data Source	Findings	Page
1.31 Suicide rates: trends over time	Intra-UK 1997–2002	ONS	Suicide rates have been fairly static since 1997, but the rate in Scotland (at 21 per 100 000 population) is almost double that of other UK countries.	46
1.32 Emergency psychiatric readmissions	England 1997–2002	Social Services Performance Assessment Framework	The number of emergency readmissions for psychiatric disorders has fallen slightly over time.	47
1.33 Surgical outcomes	Scotland 1997–2003	QIS Scotland	The percentage of patients who died within 30 days of the operation stayed fairly static at about 0.35%. Similarly, the rate of emergency readmissions following operations showed little change over time.	49
1.34 Caesarean section rates	1.34a Intra-UK and four international comparators 2000	RCOG National Sentinel Caesarean Section Audit	Caesarean section rates across the countries of the UK range from 19.3% in Scotland to 24.2% in Wales; all are outside the recommended limits. The UK results are in line with those of the US and Australia but higher than for several European comparators. Rates of caesarean sections across NHS Trusts in England range from 6% to 34%. Fifteen percent of NHS Trusts of England have a caesarean section rate of 23%.	50
	1.34b NHS Trusts in England 2002–03	Healthcare Commission (HES data)		

2 Access

Chart	Level of Analysis	Data Source	Findings	Page
2.1 Waiting for elective surgery: international comparisons	2.1a UK and four international comparators 1998, 2001	Commonwealth Fund	The UK in 1998 and 2001 had high numbers of patients waiting; and in 2000 had long waits for elective surgery, relative to comparative countries.	57
	2.1b England and three international comparators 2000	OECD		
2.2 Proportion of population waiting for inpatient admission: UK countries, 2004	Intra-UK 2004	Official statistics, Department of Health and equivalents	In September 2004, England had the lowest number of people on the inpatient waiting list (16.9 per 1000 population) and Northern Ireland had the highest (29.8).	58
2.3 Excessive waits: intra-UK comparison	Intra-UK 2004	Official statistics, Department of Health and equivalents	In September 2004, the percentage of patients on the inpatient waiting list who had been waiting more than six months ranged from 7% in Scotland to 36% in Wales (data not available for NI); the percentage waiting more than 12 months ranged from 0% in England and Scotland to 13% in Northern Ireland. Longitudinal data from England showed significant improvement from 1999.	59

Chart	Level of Analysis	Data Source	Findings	Page
2.4 Number of patients waiting for hospital admission and median length of waits	2.4a England 1999–2000 to 2004–05 2.4b England 1997–2004	Department of Health	The number of English patients who had been waiting more than six months for hospital admission fell from 275 621 in 1999 to 75 050 in 2004. Since 2003 there has been no quarter when more than 100 patients had been waiting longer than 12 months. Median waiting times also show considerable, although less dramatic, improvement from a peak of 14.2 weeks in 1998 to 10.2 in 2004.	60
2.5 Cancelled operations and rescheduling	England 1998–2004	Department of Health	The number of operations cancelled at the last minute for non-clinical reasons has made no significant sustained improvement over the past six years. The number of patients who did not have their operations rescheduled for within 28 days following a cancellation has fallen from a peak of 5437 in 2001 to 1410 in September 2004.	61
2.6 Delayed discharges	England and Scotland 2000–04	Department of Health ISD Scotland	The number of delayed discharges in English hospitals has decreased steadily from 7065 in September 2001 to 2742 in September 2004. Data for Scotland show that the number of delayed discharges has dropped since 2000; nonetheless in October 2004 there were 1908 patients affected, 1109 of which had been ready for transfer for over six weeks. The two countries use different definitions for delayed discharges.	62
2.7 Outpatient waits	2.7a Completed outpatient waits, England, Scotland, Northern Ireland 1999–2000 to 2004–05 2.7b Outpatient waiting list, Wales and Northern Ireland 2000–01 to 2003–04	Department of Health and equivalents	The percentage of patients who waited over 13 weeks for an outpatient appointment between 1999–2000 and 2004–05 fell in England (by 7.8%) but rose in Northern Ireland (by 7.9%) and in Scotland (by 8.1%). Chart 2.7b shows data for Wales and Northern Ireland and is based on waiting lists on a given day i.e. of all patients on the waiting list at the end of the month/quarter, the percentage who had been waiting over 13 weeks. Between 2000–01 and 2003–04 the percentage of patients waiting over 13 weeks increased by 5.2% in Wales and 6.9% in Northern Ireland.	63
2.8 Waiting in Accident and Emergency	UK and four international comparators 2004	Commonwealth Fund International Health Policy Survey	82% of UK respondents indicated that they were treated in A&E in less than four hours, a figure broadly in line with comparator countries (AUS 87%; CAN 74%; NZ 86%; US 87%).	64

Chart	Level of Analysis	Data Source	Findings	Page
2.9 Waits for primary care	2.9a UK and four international comparators 2.9b Intra-UK 2004	Commonwealth Fund International Health Policy Survey	Patient reports of access to primary care within 48 hours saw the UK (59%) outperform both the US (51%) and Canada (42%) although more prompt attention was reported by New Zealand (84%) and Australian (75%) respondents. Within the UK, 60% of English respondents were seen on the same or next day, compared to 45% in Scotland.	66
2.10 Waits for primary care appointments	England 2003 and 2004	Healthcare Commission patient surveys	Almost one-quarter of respondents, in both surveys, waited longer than 48 hours for a primary care appointment.	67
2.11 Using A&E for primary care	UK and four international comparators 2004	Commonwealth Fund International Health Policy Survey	In response to a question regarding whether recent A&E visits would have been necessary if appropriate primary care had been available (a proxy measure for access to primary care), the UK had the best result. About one-fifth of UK respondents that had been to A&E indicated that their visit was a result of poor access to primary care, compared to about half of American and Canadian respondents.	68
2.12 Coronary heart disease waits for diagnostic or therapeutic interventions	Scotland 2003–04	ISD Scotland	In September 2004, 88.3% of Scottish patients were waiting less than the target time of eight weeks for angiography, and 100% of patients waited less than the target 18 weeks for revascularisation surgery.	70
2.13 Cancer waits: progress against Government commitments	England 2004	Department of Health	Commitments for timeliness of cancer care were made in *The NHS Plan* (2000) and *The Cancer Plan* (2000). In September 2004, 99.5% of patients referred urgently to cancer specialists were seen within two weeks; 97.5% of breast cancer patients waited less than a month between diagnosis and commencing treatment; and 96.5% of breast cancer patients waited less than two months from urgent GP referral to treatment.	71

3 Capacity

Chart	Level of Analysis	Data Source	Findings	Page
3.1 Spending on health	UK and five international comparators 1980–2002	OECD	Spending on health has increased considerably over the past 20 years. The UK spends less than many comparable nations on health, both in terms of per capita spend and spend as a percentage of GDP. Between 2000 and 2002 spending in the UK increased by 17% (per capita $US PPP) and by 0.4% of GDP.	74

Chart	Level of Analysis	Data Source	Findings	Page
3.9 Imaging equipment	UK and four international comparators 2000, 2001–02	OECD	In 2001 Germany and the US had more than double the number (13.3 and 12.8 per million population, respectively) of computerised tomography (CT) scanners than the UK (5.8 per million). The UK also had a relatively low number of magnetic resonance imaging (MRI) units in relation to comparator countries.	82
3.10 Percutaneous coronary interventions	3.10a UK time series 1997–2003 3.10b Intra-UK comparison 2003	BCIS Audit	PCI rates for the UK increased by 122% between 1997 and 2003. Within the UK, rates of PCI per million population in 2003 ranged from 592 in Wales to 1044 in Northern Ireland. As a reference point, in 2001 the PCI rate in the US was approximately 1700 per million population.	83
3.11 Stroke units	England, Wales and Northern Ireland 2004	National Sentinel Stroke Audit CEEU, Royal College of Physicians	Of all hospitals in three UK countries, 82% in England, 45% in Wales and 85% in Northern Ireland have a dedicated stroke unit. Such units have been shown to improve stroke outcomes.	84
3.12 Acute stroke units: facilities audit	England, Wales and Northern Ireland 2004	National Sentinel Stroke Audit CEEU, Royal College of Physicians	The facilities (such as continuous physiological monitoring, access to 24-hour brain imaging) provided by acute stroke units are unevenly distributed.	85
3.13 Mental health services teams	England 2000–04	Annual Service Mapping Exercise, University of Durham	Growth in the number of mental healthcare teams in England has been considerable. The number of assertive outreach teams increased from 130 in 2000 to 271 in Spring 2004, achieving a NHS Plan target. Over the same period, 179 crisis resolution teams and 41 early intervention teams were established. In both cases, however, these figures reflect a shortfall on NHS Plan targets.	86

4 Safety

Chart	Level of Analysis	Data Source	Findings	Page
4.1 Adverse events: routine data source	England 1999–00 to 2002–03	Hospital Episode Statistics (HES)	Of all hospital episodes, 2.2% were coded for an adverse event. Underreporting of adverse events in routine data remains a concern.	92
4.2 Adverse events: case notes review	Two acute hospitals in London 1999–2000	Retrospective review of 1014 medical and nursing records	One in 10 patients experienced an adverse event during a hospital stay. About one-half of these events were judged preventable with ordinary standards of NHS care. One-third of adverse events led to moderate or greater disability or death.	93

Chart	Level of Analysis	Data Source	Findings	Page
4.3 Adverse events under surgical care	Scotland 1998–2003	Scottish Audit of Surgical Mortality	The number of surgical cases with areas of concern in management that caused or contributed to death shows a sustained reduction over five years.	94
4.4 Errors in the preparation of intravenous infusions: observational study	10 wards; 2 UK hospitals, one teaching, one non-teaching (each with about 20 wards and 400 beds) 1999	Prospective observation study of 430 intravenous drug doses	At least one error was identified in almost half of the observed intravenous infusions. Three doses (~1% of total observed) had potentially severe errors, 126 (29%) potentially moderate errors and 83 (19%) had potentially minor errors.	96
4.5 Errors in the preparation of intravenous infusions: acetylcysteine	184 infusion bags in four hospitals in England, Wales, and Scotland 1999	Prospective collection of pre- and post-infusion samples from infusion bags and subsequent assay	Just over one-third of infusions were within 10% of the ordered dose; two-thirds were within 20%. Concentration of active drug for one in 10 of the infusions was more than 50% different from the intended dose.	97
4.6 Infusion error incident study	Six pilot site hospitals in England and Wales 2003	Internal audits by pilot sites	The pilot study identified 321 infusion-related incidents occurring in six NHS Trusts over one year.	98
4.7 Healthcare-associated infections post-surgery	England, 168 hospitals 1997–2002	Health Protection Agency	Of 107 492 patients on whom an operation was performed, 4% contracted a healthcare-associated infection.	100
4.8 Healthcare-associated infections as a factor in surgical mortality	Scotland 2003	Scottish Audit of Surgical Mortality	Of 4084 audited deaths in hospital under surgical care, 344 (8.4%) patients had developed a healthcare-associated infection.	101
4.9 MRSA as a proportion of all *Staphylococcus aureus* bacteraemias	UK data, European comparators 1999–2002	European Antimicrobial Resistance Surveillance System (EARSS)	The proportion of *Staph aureus* blood culture isolates that are methicillin-resistant (MRSA) varies widely across Europe. The highest proportion of MRSA was in Greece (44.4%); the lowest was in the Netherlands (0.6%). The UK's result was among the highest at 41.5%.	102
4.10 MRSA bacteraemia rates	Intra-UK 2003–04	Health Protection Agency (and equivalents)	Rates of MRSA bacteraemia range from 0.11 cases per 1000 bed days in Wales to 0.18 cases per 1000 bed days in England.	103
4.11 Deaths involving MRSA	England and Wales 1993–2002	ONS (Health Statistics Quarterly 21)	During 1993 to 2002, MRSA mortality rates (i.e. MRSA mentioned on death certificate) in England and Wales increased more than 15-fold (from 51 to 800 deaths).	104
4.12 Hospital effectiveness at finding and addressing medical error: physicians' views	UK and four international comparators 2000	Commonwealth Fund International Health Policy Survey	Doctors in the UK rated the hospitals in which they work quite poorly in terms of their ability to find and address medical errors; only 3% of respondents rated their hospital excellent.	106

Chart	Level of Analysis	Data Source	Findings	Page
4.13 Safety views of hospital executives	UK and four international comparators 2003	Commonwealth Fund International Health Policy Survey	Almost one-quarter of hospital executives surveyed in the UK considered that their systems for finding and addressing errors were very effective; a figure that was the highest (together with that in the US) among the surveyed countries. Of respondents in the UK, 35% indicated that the physicians in their hospitals were very supportive of reporting and addressing medical errors – the highest proportion within any of the surveyed countries to do so.	107
4.14 Medical errors and their consequences: patients' perspective	UK and four international comparators 2002	Commonwealth Fund International Health Policy Survey	Almost one in five UK respondents indicated that they had experienced a mistake or error; half of those (9% of total sample) reported that these errors had serious consequences for their health. The UK had the lowest rate of reported errors and mistakes and the lowest level of health consequences resulting from those errors and mistakes.	108
4.15 Medication errors: patients' perspective	UK and four international comparators 2002 and 2004	Commonwealth Fund International Health Policy Survey	In two surveys, one of adults with health problems and one of primary care patients, the UK had the lowest level of medication errors reported by respondents. However, one in 10 adults with health problems reported a medication error.	109
4.16 Safety issues after discharge from hospital	England (inpatients and young patients) 2004	Healthcare Commission	The vast majority of patients had the purpose of their medicines clearly explained to them upon discharge from hospital. Nonetheless, 44% of inpatient respondents and 31% of young patient respondents indicated that a member of staff did *not* tell them about possible side effects. Further, 41% of inpatients and 14% of young patients were *not* told about danger signals to watch for when they got home.	110
4.17 Managing polypharmacy risks	UK and four international comparators 2004	Commonwealth Fund International Health Policy Survey	UK respondents were the least likely of the five surveyed countries to have had a thorough medications review with their general practitioners in the past two years (37% reported not having had such a review).	111

Chart	Level of Analysis	Data Source	Findings	Page
5 Patient-centredness				
5.1 Extent of change required in healthcare system	5.1a UK and four international comparators 5.1b Intra-UK	Commonwealth Fund International Health Policy Survey	UK respondents were the most satisfied with their healthcare system. Only 13% of UK respondents indicated that their healthcare system required a complete rebuild compared to 33% of US respondents. UK respondents also had the highest proportion of respondents (26%) indicating that only minor change was required. Attitudes across UK countries were fairly uniform.	117
5.2 Extent of change required in healthcare system: time series	UK 1998–2004	Commonwealth Fund International Health Policy Survey	No marked change in views about the extent of change required in the healthcare system is obvious. Consistently, about 25% of respondents indicated that minor change is required; and about 15% answered that a complete rebuild is required.	118
5.3 Getting better or worse? Public perceptions of the NHS in Scotland	Scotland 2000 and 2004	Public Attitudes to the NHS in Scotland Survey	The view of recent NHS performance was more positive in 2004 than in 2000. Of the respondents, 39% were optimistic about the future of the NHS in Scotland, 23% were pessimistic.	119
5.4 Patient ratings of hospital and mental healthcare in England	England 2002 and 2004	Healthcare Commission Patient Surveys	For the three surveys that focused on hospital care, between 74% and 79% of respondents indicated that care was excellent or good. Mental health patients were less satisfied with the care they received; 54% rated it excellent or good.	120
5.5 Public ratings of healthcare services in Northern Ireland	Northern Ireland 2004	Public Attitudes to Health and Personal Social Services in Northern Ireland Survey	The vast majority of respondents were satisfied with the care they received on an individual level; ratings of very satisfied or satisfied ranged from 95% for GP services to 90% for outpatient services and 89% for inpatient services. More than 75% indicated that they were satisfied with the health service overall.	121
5.6 Public ratings of healthcare services in Scotland	Scotland 2004	Public Attitudes to the NHS in Scotland Survey	The proportions of respondents indicating that they were very or fairly satisfied with the NHS services they had used in the previous 12 months were: 93% for GP services; 90% for inpatient services; 88% for out-of-hours services; 86% for outpatient services; and 85% for the NHS overall. The proportion of respondents who were *very* satisfied with the NHS overall was lower (37%) than that for GP, inpatient, outpatient and out-of-hours services (53–62%).	122

Chart	Level of Analysis	Data Source	Findings	Page
5.7 Importance of more choice over hospital	Britain 2004	Economist /YouGov survey	One-quarter of respondents indicated that choice of hospital was very important to them. Almost two-thirds said hospital choice was very or fairly important.	124
5.8 Choice of doctor	UK and four international comparators 2004	Commonwealth Fund International Health Policy Survey	Of all UK respondents, 80% indicated that they were satisfied with the amount of choice they had in the doctors they saw. This figure was broadly in line with responses from comparator countries.	125
5.9 Choice in referrals	England and Scotland 2004	Healthcare Commission Patient Surveys Public Attitudes to the NHS in Scotland Survey	Almost one-quarter of English inpatient survey respondents indicated that they were given a choice of admission date, as did 34% of Scottish respondents. Of English primary care respondents 74% indicated that they were not offered a choice in where they were referred. Only 16% of respondents would have welcomed such a choice but were not offered one.	126
5.10 Involvement in decision-making	England 2004	Healthcare Commission Patient Surveys	In surveys of primary care patients and of parents/ guardians of young patients, 69% indicated that they were definitely involved as much as they wanted to be in decisions about care. Rates were lower for inpatients and young patients (just over half) and even lower for mental health patients (only 41%).	127
5.11 Interactions with general practitioners	5.11a UK and four international comparators 5.11b Intra-UK 2004	Commonwealth Fund International Health Policy Survey	Results indicated a generally positive view of doctor–patient interactions. However, time pressures may be affecting patients' perceptions of quality. Only 66% of New Zealand, 63% of Australian, 58% of UK, 55% of Canadian and 44% of US respondents indicated that doctors *always* spend enough time with them. Within the UK, results were fairly uniform, except for London where scores were considerably lower.	128
5.12 Communicating about treatment options in primary care	Intra-UK and two international comparators 2004	Commonwealth Fund International Health Policy Survey	About two-thirds of respondents in each country indicated that instructions were always given clearly; about one-half were told of specific goals and plans. However, only about one-quarter (with the exception of Australia, 43%) indicated that an active dialogue always took place.	129

For more than 50 years the NHS has provided the citizens of the United Kingdom with comprehensive healthcare services that are, for the most part, free at the point of delivery. During that time, patients have benefited greatly from advances in knowledge and technology, effective public health interventions and, in recent years, a growing emphasis on patient-centredness. Despite these many benefits, concerns about the quality of healthcare are both widespread and serious.

Upon taking power in 1997, the Labour Government embarked on a 10-year reform agenda and clearly emphasised the central role of quality improvement in its drive to modernise public services. In the health arena, the quality agenda in England resulted in what we have previously described as the 'most ambitious, comprehensive, systemic and intentionally funded effort to create predictable and sustainable capacity for improving the quality of a nation's healthcare system' (Leatherman and Sutherland, 2003: p1).

Although a considerable number of programmes and organisations have focused on improving quality since 1997, there are few coherent, independent reports that provide a comprehensive, reliable, balanced and rigorous account of the strengths and weaknesses of quality in healthcare delivery in England, and none that portray the wider UK picture. Despite the fact that deficiencies in quality of care are recognised as an international problem, and that significant assets are spent on the performance of the NHS in particular, we lack the information necessary to develop a common understanding of the key problem areas, acknowledge successes from which valuable lessons can be learned, and inform health policy that will drive predictable healthcare improvements over time. This is particularly troublesome because health is a highly politicised topic in the UK. There is a maelstrom of conflicting accounts, claims and counterclaims. The press and electronic media report almost daily on concerns and problems occurring in the NHS. Opinion polls and patient surveys consistently report a paradoxical

mix of commitment to the principles of the NHS, generalised satisfaction with individual experiences, and concerns about the performance of the system as a whole. This confusion may be rooted in, and is certainly exacerbated by, the lack of a shared understanding of how the NHS is performing in terms of quality of care.

This chartbook builds on our previous report, *The Quest for Quality in the NHS: a mid-term evaluation of the ten-year quality agenda* (Leatherman and Sutherland, 2003). That work, funded by The Nuffield Trust, noted that the 10-year reform agenda in England had, at its midpoint, made considerable progress, demonstrating a number of early successes and auguring predictable capacity for more improvements in the NHS. At the same time, it sounded a note of concern regarding the 'lack of a shared robust information base that provides a common understanding of the NHS's strengths and weaknesses'. This chartbook seeks to demonstrate the feasibility and desirability of having independently and routinely reported quality of care data for the UK. The potential benefit from such data is significant, providing a basis for communication and cooperation among the many stakeholders in healthcare, in their pursuit of improving performance.

What do we mean by quality?

Quality is a multifaceted concept. The complex and intricate network of stakeholders in healthcare is populated with different perspectives, values and priorities for quality. Conceptualisations of quality range from *technical*, the appropriate application of scientific evidence to an individual health problem, to *interpersonal*, the human relationship between patient and care-giver with the underpinning values of trust, respect and compassion.

The contested and kaleidoscopic nature of healthcare quality presents considerable problems to researchers, policymakers, managers and clinicians seeking to measure accurately and compare fairly health services. In response to these difficulties, there has been a concerted effort in recent years to standardise and build international consensus about the key domains of quality in healthcare (Institute of Medicine, 2001; OECD, 2002; AHRQ, 2003). In general, the key quality domains include effectiveness, access and timeliness, safety, patient-centredness and disparities. In developing a UK chartbook, we have added a sixth domain, that of capacity, primarily because of the historical context in which the NHS operates. The last decades of the twentieth century saw the NHS subject to stringent resource constraints. As the Government embarked on its quest for quality in the late 1990s, the NHS was widely regarded as under-resourced, and plagued with shortages in both personnel and facilities. Capacity constraints were affecting quality of care, and were most visibly manifested in extensive waiting lists for treatment.

Table A summarises the principles underlying the six domains of quality, which have been used as organising schema for the chartbook, and provides illustrative measures and indicators.

Table A Six domains of quality

Domain	Principle	Examples of measures
Effectiveness	Healthcare services should be based, as far as is possible, on relevant, rigorous science and research evidence.	• Survival and mortality rates • Screening rates for cancer • Secondary prevention after heart attack
Access and timeliness	Healthcare services should be provided at the time they are needed within the appropriate setting.	• Waiting times for elective surgery and for primary care appointments • Cost barriers to accessing care • Timely referrals to specialist
Capacity	Healthcare systems should be sufficiently well resourced to enable delivery of appropriate services.	• Healthcare expenditure per capita • Number of doctors/nurses per capita • Availability of intensive care beds
Safety	Patients should not be harmed by the care that they receive or exposed to unnecessary risk.	• Number of adverse incidents • Medication errors • Nosocomial infections
Patient-centredness	Healthcare should: 1 be based on a partnership between practitioners and patients (and when appropriate, their families) 2 be delivered with compassion, empathy and responsiveness to the needs, values and preferences of the individual patient.	• Patient reports of experience with healthcare system • Patients' understanding of medical condition • Respectful behaviour of medical personnel to patient
Disparities	Healthcare should be provided: 1 on the basis of clinical need, regardless of personal characteristics such as age, gender, race, ethnicity, language, socio-economic status or geographic location, and 2 in such a way as to reduce differences in health status and outcomes across various subgroups.	• Comparison of surgical procedures provided across different sub-populations (e.g. elderly vs entire population) • Infant mortality by socio-economic status • Differential rates of preventive screening by race and ethnicity

Health policy context in the UK

The chartbook seeks to provide a comprehensive, relevant and multifaceted picture of the quality of healthcare in the UK. We provide data from different levels of analysis: UK-wide; intra-UK comparisons from England, Wales, Scotland and Northern Ireland; regional comparisons; and, for some case studies, individual NHS Trusts. International data is included for context and benchmarking.

This section provides a brief description of the differences and similarities in quality improvement efforts of the four countries of the UK. Because we are drawing comparisons between different countries, we emphasise that many factors may explain variations in relative performance, including differences in population such as genetic predisposition and various health-influencing behaviours, differences in level and distribution of resources and differences in policies and programmes. Notably, differences in policy have become more marked since devolution of political power to the Welsh Assembly and the Scottish Parliament in 1999,* with the nexus of policymaking shifting to Cardiff and Edinburgh rather than being solely focused at Westminster. Table B summarises differences in context across the countries of the UK with respect to population and healthcare expenditure.

Longitudinal trends in per capita spending on health in the countries of the UK show a sustained and substantial increase in spending across all countries (*see* Figure 1). Figure 1 also illustrates the differences between countries of the UK in terms of per capita spending on health, in 2002–03 ranging from £1085 in England to £1262 in Scotland, a 16% differential.

1 Per capita spending on health 1998–99 to 2002–03

Source: HM Treasury, 2004

Table B Population and per capita spend on health in countries of the UK 2002–03

	England	Scotland	Wales	Northern Ireland	UK
Population, mid-2003 (% of total UK population)	49.9m (83.7%)	5.1m (8.5%)	2.9m (4.9%)	1.7m (2.9%)	59.6m
Per capita public spend on health (2002–03)	£1085	£1262	£1186	£1214	£1109

Data sources: ONS, 2004; HM Treasury, 2004

* Devolution also took place in Northern Ireland where the Northern Ireland Executive took control of public services in 1999 but political events meant that power returned to Westminster in 2002.

England

> The new NHS will have quality at its heart. Without it there is unfairness. Every patient who is treated in the NHS wants to know that they can rely on receiving high quality care when they need it. Every part of the NHS, and everyone who works in it, should take responsibility for working to improve quality. This must be quality in its broadest sense: doing the right things, at the right time, for the right people, and doing them right – first time. And it must be the quality of the patient's experience as well as the clinical result – quality measured in terms of prompt access, good relationships and efficient administration.   DH, 1997: 3.2

The quality agenda in England, unveiled in 1997–98, is a broad and ambitious policy initiative encompassing a plethora of new organisations, programmes and capabilities. In its early stages, it encompassed:

- identification of priorities for improvement by clinical conditions and population subgroups
- use of standard setting through National Service Frameworks (NSFs)
- evaluation and provision of guidance for usage of health technologies through the National Institute for Clinical Excellence (NICE)
- external inspection of NHS organisations (currently conducted by the Healthcare Commission and Monitor)
- endowment of statutory responsibilities for quality upon Chief Executives of NHS organisations (labelled 'clinical governance')
- commitment to patient safety through the National Patient Safety Agency (NPSA)
- enhanced individual accountability through professional appraisal and revalidation schemes
- collection and reporting of performance data
- implementation of financial and non-financial incentives and sanctions.

As the quality reforms continue to evolve, policymakers have turned their attention to reducing health inequalities, devolving decision-making from Whitehall, and strengthening patient choice as a route to improving system performance.

Scotland

> Good quality health care delivered consistently and to a high standard must be a key objective of the NHS in Scotland. It is a shared responsibility for everyone working in the NHS, and covers all aspects of health care including the effectiveness of clinical practice, the environment in which it is delivered, and responsiveness to the needs of patients.   Scottish Office, 1997: p4

Scotland has long nurtured organisational capacity for quality assurance, endorsed the notion of clinical effectiveness, and demonstrated a high level of professional leadership and engagement. NHSScotland benefits from well established organisations for clinical audit (Clinical Resource and Audit Group, CRAG), the development of clinical guidelines (Scottish Intercollegiate Guidelines Network, SIGN) and data collection and publication (Information and Statistics Division, ISD, of the Common Services Agency). More recently, two key players were established:

- in 1999, the Clinical Standards Board for Scotland (CSBS), with a remit to assure the quality of clinical services, through the use of standards and review visits, and to promote public confidence in NHSScotland
- in 2000, the Health Technology Board for Scotland (HTBS), charged with evaluating the clinical and cost-effectiveness of new and existing health technologies, including medicines, devices, clinical procedures and healthcare settings.

In 1999 political power was devolved from the UK Parliament to Scotland. The Scottish Executive's first health plan, *Our National Health*, was published in 2000. It placed great emphasis on setting and monitoring national clinical standards and extended the remit of CSBS to include issues such as cleanliness, food and infection control. Managed clinical networks are the main mechanism used to promulgate best practice and clinical standards. January 2003 saw a rationalisation of the multiple quality organisations into a special health entity, NHS Quality Improvement Scotland (QIS).

Although many parallels exist between the Scottish approach and those of the other countries in the UK, Scotland is said to be distinctive in terms of the extent of professional leadership and clinical ownership of quality initiatives and the eschewal of star ratings and league tables (Steel, 2003).

Wales

At first glance, the health policies of Wales resonate with those of its neighbours. For example, various policy documents introduce into NHS Wales initiatives and programmes such as:

- clinical governance
- inspection (through Healthcare Inspectorate Wales)
- targets
- NICE (operates across England and Wales)
- standards (through National Service Frameworks).

Closer inspection reveals a difference in emphasis and tone. 'Quality' is less prominent as an explicit objective than in either England or Scotland. Instead, Wales places much more emphasis on health improvement in the context of social and economic renewal.

> The [Welsh] Assembly has developed and is implementing a number of strategies to counteract social exclusion and to create a socially inclusive Wales . . . the new Wales is characterised by an opening up of the policy making process . . . The [NHS] Plan is based on an understanding that the NHS, though vitally important, is but one part of the drive to improve the nation's health.
>
> NHS Wales, 2001: p5

Northern Ireland

In 1998 the publication *Fit for the Future* (DHSS, 1998) emphasised the importance of quality in Health and Personal Social Services (HPSS) in Northern Ireland and resonated with the UK-wide drive to reform and modernise public services.

With devolution, the Belfast Agreement placed a requirement on the Executive to establish an agreed annual budget linked to policies and programmes, subject to approval by the Assembly, and entitled *Programme for Government*. Since the suspension of devolution in October 2002, the process of establishing and reviewing a programme for Government in Northern Ireland has continued with the production of explicit outlines of priorities, plans, and budgets by the Secretary of State. Incorporated in the current *Priorities and Budget 2004/06* is the Department of Health, Social Services and Public Safety's Public Service Agreement (PSA). The PSA sets out the Department's overall aims, objectives, and key targets. These include:

- improvement in population wellbeing
- reduction of preventable deaths and diseases
- improvement in the quality of health and social care provided
- increased responsiveness in hospital services
- provision of accessible and effective primary care services
- increased support for those who need it in the community
- improved life chances for children
- safeguards for rights and interests of children.

It is recognised that the people of Northern Ireland expect the same level and quality of service as provided in Britain. Such expectations are seen to be a lever for the adoption and application of standards, such as those defined in England's National Service Frameworks, across Northern Ireland (McWhirter, 2002).

> The Programme for Government commits the Executive to improving the quality of care and maximising the effectiveness of both health and social services.
>
> McWhirter, 2002: p124

Development of the chartbook: purpose and methods

Measuring quality

Exploration and evaluation of the six domains of quality (as described earlier) is achieved through the use of three well-established types of measures: process measures, outcome measures and structural measures (Donabedian, 1966, 1980; Institute of Medicine, 2001; AHRQ, 2003).

Process measures focus on the services that are provided and seek to answer the question: What was done? The potential value of process measures is realised when they are based on research evidence (or in cases when evidence is lacking, on expert consensus) attesting to a link between the particular intervention or process to be measured and subsequent improvements in health status or outcomes. Then the key question becomes: Was the healthcare provided appropriate to the needs of the patient?

In assessing appropriateness, process of care measures focus on three main issues:

1 *overuse*, where services are provided that are not indicated as appropriate by the evidence base for the medical needs of a particular patient, e.g. conduct of unnecessary caesarean sections in obstetrics or the use of antibiotics for the common cold
2 *underuse*, where services are not provided to those patients whom the evidence base indicates would benefit, e.g. hip replacement surgery not provided to patients who would benefit in terms of decreased pain and increased mobility
3 *misuse*, where interventions are applied in the wrong context, e.g. use of wrong drug for treatment of specific symptoms.

Outcome measures focus on the impact of services provided and seek to answer the question: What effects have services had? Indicators may include measures of changes in health status, quality of life, satisfaction with care, and health-related behaviours. Outcome measures may be positive, such as reduction of symptoms or reduced mortality, or they may be negative, such as the occurrence of an infection in hospital or reduced functioning of the patient. It is often difficult to establish incontrovertibly a link between changes in health outcomes and quality of care because outcomes are influenced by a wide range of factors outside the control of health services.

Structural measures focus on the workforce, facilities and financial resources that are needed to provide care and seek to answer the question: What is the potential capacity of the system to deliver care? Indicators may include the number and distribution of professionals, of hospitals and of specialist facilities. Structural factors, whilst not inextricably linked to quality, are critically important because of their ability to either increase or decrease the probability that high quality services are delivered.

Process and structural components of quality are generally seen to be under the control of the healthcare system and therefore a reasonable measure of performance. Outcomes, on the other hand, are known to be affected by a variety of extraneous factors beyond the control of healthcare providers such as poverty, geography, genetics, lifestyles and patient compliance with a recommended medical regimen. However, outcomes represent the ultimate results of treatment and are compelling both to the public and policymakers. Hence the need for a mix of all three types of measures is generally accepted (AHRQ, 2003).

Data sources

With the growth in interest in quality of healthcare, both internationally and domestically, has come a corresponding increase in interest in data sources and comparisons of performance. A selection of some key information sources, arranged alphabetically, is listed in Table C. The first column lists international data sources and the second and third columns list UK-specific sources.

The chartbook aims to depict a broad view of quality in the NHS and draws on a wide range of data sources and of perspectives. In compiling the charts, we canvassed multiple sources, starting with those shown in Table C. We conducted electronic literature searches using non-specialist (e.g. Google) and specialist search

Table C A range of international and national information sources on quality of healthcare

International	UK	UK
Agency for Healthcare Research and Quality (AHRQ) www.ahrq.gov/	Audit Commission (aims to improve the quality of financial management in the NHS and releases focused reports on specific issues of interest) www.audit-commission.gov.uk	Medical Royal Colleges (in particular, coordinated clinical audits in specialist areas) www.aomrc.org.uk/; www.rcplondon.ac.uk/index.asp
Commonwealth Fund (charitable organisation publishes annual survey data for Australia, Canada, New Zealand, UK and US; also funds research into other quality issues) www.cmwf.org/	Department of Health (Hospital Episode Statistics [HES]; activity data, waiting lists) www.dh.gov.uk	National Assembly for Wales – StatsWales www.statswales.wales.gov.uk/ReportFolders/reportfolders.aspx
Organisation for Economic Cooperation and Development (OECD) (releases comparative data drawn from 30 countries annually; developing international indicator set; one-off studies) www.oecd.org	Department of Health and Social Services and Public Safety Northern Ireland www.dhsspsni.gov.uk/stats&research/index.asp	National Audit Office (NAO) (one-off focused studies into areas of interest, particularly value for money) www.nao.org.uk/
Peer-reviewed literature containing quality of care and clinical effectiveness studies (*see* PubMed at www.ncbi.nlm.nih.gov/entrez/query.fcgi)	Dr Foster (provides user-friendly reports based on HES data) www.drfoster.co.uk/	National Centre for Health Outcomes Development (NCHOD) (funded by Department of Health, develops a range of outcome indicators from various sources, including HES and ONS mortality data) http://nchod.uhce.ox.ac.uk/
World Health Organization (WHO) www.who.int/en/	Healthcare Commission (for patient surveys *see* www.nhssurveys.org; for State of Healthcare Reports, *see* www.healthcarecommission.org.uk/NationalFindings/StateOfHealthcare/fs/en?CONTENT_ID=4006361&chk=sNVkqk)	Office for Health Economics (OHE) (an independent research and consultancy organisation that focuses on health economics and associated policy issues and publishes a Compendium of Health Statistics annually) www.ohe.org/
	Information and Statistics Division (ISD), NHSScotland (comprehensive datasets across clinical and organisational domains) www.isdscotland.org/isd/	Office for National Statistics (ONS) www.statistics.gov.uk/

engines (e.g. MEDLINE®). Search terms are shown in the Technical Appendix. We also monitored electronically-collated health news summaries for reports of quality studies conducted by various organisations.

In selecting charts for inclusion, we used the following criteria:

1 **relevance:** importance to population and individual health
2 **comprehensibility:** the issue can be captured and presented in a clear and compelling way, suitable for non-expert audiences
3 **actionability:** there is clear scope for improvement
4 **methodological rigour:** the data has credence and validity
5 **balance:** contributes to a multifaceted picture of quality in healthcare
6 **timeliness:** the data presented is relevant and relatively recent, within historical and policy context (last data point in or after 1999).

The recognition of a need for standardised sets of indicators is gaining ground internationally with the development of initiatives such as the National Healthcare Quality Report (AHRQ, 2003) in the US and the OECD Health Quality Indicators Project. As far as has been possible, we have aligned our selection of quality indicators for this chartbook with wider international efforts.

The chartbook has drawn on experience in the US (Leatherman and McCarthy, 2002; 2004) and been designed with three principles in mind:

• **Accessibility:** In arraying charts that are both comprehensible and comprehensive in their coverage, the chartbook provides an accessible overview of quality in healthcare in the UK for expert and non-expert interested parties.
• **Diversity of perspectives:** Drawing on relevant datasets from general and specialist sources and combining them in a way that illustrates the multifaceted nature of healthcare quality, the chartbook presents views from different perspectives and different stakeholders within the healthcare sector.
• **Balance in presentation of data:** Presenting data in varied formats, the chartbook provides different types of information:
  – longitudinal data to show changes over time

– 'snapshot' accounts of quality at a particular point in time
– comparative data to show differences in performance across countries, regions or organisations and facilitate benchmarking.

Given the many varied sources of information about healthcare quality and performance, what contribution does the chartbook aspire to make? Its intention is to provide a coherent and compelling summary of the state of healthcare quality in the UK. In *The Quest for Quality* (Leatherman and Sutherland, 2003), which reported positively on many of the new policies and initiatives emerging from the quality agenda in England, we highlighted the paucity of independent, authoritative and credible reports on quality of care and noted that much of the current information on quality emanates from the Government. Although this arrangement may be both well intentioned and necessary for accountability, it can be seen as a potential conflict of interest with the Government acting as the funder, deliverer and evaluator of healthcare. The chartbook draws on official data but sets it alongside information drawn from wider and more disparate sources.

Data caveats

In analysing and synthesising a large and varied set of information sources, questions regarding data integrity inevitably come to the fore. The issue of reliability and accuracy is one of great contention. In compiling the chartbook, we have used datasets from official information sources, widely recognised and respected organisations, and peer-reviewed literature. We have made no attempt to check the validity of data as published in the original source. Ongoing debates about the reliability of some widely quoted data highlight our finding that, in some instances, data from different sources presents conflicting pictures of performance. For example, as Chart 2.10 highlights, patient survey data on waits for primary care appointments indicates that 25% of patients waited longer than two days for an appointment with their general practitioner (GP) – a finding that contradicts official figures that claim that more than 99% of patients see their GP within two working days.

Concerns about processes of routine data entry and the engagement of professionals in data collection are widespread (Williams and Mann, 2002). Perhaps because of the limited use historically of official data such as that collected for the Hospital Episode Statistics database (HES), professionals have tended to regard routine data collection as unimportant. The resulting datasets provided a contested (and some would assert inaccurate) interpretation of performance, thereby exacerbating the view that routine data is of little value to practising clinicians. More effective engagement of professionals and a subsequent improvement in data would benefit the quest for quality.

In any system that places credence on data, the risk of compromising data entry, collection and collation is ever-present. Often referred to as 'gaming', intentional manipulation of data has been discovered in the management of waiting lists in England (NAO, 2001), and it is suspected in the reporting of waits under 48 hours for GP appointments. Such distortions are a common feature of systems in which data submission has significant consequences in terms of rewards and sanctions.

Findings: what do the charts tell us?

The charts provide a rich and varied picture of quality in healthcare in the UK. They depict impressive successes and areas for concern, and raise important questions for future work. The following list illustrates a small selection of the most compelling accomplishments, gaps and questions needing further study.

Successes

1 Greater investment in healthcare across the UK, with a 7.4% increase in expenditure in real terms each fiscal year between 2003–04 and 2007–08. This translates into an increase in the percentage of gross domestic product (GDP) spent on healthcare from 7.7% in 2003 to 9.4% in 2008. The increased investment has been translated into increases in the numbers of nurses and doctors, more critical care beds, additional stroke units, and more community mental health teams.

2 In England, the problem of inpatient waiting lists has been tackled with great success. The inpatient waiting list has been cut by more than one-third since 1998. Maximum waiting times, which stood at 18 months in 1998, are said to be 'on course' to be reduced to six months this year (DH, 2004).

3 Across the UK, although serious disparities exist in terms of overall health status, the NHS offers equitable care across different socio-economic groups. Public surveys reveal a high level of confidence that patients receive needed healthcare, regardless of income – a finding that sets the UK apart from many comparator countries.

4 Mortality rates from the major killers (cancer, circulatory diseases) have been steadily decreasing, although the achievements in this area should be placed in context. Several comparator countries have lower mortality rates and have seen similar rates of reduction.

5 Specific care processes, which have been associated with better outcomes, have improved. Examples include use of thrombolytic therapy to improve survival following a heart attack and increased use of statins to help prevent diseases associated with high cholesterol levels.

6 NHS services, across the UK, receive high satisfaction ratings in patient surveys.

Areas of concern

1 In Wales and Northern Ireland, waiting times for inpatient care are considerably longer than those in England and Scotland.

2 Waiting times for outpatient appointments have increased in all countries except England.

3 Across the UK, capacity remains a concern, e.g. in the number of dentists and doctors, stroke service resources and radiography services.

4 Deficiencies in chronic disease management such as low levels of glycaemic control in paediatric diabetes.

5 Timely access to needed services such as revascularisation rates are lower than rates in most comparator countries, despite high mortality rates from coronary heart disease.

6 The rise in incidence of methicillin-resistant *Staphylococcus aureus* (MRSA) infections is unrelenting. International comparisons show that countries can reverse this trend.

7 Despite Government targets to reduce disparities in infant and adult mortality between different socio-economic groups, the gap in health status between rich and poor is growing.

Questions for the future

1 Improvement in a range of quality measures across the NHS has been considerable. The tendency to date, completely justifiable and understandable, has been to focus on the major health issues, in terms of morbidity and mortality, through the publication of standards and National Service Frameworks (NSFs). As progress becomes established in these areas, questions about non-NSF conditions (e.g. chronic obstructive pulmonary disease (COPD), sexually transmitted infections) and about preventive interventions arise: are they sufficiently well resourced in financial, organisational and R&D terms; is it possible to focus on these whilst maintaining momentum on the NSF issues: is there sufficient available data to monitor performance?

2 Since 1997, the quest for quality across the NHS has been an ambitious and bold undertaking. Several important interventions designed to improve quality and performance have however started relatively recently. Therefore, the data does not reflect the potential impact of such pivotal levers for change as pay for performance contracts with physicians, a fully implemented programme of patient choice, new requirements for professional revalidation and huge investment in information technology.

3 The increased health expenditures that came on stream in 2003–04 have not yet been rigorously evaluated in terms of identifying where the extra resource has been spent, assessing value for money, or delineating wider relationships between cost and quality. Looking ahead, there are also important questions to be answered about resourcing levels once the current commitments for significant year-on-year increases in NHS investment come to an end in 2007–08.

Moving forward

This chartbook provides a multifaceted compilation of a broad range of indicators of quality in the NHS. The production of an integrated picture of quality should not however be a one-off effort. There is an ongoing need for an independently collated, regular report that charts the progress over time of the NHS in its quest for quality.

Given the breadth of its coverage, the chartbook has not addressed in any depth the quality concerns particular to any one disease area or patient group. We plan to undertake more focused studies in areas such as primary care, child health and mental health.

Moving forward, we reiterate the need to monitor the progress of the considerable efforts that aim to enhance the NHS. This is necessary in order to build a common understanding of the state of quality, identify the extent to which specific initiatives and programmes are successful, and inform the development of future policy and management decisions. At the same, time we acknowledge the limitations of data monitoring in isolation. Knowledge and awareness alone are not sufficient to improve quality; they are a prerequisite to focusing attention and galvanising collective action.

References

AHRQ (2003) *National Healthcare Quality Report*. Pre-publication copy. Agency for Healthcare Research and Quality, Rockville MD. Available online at: http://qualitytools.ahrq.gov/qualityreport/documents/quality_report.pdf [last accessed 31 January 2005].

Department of Health (1997) *The New NHS – Modern, Dependable: A National Framework for Assessing Performance*. Stationery Office, London. Available online at: www.archive.official-documents.co.uk/document/doh/newnhs/newnhs.htm [last accessed 31 January 2005].

Department of Health and Social Services (1998) *Fit for the Future*. DHSS, Belfast.

Department of Health (2004) *Chief Executive's Report to the NHS, December 2004 – Statistical supplement*. DH, London. Available online at: www.dh.gov.uk/assetRoot/04/09/75/40/04097540.pdf [last accessed 31 January 2005].

Donabedian A (1966) Evaluating the quality of medical care. *Milbank Memorial Fund Quarterly*. **44**(July supplement, Part 2): 166–206.

Donabedian A (1980) *The Definition of Quality and Approaches to its Assessment, Volume 1*. Health Administration Press, Michigan.

HM Treasury (2004) Public Expenditure: statistical analyses 2004. HM-Treasury, London. Available online at: www.hm-treasury.gov.uk/media/D27/4A/pesa04_complete_190404.pdf [last accessed 2 February 2005].

Institute of Medicine (2001) *Crossing the Quality Chasm: a new health system for the 21st century*. National Academies Press, Washington, DC.

Leatherman S and McCarthy D (2002) *Quality of Health Care in the United States: a chartbook*. The Commonwealth Fund, New York.

Leatherman S and McCarthy D (2004) *Quality of Health Care for Children and Adolescent: a chartbook*. The Commonwealth Fund, New York.

Leatherman S and Sutherland K (2003) *The Quest for Quality in the NHS: a mid-term evaluation of the ten-year quality agenda*. TSO, London.

McWhirter L (2002) *Health and Social Care in Northern Ireland: a statistical profile*. Northern Ireland Statistics and Research Agency, Belfast. Available online at: www.dhsspsni.gov.uk/publications/2002/FINALHEALTHSOCIALCAREREPORT26NOV.pdf [last accessed 31 January 2005].

National Audit Office (2001) *Inappropriate Adjustments to NHS Waiting Lists: report by the comptroller and auditor general*. The Stationery Office, London.

NHS Wales (2001) *Improving Health in Wales: a plan for the NHS and its partners*. The National Assembly for Wales, Cardiff. Available online at: www.wales.gov.uk/healthplanonline/health_plan/content/nhsplan-e.pdf [last accessed 31 January 2005].

OECD (2002) *Measuring Up: improving health system performance in OECD countries*. Organisation for Economic Cooperation and Development, Paris.

ONS (2004) *Population Estimates*. Office for National Statistics, London. Available online at: www.statistics.gov.uk/cci/nugget.asp?id=6 [last accessed 2 February 2005].

Scottish Office (1997) *Designed to Care: renewing the National Health Service in Scotland*. TSO, London. Available online at: www.scotland.gov.uk/library/documents1/care-00.htm [last accessed 31 January 2005].

Steel D (2003) Quality health care in Scotland. In: K Woods and D Carter (eds) *Scotland's Health and Health Services*. TSO, London.

Williams JG and Mann RY (2002) Hospital episode statistics: time for clinicians to get involved? *Clinical Medicine*. **2**(1): 34–7.

The charts contain a vast amount of data, drawn from a wide range of sources, and utilising a multitude of research methodologies. To simplify the presentation of such complex data, each chart has a corresponding:

- entry in the Technical Appendix (*see* p. 159), which outlines background information that underpins the chart such as sample size, confidence intervals, standardisation techniques, as well as hyperlinks, where available, to the site from which the source material has been drawn
- entry in the Summary Chart (*see* p. vi), which briefly describes the findings illustrated in the chart, facilitating comparisons across different charts and datasets
- cross-reference, where appropriate, to other related charts that appear elsewhere in the chartbook.

A statistical glossary (*see* p. 172) explains the statistical methods and approaches that charts refer to and lists the acronyms (*see* p. 174) included in the document.

The chartbook draws on a wide range of source material and methodologies. We have therefore taken great care to highlight different approaches when we juxtapose different datasets. However, the reader should be aware that different datasets may appear to provide a conflicting picture of performance that, on closer inspection, is found not to be contradictory but instead grounded in variations in methodology such as age standardisation, level of aggregation and data definitions.

The selection of charts for inclusion has been driven by a concern to be fair and rigorous. This has meant that we have excluded interesting data because of time lags that occur in publication. For example, we chose not to use recently published studies on age-based and gender-based bias in the treatment of coronary heart disease (CHD) because the data they contained was more than five years old.* Given the evidence that treatment of CHD has improved dramatically in that time, their inclusion was considered to be potentially misleading and indefensible.

On a stylistic note, the process of compiling the chartbook has highlighted areas of dispute in grammar and syntax. For example, American readers may be discomfited by the use of 'healthcare' as a single word but this is increasingly used in the UK and so it has been adopted throughout the text. International readers may find the use of terms such as 'routine and manual groups' anachronistic but they reflect methodologies used to collect data on socio-economic status in the UK and so have been used in the charts. On the other hand, readers from the UK may find the unhyphenated 'chartbook' jarring but the utility and aptness of the term has persuaded us to adopt it. Those from a scientific background may object to our use of data as a mass noun but, in the UK at least, that usage is seen as more accessible language and so we have adopted the populist rather than the classical application. We recognise that such discrepancies may be unsettling to some readers, and they have been the subject of long debate in the production of the chartbook. They are however, the result of deliberate decisions rather than random error.

---

* e.g. Majeed A, Moser K and Maxwell R (2000) Age, sex and practice variations in the use of statins in general practice in England and Wales. *Journal of Public Health Medicine.* **22**(3): 275–9 (data from 1996); Reid FDA, Cook DG and Whincup PH (2002) Use of statins in the secondary prevention of coronary heart disease: is treatment equitable? *Heart.* **88**: 15–19 (data from 1998); DeWilde S, Carey IM, Bremner SA *et al.* (2003) Evolution of statin prescribing 1995–2001: a case of ageism but not sexism? *Heart.* **89**: 417–21 (data on age disparities from 1998).

Effectiveness refers to the extent to which an intervention produces its intended result. Effectiveness in the context of the quality of healthcare also encompasses the concept of *appropriateness*, the extent to which interventions or services, based on scientific knowledge, are provided to all those who could benefit and withheld from those who would not (Hurtado *et al.*, 2001). Effectiveness indicators can focus on *outcomes* such as mortality or survival rates that reflect the success of preventive measures, diagnosis and treatment; or on *processes* that have been proven to affect those outcomes and can be used as more immediate measures of quality, for example the use of thrombolysis in the treatment of heart attacks.

We have organised the effectiveness charts into six sections, primarily on the basis of five disease groups and one type of service. They are:

1 cancer

2 circulatory disease

3 diabetes

4 infectious disease

5 mental health

6 surgery.

Preceding those sections is a chart that focuses on avoidable mortality which reflects quality across the entire healthcare sector.

The Quest for Quality in the NHS: a chartbook on quality of care in the UK

1

Chart 1.1 Mortality from causes considered amenable to healthcare

The Quest for Quality in the NHS: a chartbook on quality of care in the UK

Measures of avoidable mortality are used to gauge the extent to which healthcare services save lives and contribute to population health. *Avoidable mortality* is the number of deaths that should not occur in the presence of effective and timely healthcare (Nolte and McKee, 2004). It tallies deaths from conditions that are *amenable* to treatment and medical care (i.e. with appropriate treatment there should be no deaths, e.g. appendicitis) and those that are preventable (i.e. there are effective means to prevent the condition occurring, often through behavioural and lifestyle changes, e.g.

smoking-related lung cancer). Chart 1.1a shows international comparisons on amenable death rates for those aged 0–74 (both including and excluding figures for ischaemic heart disease (IHD)). The UK had the highest rates of the five countries shown. Chart 1.1b shows a time series of mortality rates in England and in Wales (data include IHD). Wales has had a consistently higher mortality rate, but both countries have seen a steady decline in rates, reflecting improvements in healthcare over time.

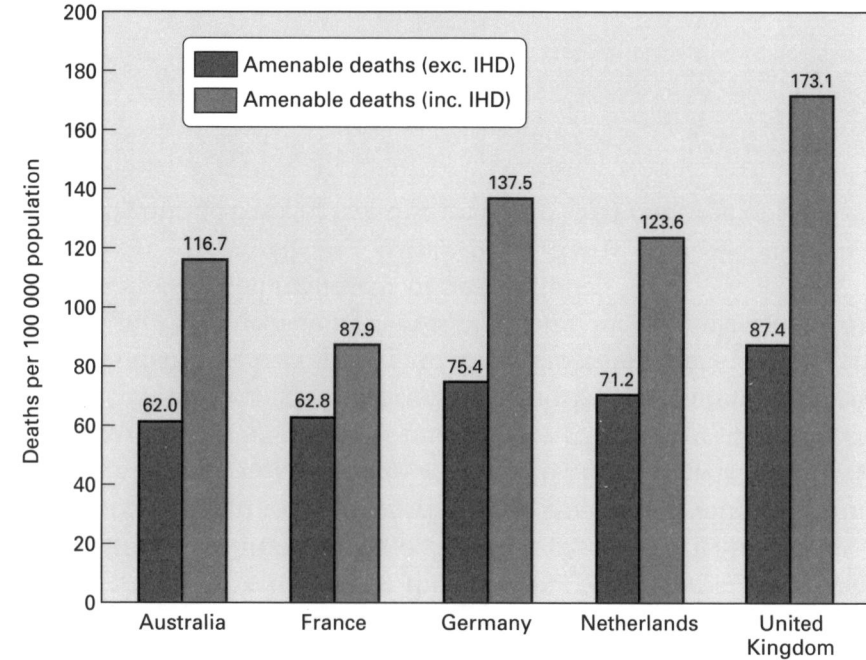

1.1a Mortality from causes considered amenable to healthcare (ages 0–74), international comparison 1998

Legend:
- Amenable deaths (exc. IHD)
- Amenable deaths (inc. IHD)

Australia: 62.0, 116.7
France: 62.8, 87.9
Germany: 75.4, 137.5
Netherlands: 71.2, 123.6
United Kingdom: 87.4, 173.1

Source: Nolte and McKee, 2004; Korda and Butler, 2004.

1.1b Mortality from causes considered amenable to healthcare (ages 0–74), England and Wales 1993–2003

Legend: Wales, England

Source: ONS; NCHOD (analysis by Lakhani, Eayres and Coles).

Cancer overview

Cancer arises from abnormal and uncontrolled cell division. The proliferating cells subsequently invade and destroy the surrounding tissues. Spread of cancer (metastasis) may occur via the bloodstream or the lymphatic system or across body cavities such as the pleural and peritoneal spaces, resulting in secondary tumours.

In 1999–2001, the average annual number of new cancer cases registered in the UK was 269 631 (133 697 for males; 135 934 for females). Incidence rates varied within the countries of the UK with the highest incidence for males occurring in Wales and for females occurring in Scotland (*see* Table 1.1).

One in three people develop cancer at some time in their lives (Summerfield and Babb, 2004). Cancer is responsible for around one-quarter of all deaths in the United Kingdom. In England and Wales, there were 136 777 cancer deaths in 2002 (ONS, 2004a: pp128–9); and in Scotland 15 063 cancer deaths in 2003 (ISD Scotland, 2004).

Cancer is predominantly a disease of the elderly. Only 0.5% of cases registered in 2001 were in children (aged under 15) and 25% were in people aged under 60 (ONS, 2004c).

The charts in this section display data on mortality, survival and screening rates for the most common types of cancer.

Table 1.1 Incidence per 100 000 population (age-standardised, average rates 1999–2001)

	Males	*Females*
UK	403.4	343.0
England	398.6	339.1
Wales	437.8	357.6
Scotland	431.2	370.1
Northern Ireland	392.1	345.0

Source: ONS, 2004b.

1 Effectiveness

Chart 1.2 Cancer mortality rates

Comparisons of mortality rates can give some indication of quality of healthcare, but should be interpreted carefully because many other factors, such as lifestyle, genetics and behaviour, also contribute to mortality rates. Comparative data can however give insight into the extent to which deaths may be amenable to healthcare or preventable. The chart shows that since 1990 mortality rates from cancer have fallen more sharply in the UK than in many other countries, a 12% drop compared to 9% in Australia, 7% in the US and Germany, and 5% in Sweden and France. However, the most recently available OECD data shows that the UK mortality rate was still high relative to comparator countries. In 1999 184.7 deaths per 100 000 were attributed to cancer in the UK, compared to 151.3 deaths per 100 000 in Sweden.

Source: OECD, 2004.

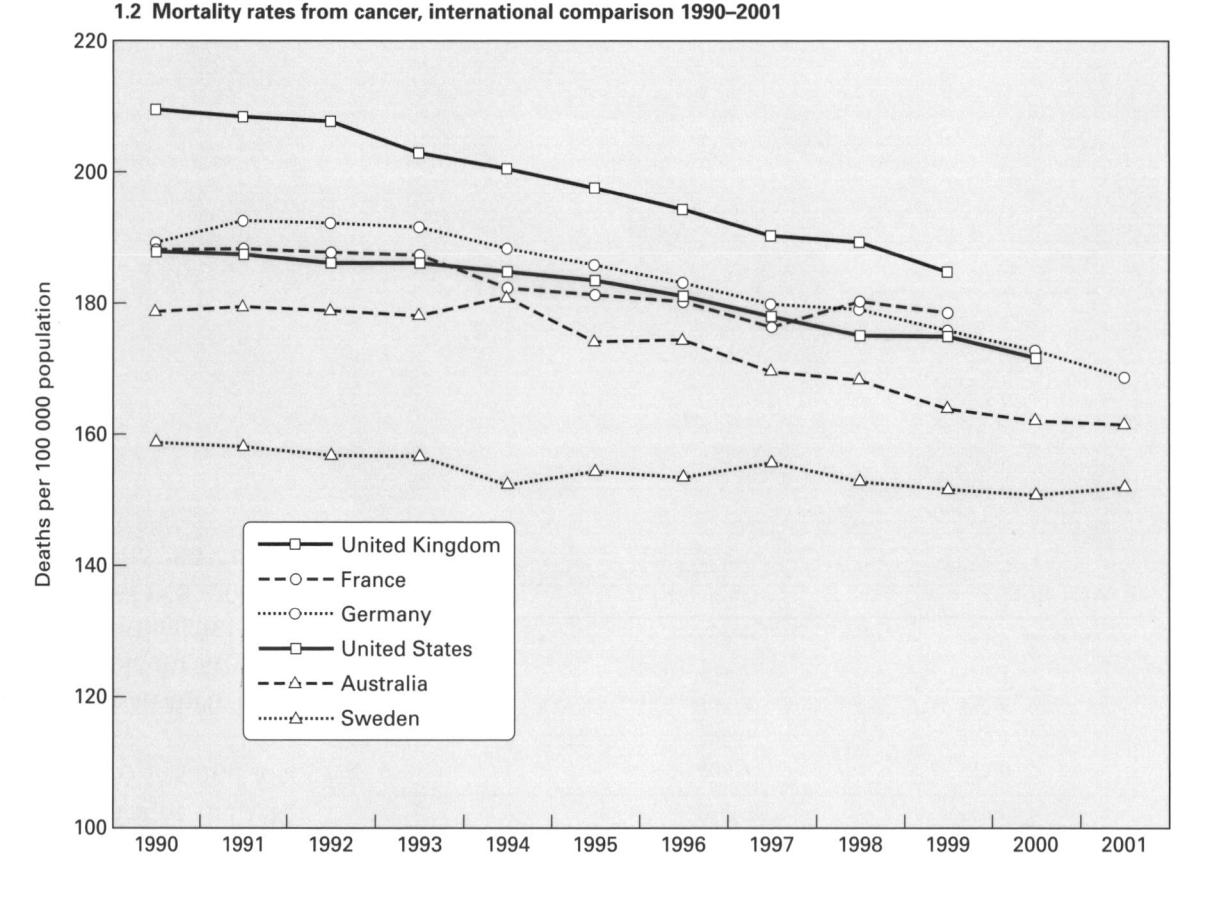

1.2 Mortality rates from cancer, international comparison 1990–2001

The Quest for Quality in the NHS: a chartbook on quality of care in the UK

Chart 1.3 Mortality rates from common cancers, UK time series

The four most common cancers – colorectal, lung, breast and prostate – account for more than half of all cancers registered each year (ONS, 2004c). These charts show that mortality rates for these cancers have declined since 1990. Particularly noteworthy is the data on lung cancer; with a marked decrease in the death rate among males (from 87.9 deaths per 100 000 in 1990 to 58.3 deaths per 100 000 in 2002) and little change among females (from 30.6 deaths per 100 000 in 1990 to 29.9 deaths per 100 000 in 2002). The decrease in lung cancer mortality overall echoes a similar decrease in smoking rates, attesting to the major influence that lifestyle changes have on mortality (Summerfield and Babb, 2004).

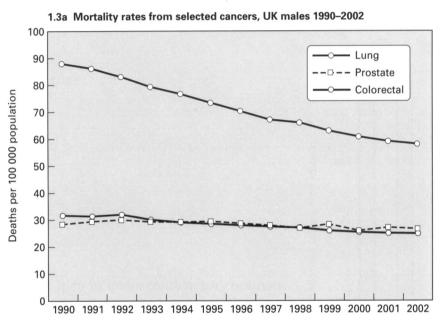

1.3a Mortality rates from selected cancers, UK males 1990–2002

Source: ONS.

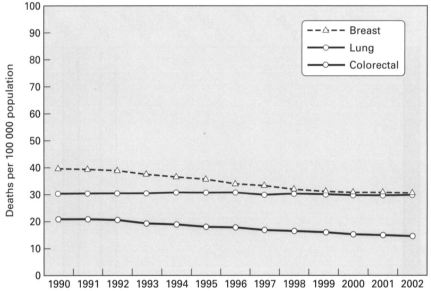

1.3a Mortality rates from selected cancers, UK females 1990–2002

Source: ONS.

The Quest for Quality in the NHS: a chartbook on quality of care in the UK

Chart 1.4 Premature deaths from cancer: progress against a target

The Government set a target in 1999 to reduce by 20% the death rate from cancer in people under age 75 by 2010, using 1995–97 data as a baseline (DH, 1999a). As of 2002, a 10% reduction in the rate of deaths had been achieved. A decline in mortality rates has been seen across all developed healthcare systems although, as Chart 1.2 illustrates, the decrease in the UK has been steeper than in many comparator countries.

Source: ONS.

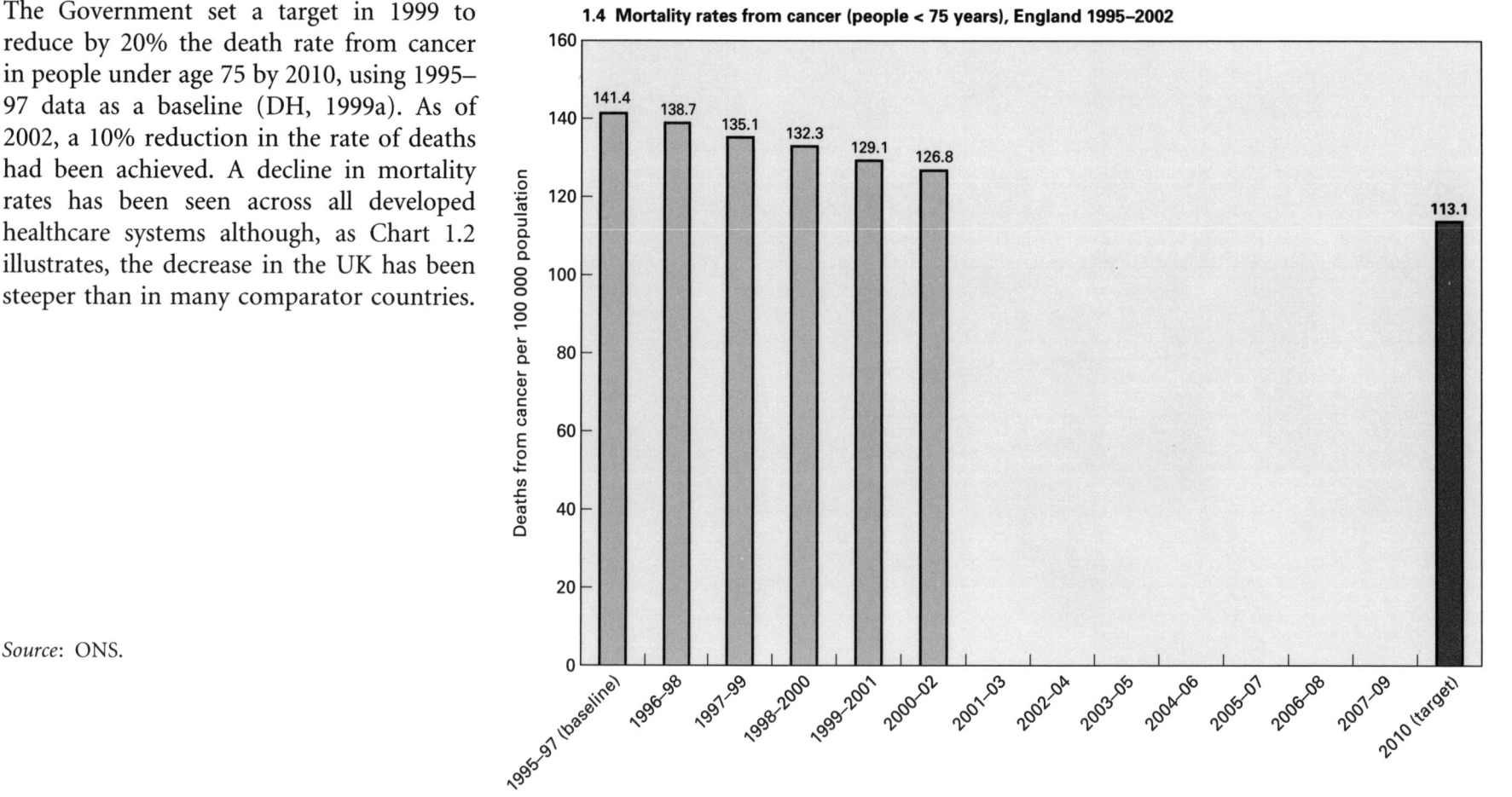

1.4 Mortality rates from cancer (people < 75 years), England 1995–2002

The Quest for Quality in the NHS: a chartbook on quality of care in the UK

Chart 1.5 Five-year relative survival rates for common cancers

Five-year survival rates, the proportion of patients with cancer who are alive five years after diagnosis, can reflect quality of healthcare as well as features of the disease and its interaction with patient characteristics. These charts show five-year survival rates for the most common cancers in England and Wales (Chart 1.5a) and in Scotland (Chart 1.5b) over two consecutive five-year periods (note slightly different time frames). Survival rates increased over time for all the cancers shown. The greatest improvement was in prostate cancer survival rates, which increased by 9.4% in Scotland between 1992–96 and 1997–2001 and by 11.2% in England between 1991–95 and 1996–99. There was little difference between England and Wales and Scotland in terms of survival rates.

1.5a Five-year relative survival rates for adults diagnosed 1991–95 and 1996–99, England and Wales

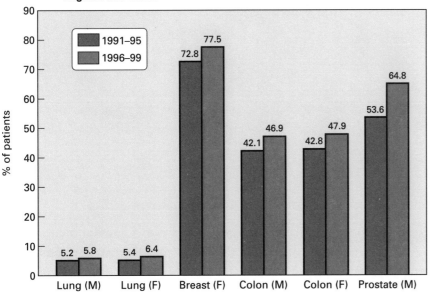

Source: ONS.

1.5b Five-year relative survival rates for adults diagnosed 1992–96 and 1997–2001, Scotland

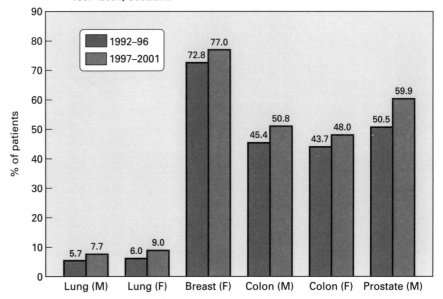

Source: ISD Scotland.

The Quest for Quality in the NHS: a chartbook on quality of care in the UK

Breast cancer

Worldwide, around one million women develop breast cancer each year. In the UK, breast cancer accounts for around 30% of all cancers in women. One in nine women will develop breast cancer at some time in their life. The World Health Organization's International Agency for Research on Cancer (IARC) calculated that there is a 35% reduction in mortality from breast cancer among women aged 50–69 years who choose to participate in screening programmes. This translates into one life saved per 500 screened (IARC, 2002).

Breast screening programmes were set up in the UK in the early 1990s. The NHS Breast Screening Programme provides free breast screening every three years for all women aged between 50 and 64, and there are plans to extend the programme to women up to and including the age of 70. About 1.5 million women are now screened in the UK each year. In 2002–03 for every 1000 women screened, 7.5 cancers were detected. In England, the budget for the breast screening programme is approximately £52 million. This corresponds to £40 per woman screened (NHS Breast Screening Programme, 2004).

Chart 1.6 Breast cancer mortality rates

Since 1990 the rate of deaths from breast cancer in developed countries has generally dropped. This reduction has been linked to advances in treatment and to the introduction of national screening programmes (Summerfield and Babb, 2004). Despite a 21% reduction between 1990 and 1999, England continued to have the highest breast cancer mortality rates among these comparator countries with 28.9 deaths per 100 000 as compared to Australia, with the lowest rate, 21.9 per 100 000.

Source: Commonwealth Fund, 2004a.

1.6 Breast cancer mortality rates, international comparison 1990 and 1999

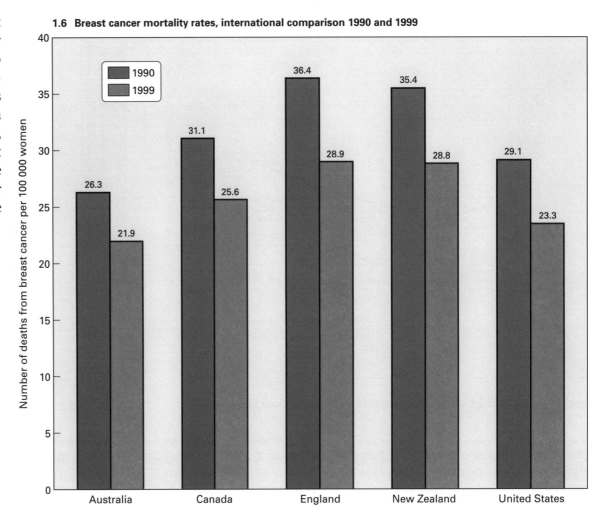

The Quest for Quality in the NHS: a chartbook on quality of care in the UK

9

Chart 1.7 Breast cancer survival and screening rates

The Quest for Quality in the NHS: a chartbook on quality of care in the UK

These charts provide comparative data on screening coverage and five-year survival rates for breast cancer. Chart 1.7a illustrates that, of the five countries shown, the US had the highest survival rates, with 86% of women with breast cancer alive five years after diagnosis; England had the lowest rate with 75%. The same chart shows that the US had one of the lowest rates of breast cancer screening. Although this combination of high survival and relatively low screening rate seems paradoxical given the strong research evidence on improvements in survival that result from early detection and treatment made possible by screening programmes

(NHS Breast Screening Programme, 2004), they may be a reflection of differences between the countries in terms of age bands within which screening is offered (e.g. US data is for women aged 40 and over screened in the preceding two years, England data is for women aged 50–64 screened in the preceding three years); concerns about affordability in the US affecting screening rates; or differences in treatment regimes across the countries. Chart 1.7b compares screening rates of women aged 50–64 years within the countries of the UK, showing that in 2002, Scotland had the highest coverage (75%) and Wales the lowest (67%).

1.7a Breast cancer survival (~1992–97) and screening rates (~2000), international comparison

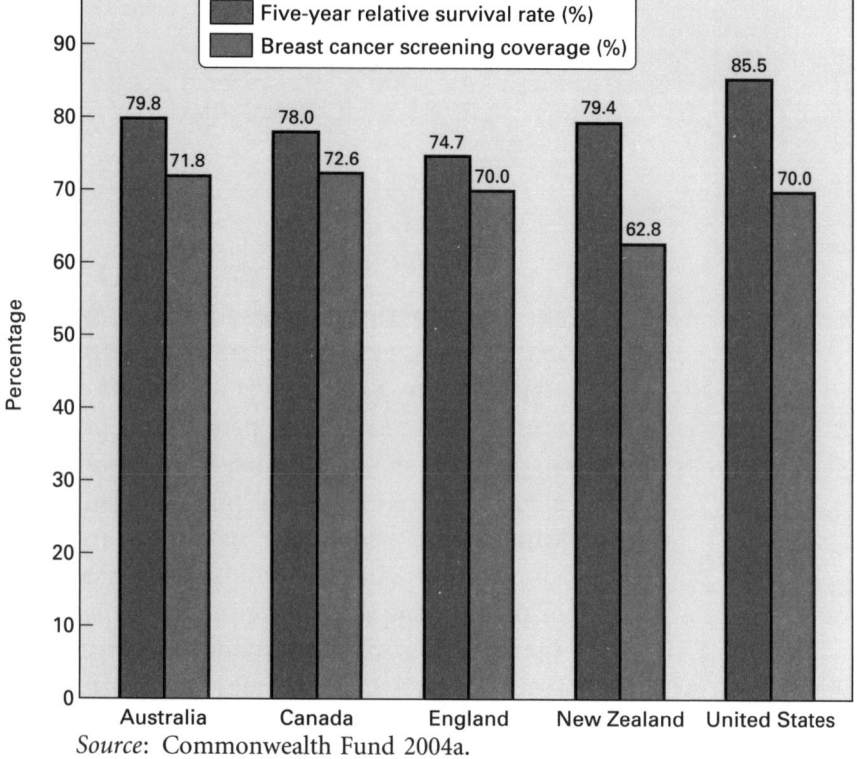

Source: Commonwealth Fund 2004a.

Note: Countries in the Commonwealth Fund dataset differ in the date and methodology of data collection, screened population and screening interval. For details, *see* Technical Appendix.

1.7b Breast sceening coverage on women aged 50–64, UK countries 1992–2002

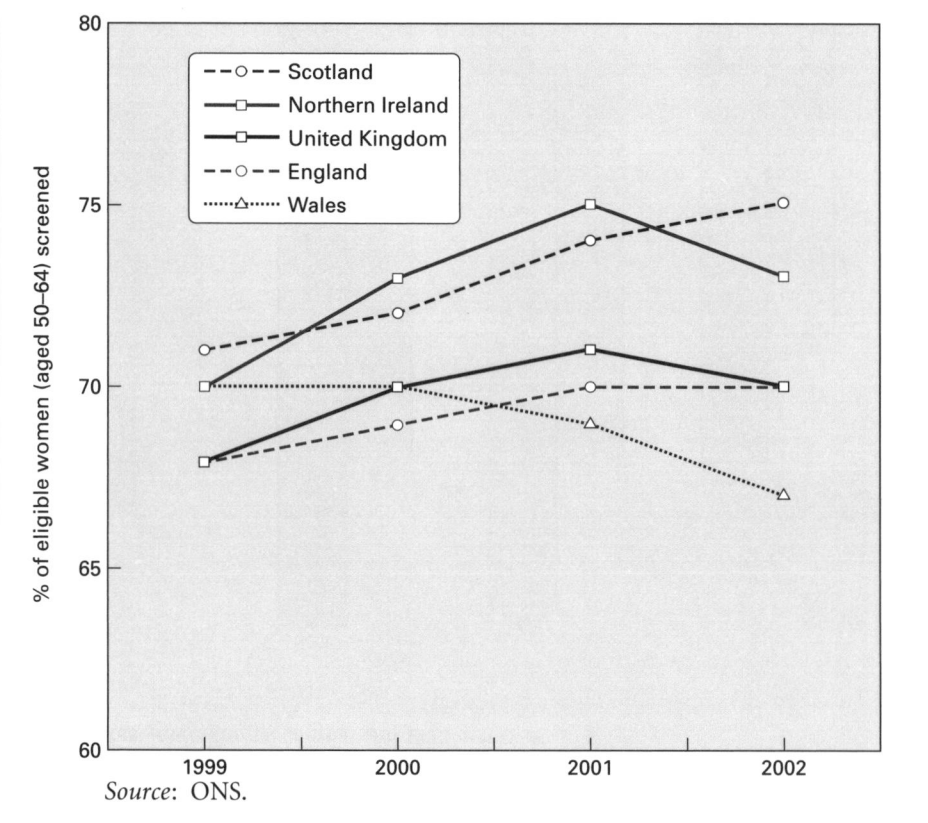

Source: ONS.

Colorectal cancer

In the UK, colorectal (bowel) cancer is the third most common cancer in men, and the second most common cancer in women. Each year, about 18 400 new cases of colorectal cancer are diagnosed in men, and 16 000 cases in women. In England and Wales, this number is increasing by 1% every year for men although it is remaining steady for women. Colorectal cancer is the second most common cause of cancer death in the UK and some 16 000 people die of the disease every year (ONS, 2004b).

Survival rates in the UK have improved over the past 25 years. Today, approximately half of the people diagnosed with bowel cancer will still be alive in five years' time (NHS Cancer Screening Programme, 2005).

In 2001, England's Department of Health began pilots of a screening method that involves looking for hidden blood in stools (faecal occult blood test or FOBT). These pilot studies and other research (Hardcastle *et al.*, 1996) indicate that using this method would reduce the mortality rate from bowel cancer by 15% (DH, 2004a). A national screening programme for bowel cancer using FOBT will be phased in across England among men and women in their sixties from April 2006.

According to recent reviews, however (Weitz *et al.*, 2005; Pignone *et al.*, 2002), the choice of screening method for colorectal cancer remains controversial. FOBT is not regarded to be unequivocally better than flexible sigmoidoscopy, double contrast barium enema or colonoscopy, although it is less expensive and less invasive than the alternative tests.

Chart 1.8 Colorectal cancer mortality rates

The Quest for Quality in the NHS: a chartbook on quality of care in the UK

Chart 1.8a shows that, between 1990 and 1999, deaths from colorectal cancer fell significantly. In 1999, New Zealand had the highest mortality rate (28.0 per 100 000 population) of the countries shown and the US had the lowest (17.4 per 100 000). Chart 1.8b shows the variation in mortality rates within the countries of the UK – England having the lowest rate and Scotland the highest. It also illustrates the discrepancy between male and female colorectal cancer mortality rates in the UK – at its widest in Scotland where the male mortality rate is 78% higher than the female rate.

1.8a Mortality rates from colorectal cancer, international comparison 1990 and 1999

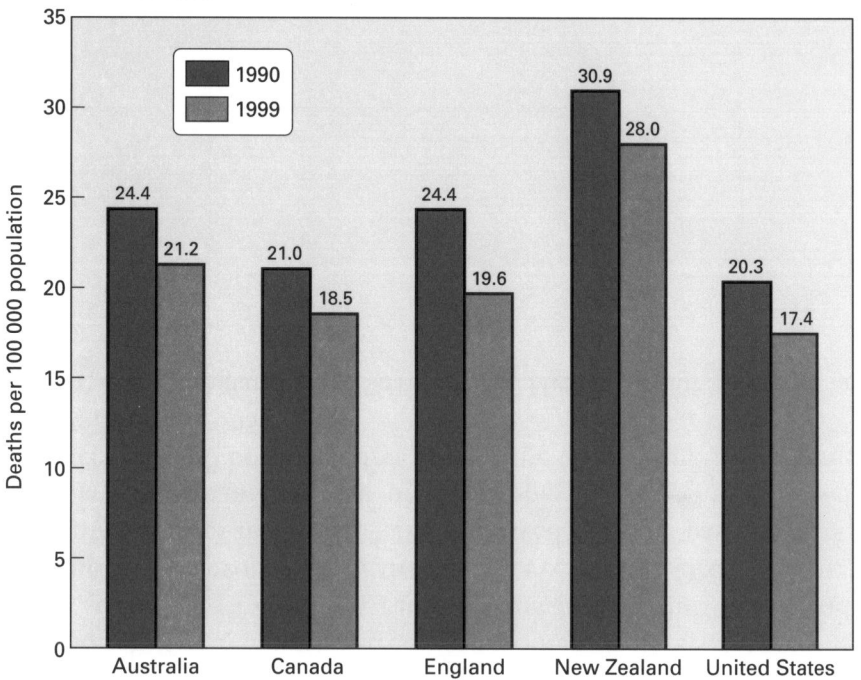

Source: Commonwealth Fund, 2004a.

1.8b Mortality rates from colerectal cancer, UK countries 2002

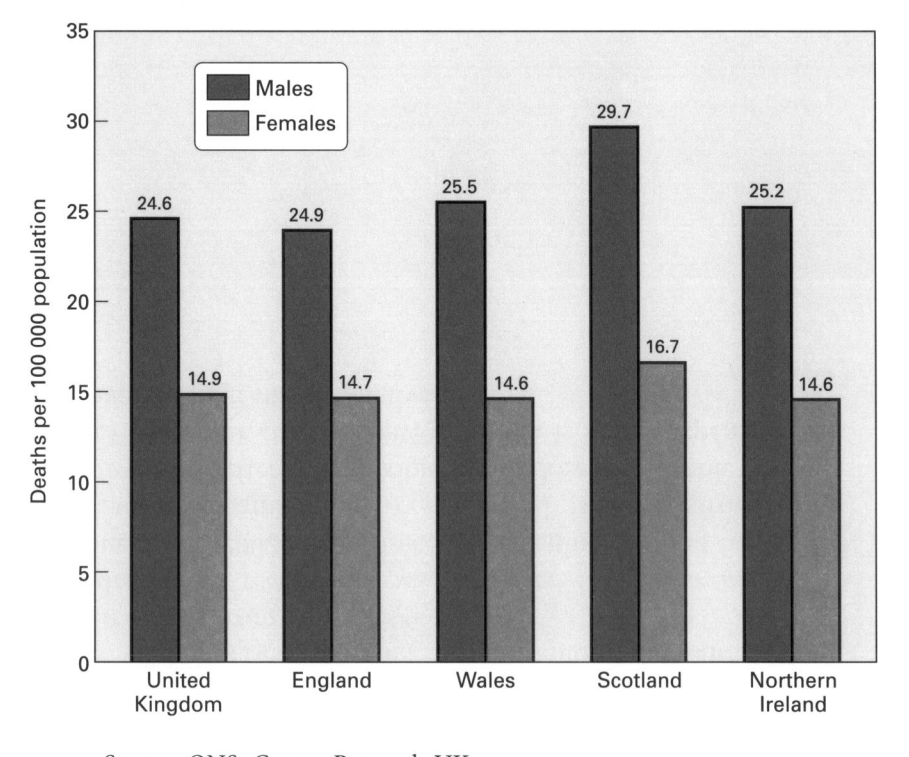

Source: ONS; Cancer Research UK.

Chart 1.9 Colorectal cancer survival rates

These charts provide a time series of relative survival rates from colorectal cancer in Scotland. For both males and females (aged 15–74 years), the improvement in survival rates has been sustained and substantial. The percentage of people surviving 10 years following a diagnosis of colorectal cancer in the most recent dataset, 1992–96 (37.2% for males, 39.8% for females), was greater than the percentage surviving at three years in 1977–1981 (29.7% for males; 31.1% for females). That is, more people survived for 10 years following a diagnosis in the early 1990s than survived for three years following a diagnosis in the late 1970s. Female survival rates are generally higher than male survival rates.

1.9a Relative survival rates at 1, 3, 5 and 10 years, males, Scotland 1977–81 to 1997–2001

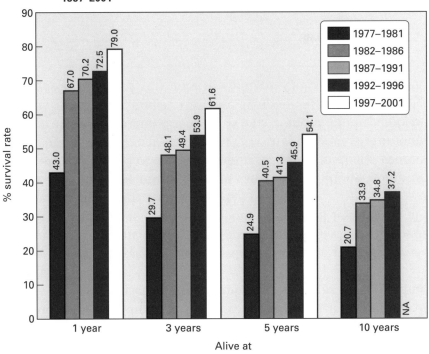

Source: Scottish Cancer Registry, ISD, 2002

1.9b Relative survival rates at 1, 3, 5 and 10 years, females, Scotland 1977–81 to 1997–2001

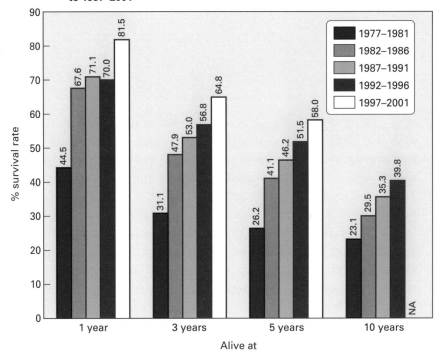

Source: Scottish Cancer Registry, ISD.

The Quest for Quality in the NHS: a chartbook on quality of care in the UK

1 Effectiveness

Childhood leukaemia

Leukaemia is a cancer of the white blood cells characterised by the production of large numbers of abnormal white blood cells in the bone marrow. These abnormal white cells do not function properly and cannot perform their normal protective role against disease. As leukaemia progresses, the production of other types of blood cells, including red blood cells and platelets, is disrupted. This results in anaemia (low numbers of red cells) and bleeding problems.

In general, leukaemias are classified into acute (rapidly developing) and chronic (slowly developing) forms. In children, about 98% of leukaemias are acute. About 80% of all leukaemias are acute lymphoblastic leukaemia (ALL).

Leukaemia is the most common cancer of childhood, comprising around a third of all cases; another 25% of childhood cancers are brain and spinal tumours; 15% are embryonal tumours (neuroblastoma, retinoblastoma, Wilms' tumour and hepatoblastoma); and just under 10% are lymphomas. On the whole, however, cancer is very rare in children. Only around 1 in 200 (0.5%) of all cancers occur in children aged under 15 years. The incidence of childhood cancer has not changed very much over the past 40 years. In 2000, there were approximately 1400 new cases diagnosed in Great Britain. However, cancer accounted for around 20% of all deaths in children aged 1–14 years.

Since the 1960s, the treatment of most childhood cancers has made great advances, resulting in markedly higher survival rates. By the mid-1990s, some 75% of children with cancer survived at least five years after diagnosis (five-year survival rate). For the main type of childhood leukaemia (ALL), five-year survival was above 80%, and it exceeded 50% for every main type of childhood cancer.

The number of adult survivors of childhood cancer has greatly increased, from around 1400 in 1971 to almost 15 000 in 2000. In 1971, only around 100 adult survivors were 30 years or over compared with 7000 (over 45%) in 2000 (all figures from ONS, 2004d).

Chart 1.10 Childhood leukaemia survival rates

Survival rates for childhood leukaemias are high. In England and Wales three-quarters of children diagnosed with leukaemia in the 1990s were alive five years after their initial diagnosis. This rate is in line with other comparable countries. For those countries shown here, the rates range from 68.7% in Australia to 81.1% in Canada.

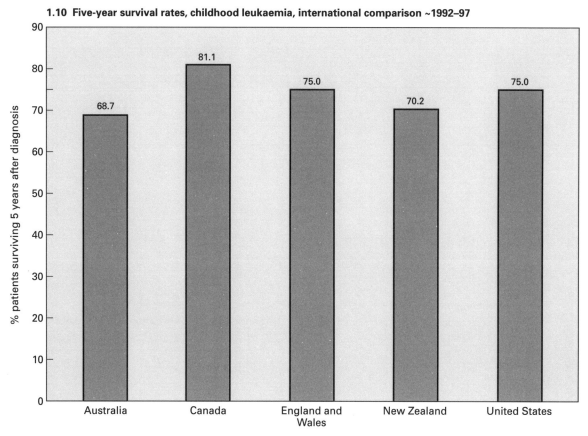

1.10 Five-year survival rates, childhood leukaemia, international comparison ~1992–97

Source: Commonwealth Fund, 2004a.

Note: Countries used slightly different time frames; *see* Technical Appendix for details.

The Quest for Quality in the NHS: a chartbook on quality of care in the UK

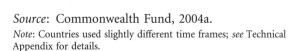

1 Effectiveness

Circulatory disease overview

According to the Office for National Statistics, circulatory diseases have been the most common causes of death in the UK for almost all of the last century. Circulatory disease encompasses both heart disease and stroke. The highest mortality rates are in people aged 85 and over. Circulatory disease in 2002 accounted for 209 433 deaths, which equated to 39% of all deaths in England and Wales (ONS, 2004e).

Male death rates from circulatory disease are higher than those for females: 312 per 100 000 males and 194 per 100 000 females in 2002. Within these, death rates were higher for heart disease than for stroke among both males and females (ONS, 2004e).

The charts concerned with circulatory disease display data for both heart disease and cerebrovascular disease which includes stroke.

Chart 1.11 Circulatory disease mortality rates

These charts illustrate a marked decrease in circulatory disease mortality rates in the UK and internationally. Chart 1.11a shows that the steepest decreases in mortality rates between 1990 and 1999 were seen in Australia (31% decrease) and the UK (25% decrease), although the UK's rates are among the highest of the countries displayed here. Wider comparisons have shown that the UK rate in 1999 of 351 per 100 000 population for males and 214 per 100 000 population for females was around the European Union (EU-15) average of 326 per 100 000 in males and 208 per 100 000 in females (*see* Summerfield and Babb, 2004: p109). Chart 1.11b provides more detail on the extent of change over time and shows a decrease in mortality rates of 55% in both males and females in the 30 years between 1971 and 2002.

1.11a Mortality rates from circulatory disease, international comparison 1990–2001

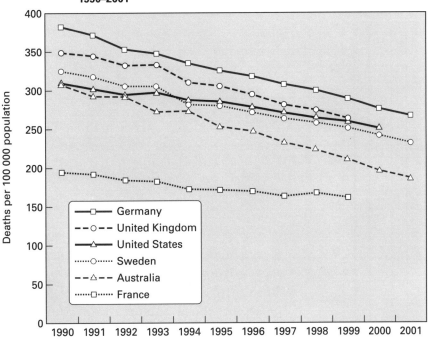

Source: OECD Health Data, 2004.

1.11b Mortality rates from circulatory disease, UK 1971–2002

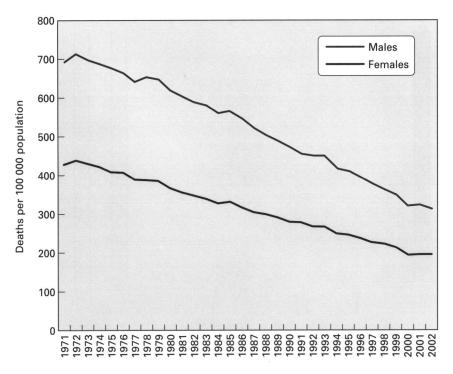

Source: ONS (Summerfield and Babb, 2004).

Chart 1.12 Premature deaths from circulatory disease: progress against a target

Circulatory disease accounted for 60 000 of 170 000 premature deaths (i.e. under 75 years of age) in England in 2001 (ONS, 2004e). *Our healthier nation* (DH, 1999a) set a target to reduce the death rate from circulatory disease among people under 75 years of age by at least 40% by 2010, using 1995–97 as a baseline. As of 2002, a 23% reduction in the rate of deaths had been achieved.

Source: ONS.

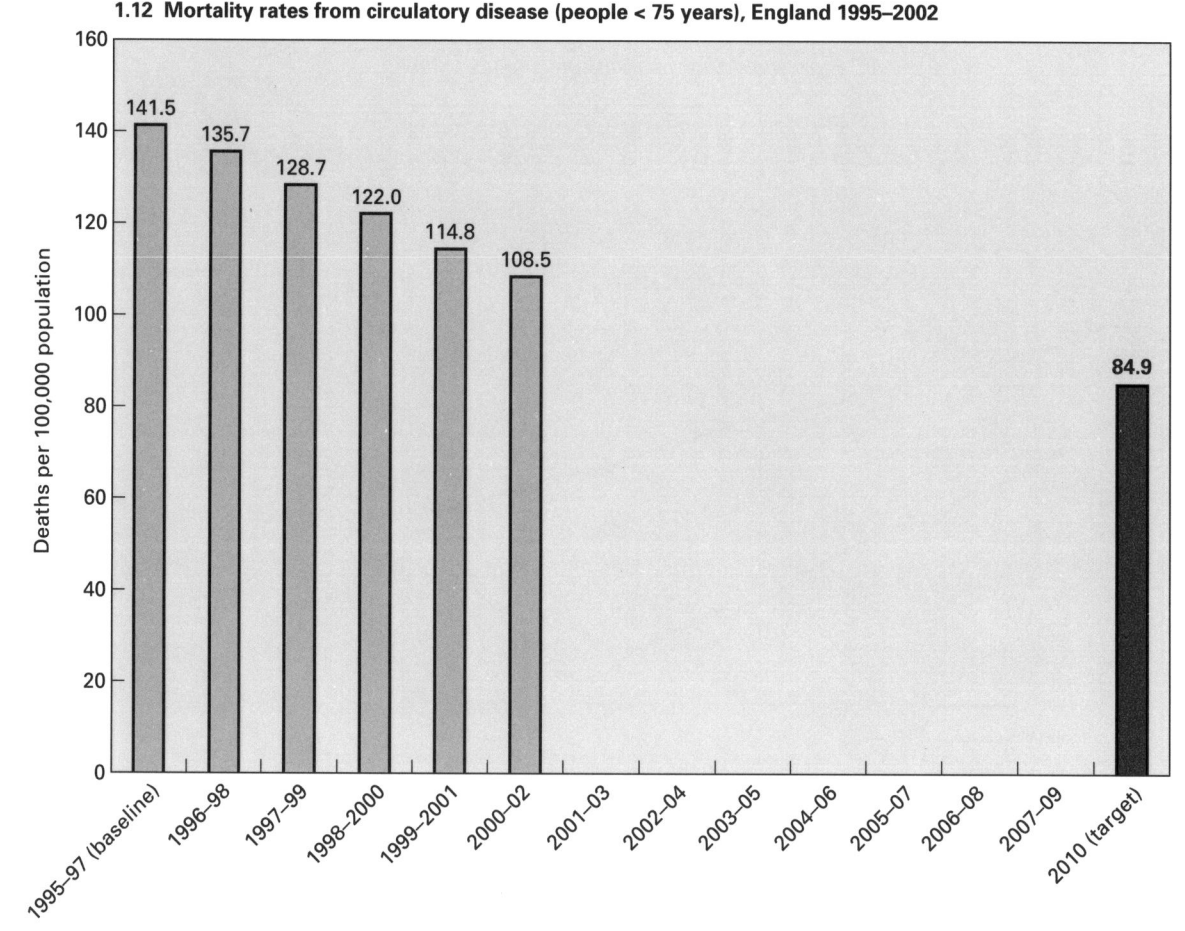

1.12 Mortality rates from circulatory disease (people < 75 years), England 1995–2002

Deaths per 100,000 population

- 1995–97 (baseline): 141.5
- 1996–98: 135.7
- 1997–99: 128.7
- 1998–2000: 122.0
- 1999–2001: 114.8
- 2000–02: 108.5
- 2010 (target): 84.9

The Quest for Quality in the NHS: a chartbook on quality of care in the UK

Coronary heart disease (CHD) is the single most common cause of premature death in the UK. It is caused by narrowing of the arteries that supply the heart. When the coronary arteries become narrowed or clogged by cholesterol and fat deposits, insufficient oxygenated blood reaches the heart, causing chest pain (often referred to as angina). If the blood supply to a portion of the heart is completely cut off by total blockage of a coronary artery by a blood clot, the result is a myocardial infarction or heart attack. The burden of CHD is not distributed equally in society. The death rate is 40% higher for males who are manual workers than for non-manual workers. The disease also varies by ethnicity. For people born on the Indian subcontinent, the death rate from heart disease is 38% higher for men and 43% higher for women than rates for England as a whole (DH, 2000a).

Risk factors for CHD include:

- age (45 years or older for men; 55 years or older for women)
- family history of early heart disease (father or brother affected before age 55; mother or sister affected before age 65)
- high total cholesterol
- smoking
- high blood pressure
- diabetes
- obesity
- physical inactivity.

Chart 1.13 Mortality from coronary heart disease

The Quest for Quality in the NHS: a chartbook on quality of care in the UK

This chart presents mortality rates from 1999 for people aged 35–74 years of age. The UK had the highest mortality rate among these comparator countries. Compared to France, mortality rates in the UK were four times higher for females and three times higher for males.

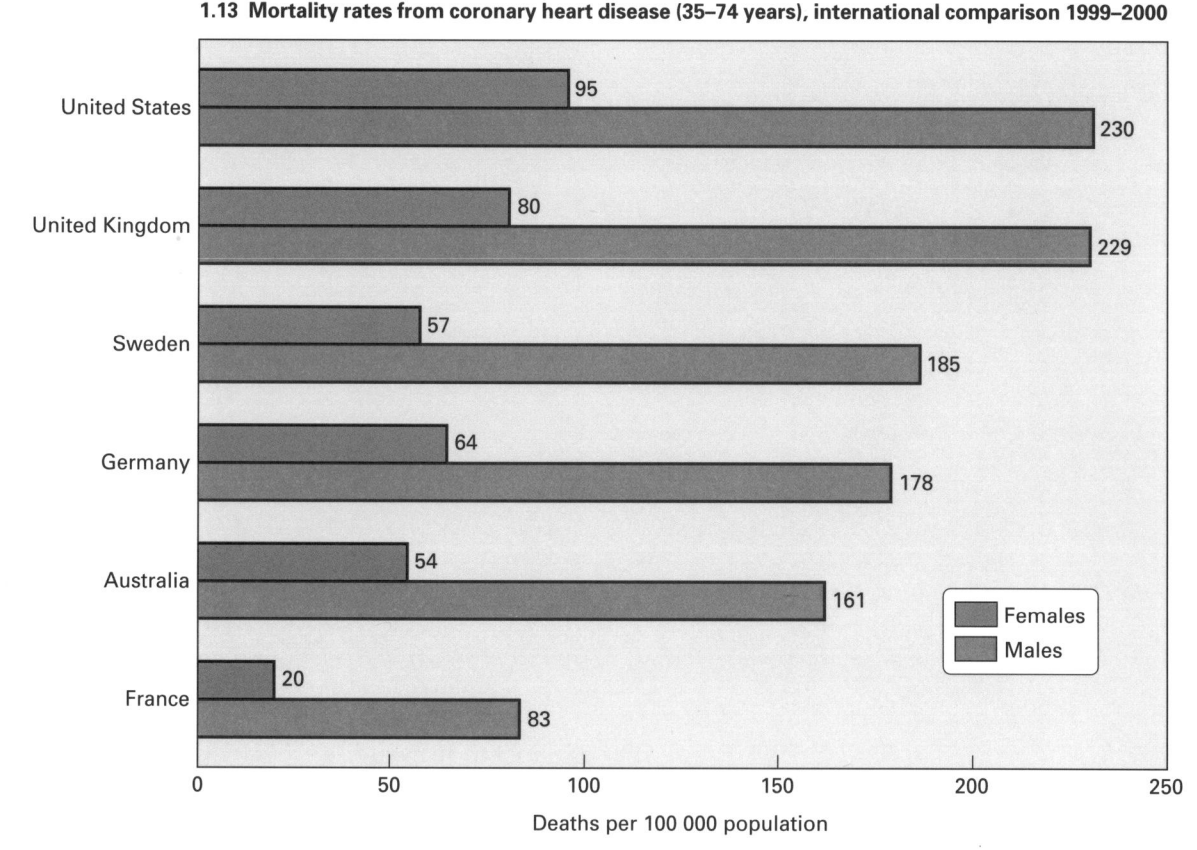

1.13 Mortality rates from coronary heart disease (35–74 years), international comparison 1999–2000

United States — Females 95, Males 230
United Kingdom — Females 80, Males 229
Sweden — Females 57, Males 185
Germany — Females 64, Males 178
Australia — Females 54, Males 161
France — Females 20, Males 83

Deaths per 100 000 population

Source: WHO mortality database.

Chart 1.14 Mortality rates from coronary heart disease: UK countries time series

These charts illustrate the relative rates of coronary heart disease (CHD) within the countries of the UK, and how they have changed over time. For both males and females, Scotland has the highest mortality rate. In 2002, there were 246 male deaths and 96 female deaths per 100 000 population due to CHD in Scotland, compared to 192 male and 65 female deaths per 100 000 in England, which had the lowest rates.

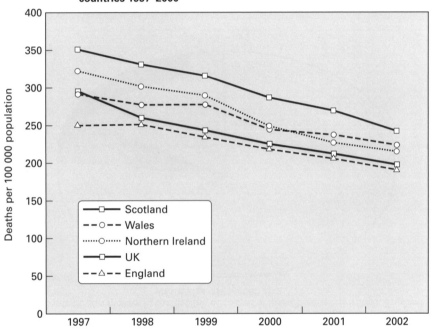

1.14a Mortality rates from coronary heart disease, males 35–74 years, UK countries 1997–2000

Source: Heartstats, ONS data

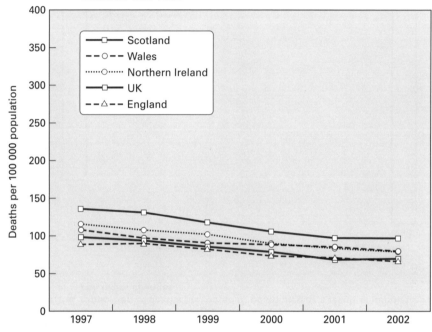

1.14b Mortality rates from coronary heart disease, females 35–74 years, UK countries 1997–2002

Source: Heartstats, ONS data.

The Quest for Quality in the NHS: a chartbook on quality of care in the UK

Chart 1.15 Explaining the decline in CHD mortality in England and Wales between 1981 and 2000

As Chart 1.14 illustrates, the fall in CHD mortality in recent years has been marked. Chart 1.15a presents research findings on the underlying factors that contributed to that decrease. Medical treatment and healthcare services were found to contribute 41.8% of the overall deaths prevented or postponed whereas changes in risk factors or behaviour (such as smoking cessation and lifestyle-mediated reductions in blood pressure and cholesterol) contributed 58.2%. Chart 1.15b provides a breakdown of the effects of various behavioural changes that contributed to improved mortality figures (chiefly smoking cessation) and gives estimates of risk factors that worsened mortality rates (such as decreased physical activity and obesity).

1.15a Contributing factors in the decline in coronary heart disease mortality, England and Wales 1981–2000 (%)

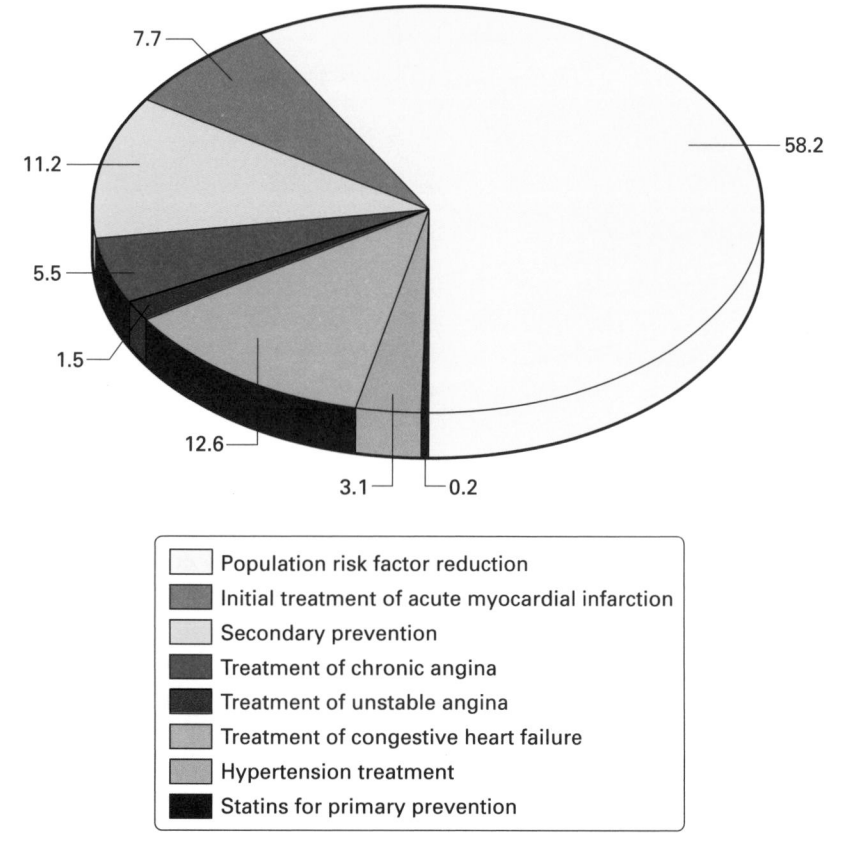

Legend:
- Population risk factor reduction
- Initial treatment of acute myocardial infarction
- Secondary prevention
- Treatment of chronic angina
- Treatment of unstable angina
- Treatment of congestive heart failure
- Hypertension treatment
- Statins for primary prevention

Source: Unal *et al.*, 2004.

1.15b Proportion of deaths prevented or postponed as a result of population risk factor changes

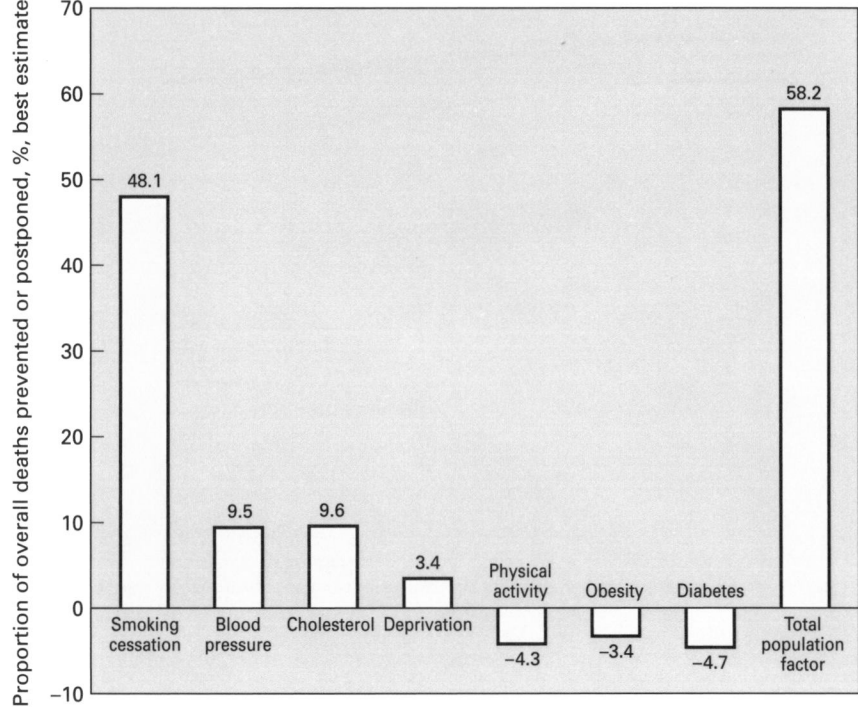

Source: Unal *et al.*, 2004.

Coronary heart disease: acute myocardial infarction

An acute myocardial infarction (AMI) or heart attack occurs when a clot or thrombus suddenly develops within an artery that supplies the heart muscle. If the blood supply is not restored quickly, the heart muscle suffers permanent damage. The restoration of blood supply via thrombolysis (the use of clot-dissolving drugs) or via revascularisation (the use of surgical procedures) have been proven to be effective treatments for AMI. In the UK, thrombolysis is recommended treatment post AMI. It is effective up to about 12 hours after the onset of symptoms but is most effective when given very early. If patients are treated in the first hour after symptoms develop, 65 lives are saved per 1000 patients, whereas after six hours have elapsed, this figure falls to 29 lives saved per 1000 treated (Boersma *et al.*, 1996).

In the US, the current guidelines from the American Heart Association and American College of Cardiology for a subset of AMI, STEMI (ST-elevated myocardial infarction),* recommend either thrombolysis within 30 minutes of arrival at the hospital *or* revascularisation within 90 minutes. Further, the guidelines state that

- Patients with STEMI who have cardiogenic shock and are less than 75 years of age should be brought immediately or secondarily transferred to facilities capable of cardiac catheterisation and rapid revascularisation (percutaneous coronary intervention (PCI) or coronary artery bypass graft surgery (CABG)) if it can be performed within 18 hours of onset of shock.
- It is reasonable that patients with STEMI who have cardiogenic shock and are 75 years of age or older be considered for immediate or prompt secondary transfer to facilities capable of cardiac catheterisation and rapid revascularisation (PCI or CABG) if it can be performed within 18 hours of onset of shock.
- It is reasonable that patients with STEMI who are at especially high risk of dying, including those with severe congestive heart failure (CHF), be considered for immediate or prompt secondary transfer (i.e. primary-receiving hospital door-to-departure time less than 30 minutes) to facilities capable of cardiac catheterisation and rapid revascularisation (PCI or CABG) (Anbe *et al.*, 2004).

After a patient has had one heart attack, there are several drugs which have been shown in large clinical trials to reduce the risk of another attack. This treatment is called secondary prevention and includes:

- aspirin, which helps to prevent the blood from clotting
- beta-blockers, which slow the heart rate and lower blood pressure, increasing the supply of blood and oxygen to the heart
- angiotensin-converting enzyme inhibitors (ACE inhibitors), which block an enzyme in the body that causes blood vessels to tighten, and therefore relax blood vessels and lower blood pressure
- statins, which reduce both total cholesterol and low-density lipoprotein (LDL or 'bad') cholesterol levels in the blood and thereby reduce the relative risk of coronary events.

* Refers to elevated ST segment on electrocardiogram (ECG).

The Quest for Quality in the NHS: a chartbook on quality of care in the UK

1 Effectiveness

Chart 1.16 Mortality from acute myocardial infarction

The Quest for Quality in the NHS: a chartbook on quality of care in the UK

Mortality rates from acute myocardial infarction (heart attack) have fallen significantly in recent years. This chart shows that England's mortality rate fell by 42% between 1990 and 1999. Despite this considerable progress, mortality rates in England remain high in comparison to those in Australia, Canada, and the United States.

1.16 Mortality rates from acute myocardial infarction, international comparison 1990 and 1999

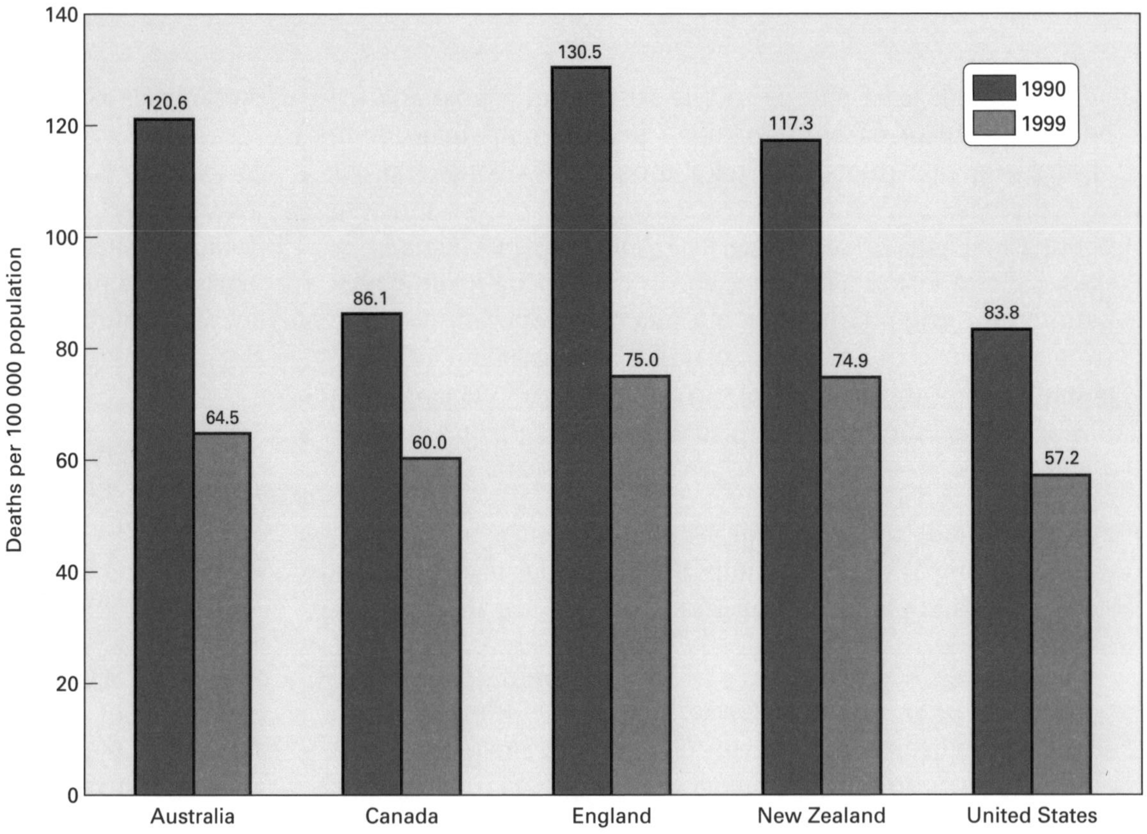

Source: Commonwealth Fund 2004a.

Chart 1.17 Managing acute myocardial infarction

The Myocardial Infarction National Audit Project (MINAP) was established in 2002 to gauge hospitals' performance in England against National Service Framework (NSF) standards for treatment of acute myocardial infarction (AMI). In 2004, data from Wales was included for the first time. The NSF standards are shown in Table 1.2.

Chart 1.17a shows the percentage of hospitals achieving the targets for timely thrombolysis (DTN30 standard) and secondary prevention of AMI. It shows great improvement in all areas with almost all hospitals achieving the NSF target that 80–90% of their heart attack patients should receive secondary prevention. For door-to-needle times, 71% of hospitals achieved the 30-minute target. Chart 1.17b compares the performance of Welsh and English hospitals in 2004. Welsh hospitals performed extremely well in secondary prevention measures but did less well in the thrombolysis measures. No Welsh

hospital achieved the 60-minute call-to-needle time (CTN60) standard. However, CTN performance is not only a reflection of hospital care; responsibility is shared with ambulance services and primary care.

Table 1.2

Standard (DH 2000a)	Target for each hospital
Patients should receive thrombolysis within 30 minutes of arriving at hospital (door-to-needle time – DTN30)	75% of patients
Patients should receive thrombolysis within 60 minutes of calling for professional help (call-to-needle time – CTN60)	48% of patients
Patients discharged from hospital following a heart attack should be given secondary prevention drugs (e.g. aspirin, beta-blockers, statins)	80–90% of patients

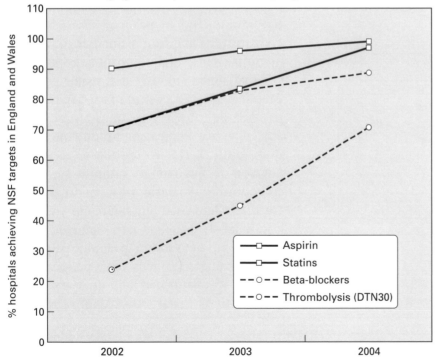

1.17a Managing acute myocardial infarctions, England and Wales 2002–04

Source: CEEU (2003; 2004); Royal College of Physicians.

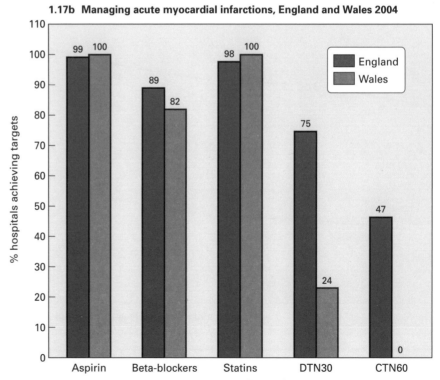

1.17b Managing acute myocardial infarctions, England and Wales 2004

Source: CEEU (2003; 2004); Royal College of Physicians.

The Quest for Quality in the NHS: a chartbook on quality of care in the UK

1 Effectiveness

Chart 1.18 Thrombolysis rates after acute myocardial infarction

The Quest for Quality in the NHS: a chartbook on quality of care in the UK

This chart differs from Chart 1.17 in that it is concerned with the percentage of *patients* who received care that conformed to the prescribed standard, rather than the percentage of hospitals that achieved target times. The chart illustrates the percentage of heart attack patients who received thrombolysis within 30 minutes of arriving at hospital (the door-to-needle or DTN time) and within 60 minutes of calling for help (the call-to-needle-time or CTN). The original National Service Framework (NSF) standard for DTN stated that 75% of eligible patients should receive thrombolytic drugs within 30 minutes of arriving at hospital. In April 2003 the target was reduced to 20 minutes. To provide longitudinal data, the Myocardial Infarction National Audit Project continues to collect data on the 30-minute time limit. In March 2002, 59% of patients were treated within 30 minutes of arriving at hospital. By September 2004 this figure had risen to 84%. The proportion of people being thrombolysed within one hour of calling for professional help, which is clinically more meaningful, was 32% in March 2002 and 54% in September 2004.

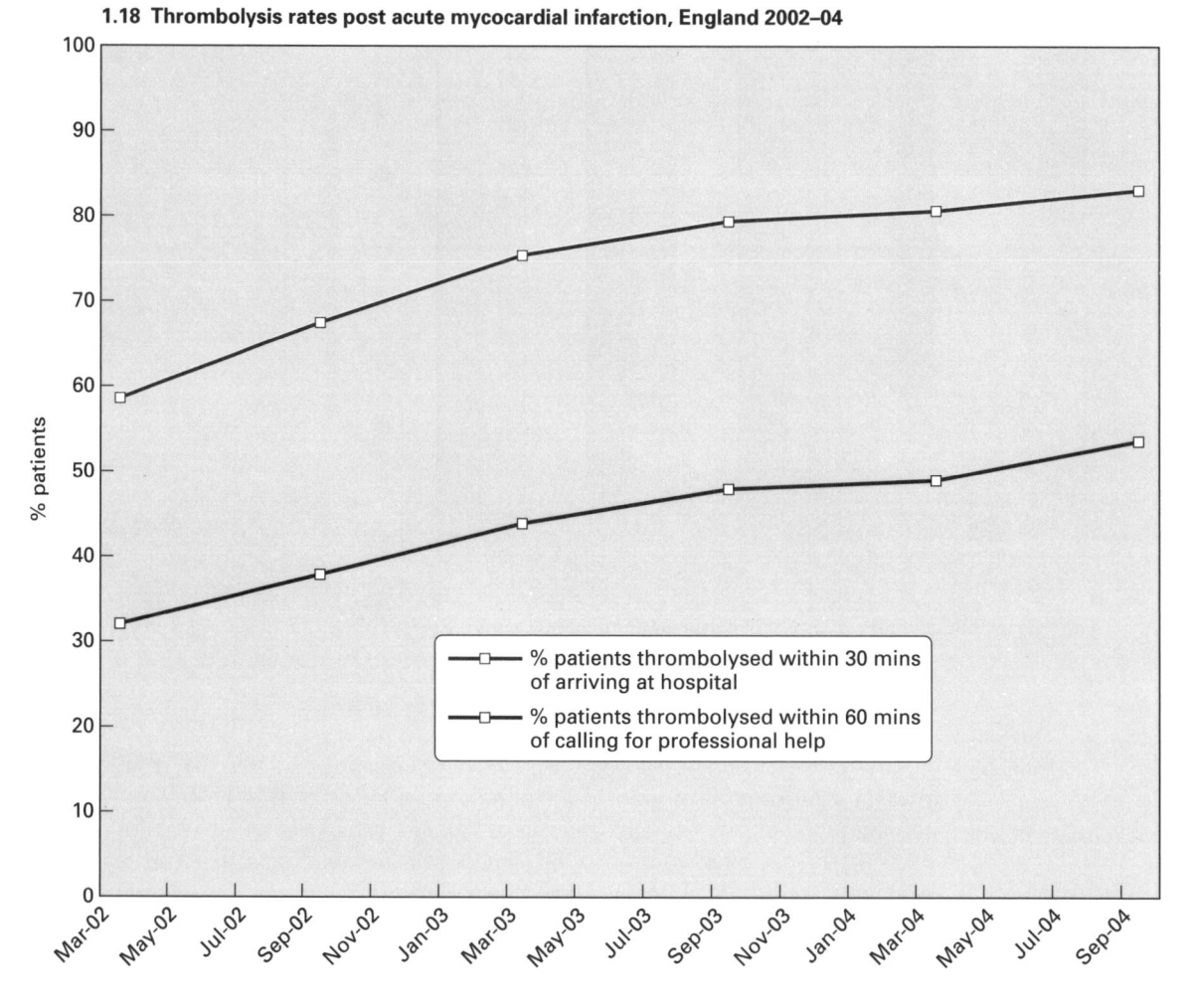

1.18 Thrombolysis rates post acute mycocardial infarction, England 2002–04

Legend:
— % patients thrombolysed within 30 mins of arriving at hospital
— % patients thrombolysed within 60 mins of calling for professional help

Source: CEEU (2003; 2004), Royal College of Physicians.

Revascularisation means making the blood vessels wider or replacing blocked arteries with grafts. Several different types of revascularisation treatment are used to treat coronary heart disease (CHD). They include:

- percutaneous transluminal coronary angioplasty (PTCA): a catheter is inserted through the upper leg, groin or upper arm and threaded through to the coronary artery. A device like a small balloon is inserted into the artery and inflated until the artery is open enough to allow a good blood supply. The balloon is then deflated and taken out
- angioplasty with stenting: following angioplasty, a steel mesh tube, called a stent, is inserted to keep the artery open
- coronary artery bypass graft (CABG): an open-heart operation which uses a blood vessel (called a graft) taken from the arm, leg or chest to bypass a narrowed or blocked coronary artery
- other forms of heart surgery, such as transmyocardial laser revascularisation and percutaneous laser revascularisation.

There are evidence-based indications for each method of revascularisation, which are not necessarily mutually exclusive (*see* www.sign.ac.uk/guidelines/fulltext/32/index.html).

The CHD National Service Framework (NSF) noted that by international standards the UK has high rates of CHD but low rates of coronary artery revascularisation. This does not appear to be because most other countries are overusing revascularisation but rather because there has been underprovision of revascularisation in the UK (DH, 2000a).

Not only are the overall rates of coronary revascularisation in the UK low, but provision is unequal. There are geographical, gender and racial variations in revascularisation rates, which are not closely correlated with measures of the level of heart disease in the community – suggesting inequities of provision or inappropriate use.

Chart 1.19 Revascularisation rates and mortality from heart disease

Use of technologies and treatments varies widely both across and within developed healthcare systems, suggesting that interventions are both overused and underused in different contexts (OECD Health Project, 2004). This is clearly illustrated when examining international data comparing revascularisation rates and mortality rates from ischaemic heart disease (IHD). Chart 1.19 illustrates a weak relationship between the mortality rates from heart disease and the rate of revascularisation. Most noteworthy are the results of the UK where, uniquely among the countries shown, mortality rates exceed revascularisation rates, suggesting underuse of the procedure.

Source: OECD Health Project, 2004.

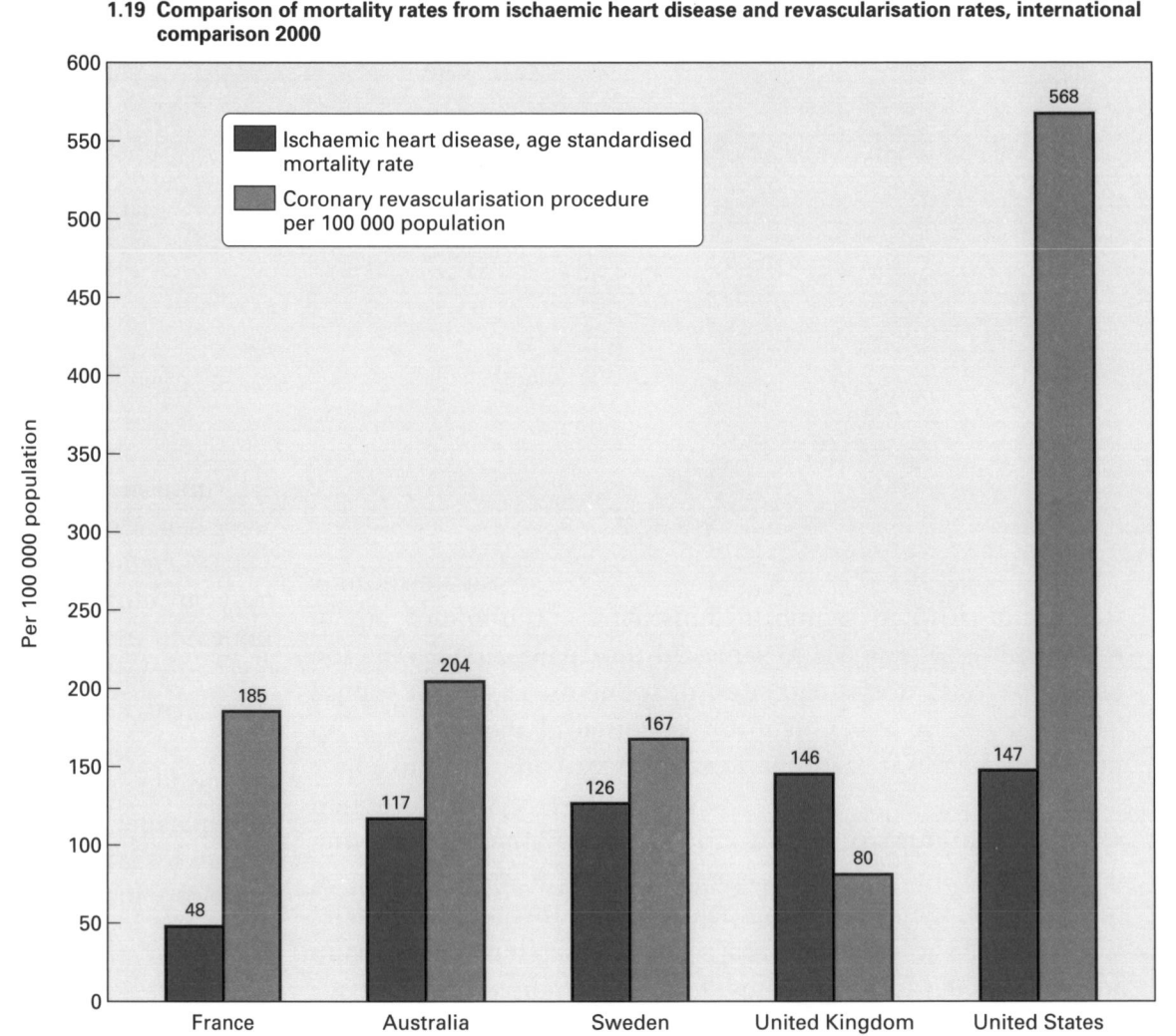

1.19 Comparison of mortality rates from ischaemic heart disease and revascularisation rates, international comparison 2000

Legend:
- Ischaemic heart disease, age standardised mortality rate
- Coronary revascularisation procedure per 100 000 population

Per 100 000 population

France: 48, 185
Australia: 117, 204
Sweden: 126, 167
United Kingdom: 146, 80
United States: 147, 568

The Quest for Quality in the NHS: a chartbook on quality of care in the UK

Chart 1.20 Appropriateness of revascularisation procedures: three London hospitals

For a prospective study of consecutive patients undergoing coronary angiography at three London hospitals, a nine-member expert panel rated the appropriateness of percutaneous transluminal coronary angioplasty (PTCA) and coronary artery bypass graft (CABG) for specific clinical conditions. These ratings were then applied to a population of patients with coronary artery disease. Treatment decisions were made without reference to the expert ratings. Chart 1.20a shows that underuse of PTCA was substantial: only 36% of patients (327 of 908) who could have benefited from PTCA received it, whereas 6% of patients (34 of 568) received PTCA when not clinically indicated. Chart 1.20b shows that CABG was used more appropriately although underuse was still appreciable: 57% of patients (765 of 1353) who could have benefited from CABG actually received it, and 8% of patients (15 of 186) for whom CABG was not appropriate received it. The group of patients for whom the expert panel indicated PTCA was appropriate but who received only medical treatment were more likely to have subsequent angina than those who received PTCA. Similarly, those patients for whom the expert panel recommended CABG but who received only medical treatment were more likely to have angina or to die or have a non-fatal heart attack than those who received CABG.

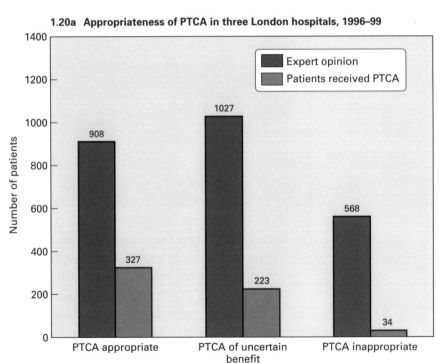

1.20a Appropriateness of PTCA in three London hospitals, 1996–99

Source: Hemingway *et al.*, 2001.

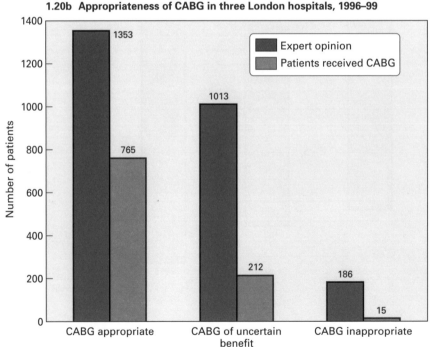

1.20b Appropriateness of CABG in three London hospitals, 1996–99

Source: Hemingway *et al.*, 2001.

Chart 1.21 Deaths within 30 days of coronary artery bypass graft (CABG)

The Quest for Quality in the NHS: a chartbook on quality of care in the UK

This chart illustrates the mortality rate within 30 days of CABG and includes patients who have been discharged and those remaining in hospital. It illustrates significant improvement in the mortality rate with a 26% decrease between 1998–99 and 2002–03. Care must be taken in interpreting postoperative mortality rates when they are not adjusted to account for any differences in patient characteristics (e.g. severity of illness) that might affect outcomes.

Source: NCHOD (analysis by Lakhani, Eayres and Coles using HES data).

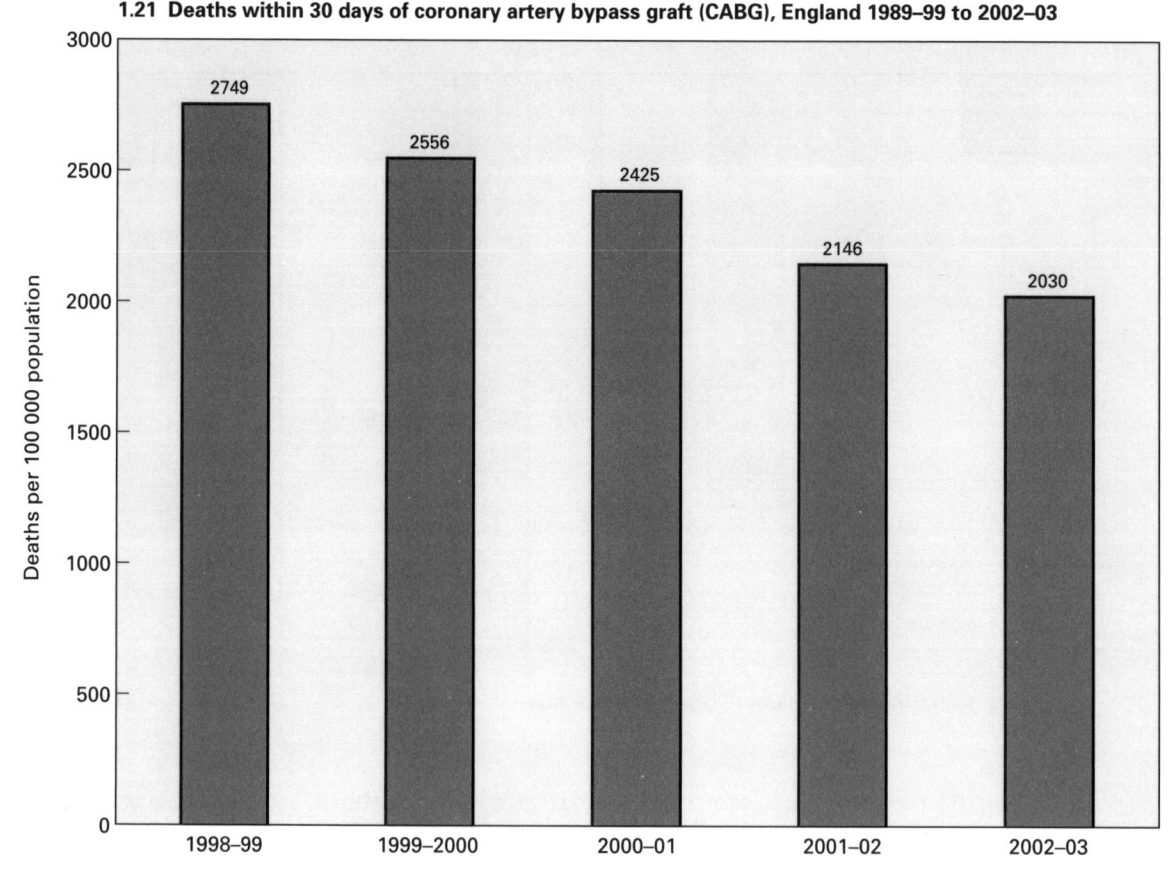

1.21 Deaths within 30 days of coronary artery bypass graft (CABG), England 1989–99 to 2002–03

Deaths per 100 000 population

Year	Value
1998–99	2749
1999–2000	2556
2000–01	2425
2001–02	2146
2002–03	2030

Coronary heart disease: use of statins

High total cholesterol is a risk factor for coronary heart disease (CHD). Results of the Framingham study (www.framingham.com/heart/) showed that the higher the cholesterol level, the greater the CHD risk. Cholesterol is a waxy, fat-like substance that occurs naturally in all parts of the body. It is present in cell walls or membranes everywhere in the body, including the brain, nerves, muscle, skin, liver, intestines and heart. Cholesterol is necessary for the production of many hormones, vitamin D and the bile acids that help to digest fat. It takes only a small amount of cholesterol in the blood to meet these needs. If there is an excess of cholesterol in the blood, it is deposited in arteries, including the coronary arteries, where it contributes to the narrowing and blockages that cause the signs and symptoms of heart disease.

A direct link between high blood cholesterol and CHD was established by the Lipid Research Clinics Program (1984) which showed that lowering total and low density lipoprotein (LDL or 'bad') cholesterol levels significantly reduces CHD. Subsequent trials of cholesterol reduction using a class of drugs collectively referred to as statins have demonstrated conclusively that lowering total cholesterol and LDL-cholesterol reduces the chance of having a heart attack, the need for bypass surgery or angioplasty, and death from CHD-related causes (Shepherd *et al.*, 1995; Downs *et al.*, 1998; Scandinavian Simvastatin Survival Study Group, 1994; Heart Protection Study Collaborative Group, 2002). Following a heart attack or stroke, statins can reduce the chance of dying in the subsequent five years by about a third (Miettinen *et al.*, 1997; Serruys *et al.*, 2002). More recent research has shown that statin therapy also rapidly reduces the incidence of ischaemic strokes, with no apparent effect on cerebral haemorrhage, even among individuals who do not have high cholesterol concentrations (Heart Protection Study Collaborative Group, 2004).

In the 10 years between 1994 and 2004, the number of statin prescriptions dispensed in the community in England increased from 800 000 to 26.4 million, a 33-fold increase (DH, 2004b).

Chart 1.22 Statin use in Europe

The use of statins across Europe is extensive but variable. Chart 1.22a shows that, in 2000, about 24 defined daily doses were prescribed per 1000 population per day in England. A defined daily dose (DDD) is the average maintenance dose per day for a drug's main indication in adults. In 2000, Norway dispensed two and a half times more DDDs of statins than England. Chart 1.22b shows that prescribing rates in England in 2003 were double those in 2000. In 2003 Wales dispensed the most statins (86.2 DDDs) and England the least (50.9 DDDs). Increasing rates of usage suggest improved quality of care, and are thought to be contributing to the falling mortality rates from coronary heart disease, but this data only indicates prescribing volume, not the appropriateness of prescribing for individual patients.

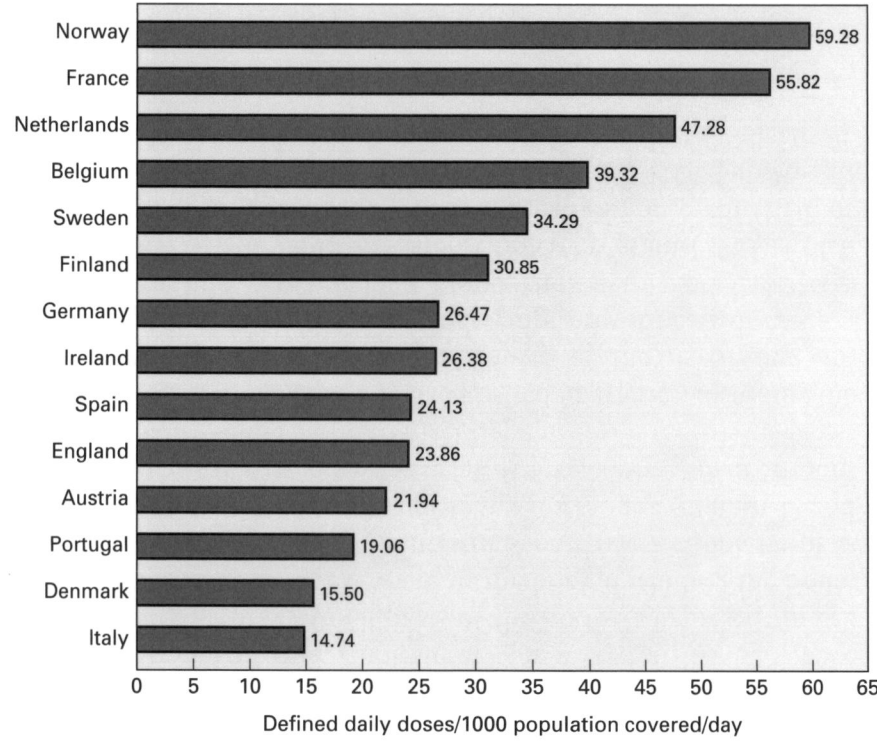

1.22a Statin prescriptions, international comparison 2000

Country	Defined daily doses/1000 population covered/day
Norway	59.28
France	55.82
Netherlands	47.28
Belgium	39.32
Sweden	34.29
Finland	30.85
Germany	26.47
Ireland	26.38
Spain	24.13
England	23.86
Austria	21.94
Portugal	19.06
Denmark	15.50
Italy	14.74

Defined daily doses/1000 population covered/day

Source: Walley *et al.*, 2004.

1.22b Statin prescriptions, UK countries 2003

Defined daily dose (DDD) per head population per day

Country	DDD
England	50.9
Scotland	85.4
Wales	86.2
Northern Ireland	72.5
United Kingdom	56.2

Source: DHSSPS, 2004

A stroke occurs when blood flow to the brain is interrupted or severely reduced and brain tissue is deprived of oxygen and nutrients. Within a few minutes to a few hours of the interrupted blood flow, brain cells begin to die. There are two different kinds of stroke. The first, ischaemic stroke, is caused by a blood clot that blocks or plugs a blood vessel or artery in the brain. The second type, haemorrhagic stroke, is caused by a breakage and subsequent leakage from a blood vessel in the brain. Roughly 80% of all strokes are ischaemic and 20% are haemorrhagic. Although stroke is a disease of the brain, it can affect the entire body. The effects of a stroke range from mild to severe and involve physical, cognitive and psychosocial functions.

Each year more than 130 000 people in England and Wales have a first stroke. About 10 000 of these are under retirement age. Stroke is the third most common cause of death in England and Wales, after heart disease and cancer. It accounts for about 60 000 deaths each year, representing 8% of all deaths in men and 13% of deaths in women in England. Stroke has a greater disability impact than any other medical condition. A quarter of a million people are living with long-term disability as a result of stroke in the UK. The cost of stroke to the NHS is estimated to be over £2.3 billion. Stroke patients occupy 20% of all acute hospital beds and 25% of long-term beds (Stroke Association, 2004).

In a prospective study of stroke in 1220 London-based patients, Wolfe (2002) found the incidence of stroke to be higher in the black ethnic group, in males, in older people, and in people from lower socio-economic groups. The incidence in the black group was twice that in the white group and occurred 10 years earlier. This increase was independent of age, sex and socio-economic status. The case fatality rate was found to be higher in the white group, after allowing for age, sex and type of stroke. At six months after stroke 37% of patients had died. For a subgroup of this cohort, long-term follow-up (mean 4.9 years; 291 patients, 123 still alive, 106 interviewed) indicated that 29% of survivors were severely or moderately disabled, 37% mildly disabled, 34% functionally independent and 36% were depressed. Many patients received little health or social service support, and coordination of follow-up was poor. Secondary prevention of risk factors was often inadequate (Wolfe, 2002).

Chart 1.23 Stroke mortality rates

Chart 1.23a shows that in 2001 England's mortality rate from stroke was lower than that in Australia but higher than that in the US and New Zealand. Chart 1.23b shows that mortality rates in the countries of the UK have declined over the past 10 years. Scotland has consistently had the highest mortality rates but has shown the most rapid rate of improvement with a 37% decrease in mortality rates between 1994 and 2003.

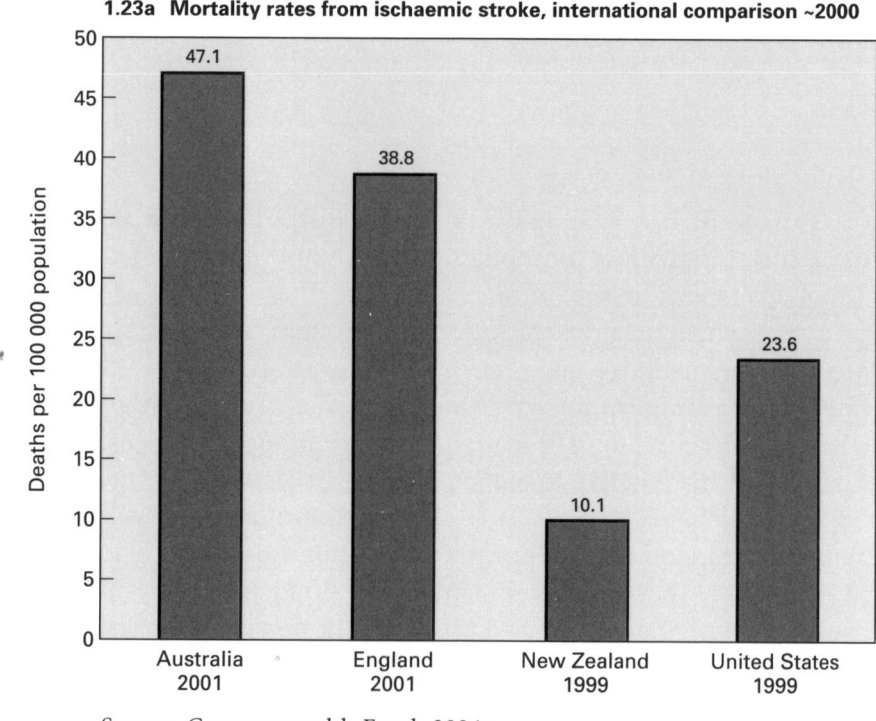

1.23a Mortality rates from ischaemic stroke, international comparison ~2000

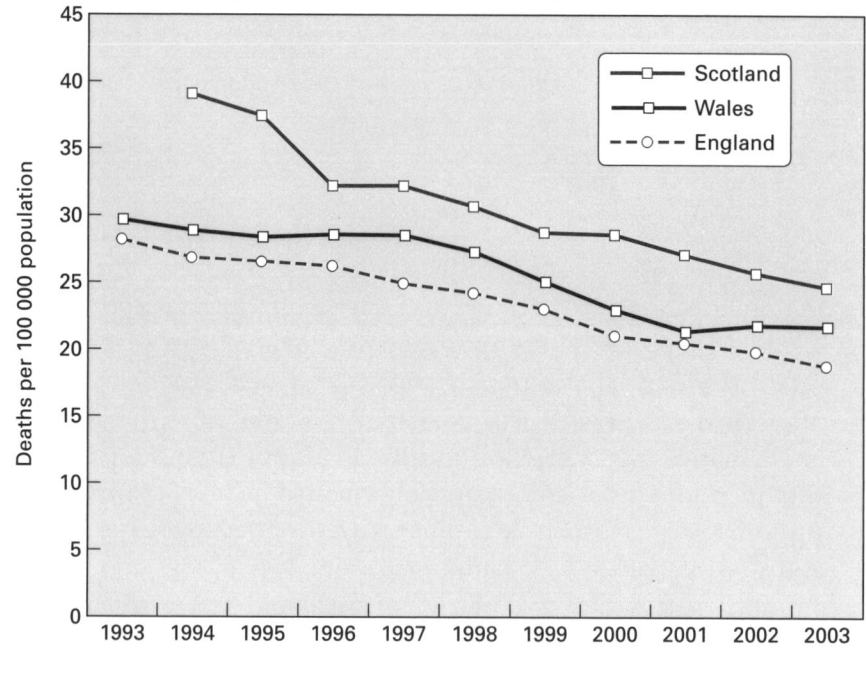

1.23b Mortality rates from stroke (people < 75 years), UK countries 1993–2003

Source: Commonwealth Fund, 2004a.

Sources: NCHOD, 2003; ONS; ISD Scotland.

Note: The Commonwealth Fund study used 1980 OECD population to standardise its data; ONS, NCHOD, and ISD Scotland all use the European standard population. This difference may explain the discrepancy in mortality rates between the two charts.

The Quest for Quality in the NHS: a chartbook on quality of care in the UK

Diabetes mellitus is a disease in which the body does not produce or properly use insulin. Insulin, a hormone produced by the pancreas, is needed to convert sugar, starches and other food into energy. The result of this deficiency is the high blood sugar levels characteristic of diabetes. There are two main forms of diabetes: type 1 diabetes results from the body's failure to produce insulin, and type 2 diabetes results from insulin resistance (suboptimal use of insulin). Obesity is closely linked with type 2 diabetes. Diabetes is associated with serious chronic ill health, disability and premature mortality. Long-term complications include heart disease, stroke, blindness, kidney disease and amputations, and they make a substantial contribution to the costs, both personal and financial, of diabetes care. Many of the long-term effects of diabetes could be avoided with effective control of blood pressure and blood sugar levels (DCCT, 1993; UK Prospective Diabetes Study Group, 1998).

Diabetes currently affects 5% of the world's population (Marso, 2003). Type 1 diabetes is almost always diagnosed under the age of 40. Type 2 diabetes tends to occur in those over the age of 40 although the prevalence of type 2 diabetes in children is increasing (National Paediatric Diabetes Audit, 2004). In the UK, almost 1.8 million people or some 3% of the population are diagnosed diabetics (Watkins, 2003). Of this, close to 250 000 people have type 1 diabetes and more than 1.5 million have type 2 diabetes. Prevalence differs markedly across ethnic groups: 20% of people with South Asian origins and 17% with African-Caribbean origins have type 2 diabetes as compared to 3% of the population as a whole (Watkins *et al.*, 2003).

The economic costs of diabetes are substantial. An estimated 5% of the NHS budget (~ £3.5bn) is spent on treating diabetes and its complications (DH, 2001). This figure is expected to rise to 10% by 2011.

Chart 1.24 Mortality from diabetes

Using data from death certificates from England and Wales, Chart 1.24 presents mortality rates from diabetes, differentiating between deaths for which diabetes was identified as the underlying cause of death; and deaths from any cause with diabetes mentioned on the death certificate. In the latter, more common case – where diabetes was mentioned as part of a patient's multifactorial health status – one cannot ascertain the precise role that diabetes has played in the death. Mortality rates in both cases remained fairly static between 1993 and 2003. Mortality rates in both categories were higher in Wales than in England although the difference was more marked in any-cause mortality.

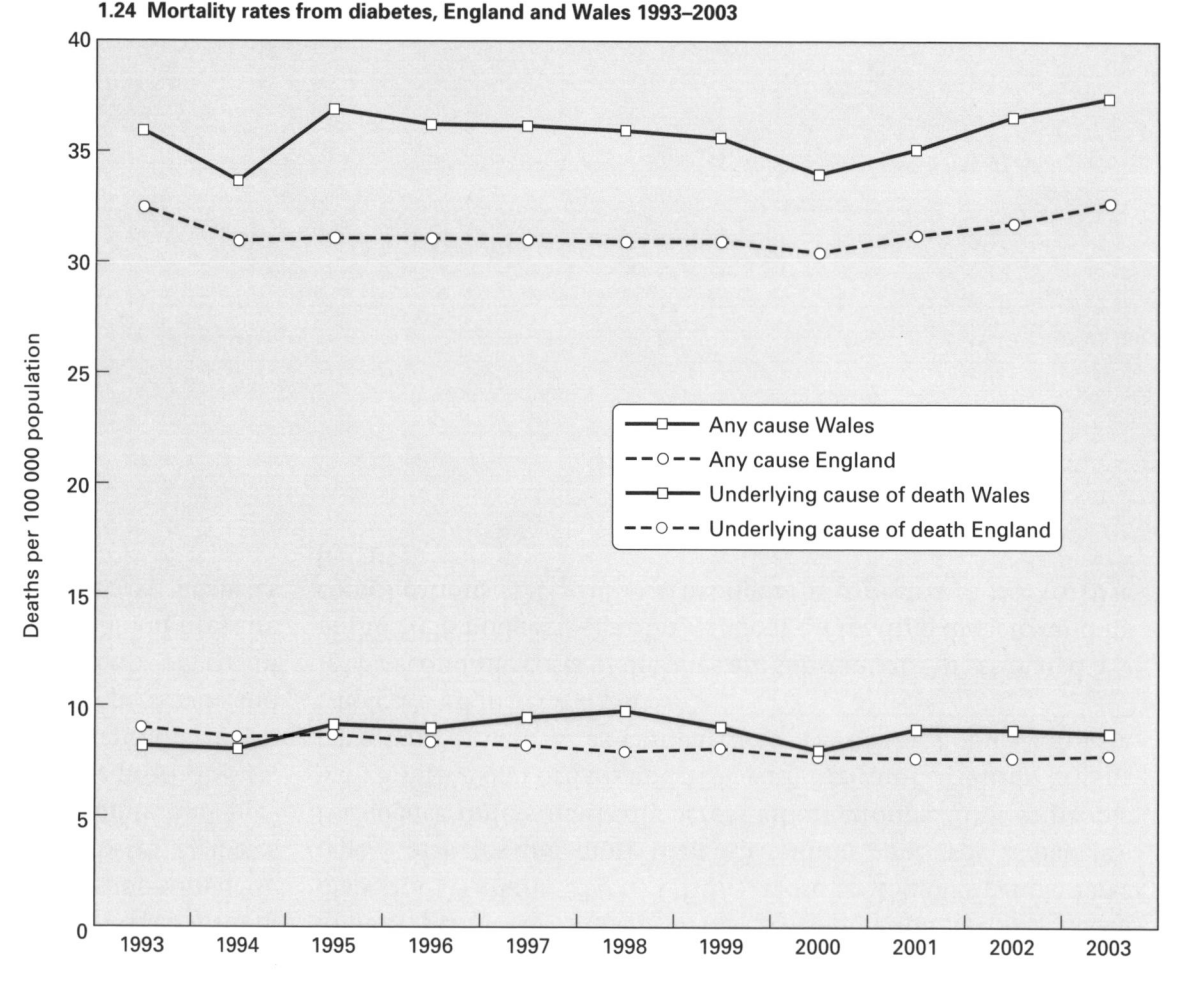

1.24 Mortality rates from diabetes, England and Wales 1993–2003

Source: DH Mortality Extracts 1993–2003, ONS; Mid-year population estimates 1993–2003; NCHOD (analysis by Lakhani, Eayres, and Coles).

The Quest for Quality in the NHS: a chartbook on quality of care in the UK

Chart 1.25 Diabetic control in children

Maintaining controlled blood glucose levels (glycaemic control) reduces the risk of long-term sequelae of diabetes such as blindness, kidney failure and nerve damage (DCCT,1993). Glycated haemoglobin (HbA1c) provides a measure of average blood sugar over the 60–90 days preceding the test and so is an indicator of glycaemic control. NICE clinical guidelines for type 1 diabetes recommend that the HbA1c level should be less than 7.5%.* Chart 1.25a shows that levels of control in diabetic children in England, Wales and Northern Ireland are poor; fewer than one in five diabetic children and young people (aged 0–16 years) maintain their blood glucose readings within the recommended level. Chart 1.25b shows the rate of emergency admissions for diabetes in Scottish children and adolescents (aged 10–19 years). Such admissions may be an indication of poor glycaemic control, which reflects on quality of primary care and levels of patient compliance (Giuffrida *et al.*, 1999). The rate of emergency admissions increased by 16% between 1993 and 2003.

1.25a Diabetic control in children, England, Wales and Northern Ireland 2002

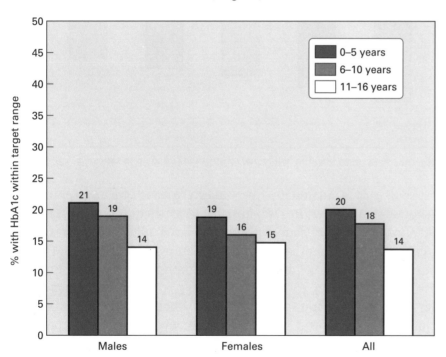

Source: National Paediatric Diabetes Audit (2004).

1.25b Emergency admissions for diabetes in children and adolescents (10–19 years), Scotland 1993 and 2003

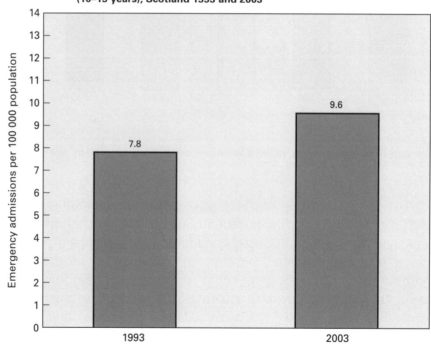

Source: ISD Scotland (Health Indicators Report, 2004).

* However, targets should be individualised to the lowest achievable HbA1c without inducing severe hypoglycaemia.

The Quest for Quality in the NHS: a chartbook on quality of care in the UK

Chart 1.26 Measures indicating poor diabetic control

These charts provide data on adverse health outcomes that may indicate suboptimal primary care, poor patient compliance, or both. Chart 1.26a shows the number of hospital episodes of ketoacidosis in England. People with diabetes lack sufficient insulin and are unable to process glucose for energy. When glucose is not available, body fat is broken down instead. The by-products of fat metabolism are ketones; if allowed to build up, they result in ketoacidosis where the blood becomes more acidified (Medline-plus Encyclopaedia, 2005). If untreated, the high level of acidic ketones, and accompanying dehydration and imbalance of electrolytes, can lead to unconsciousness and, ultimately, death. Chart 1.26a documents a 19% increase

in the number of episodes of ketoacidosis from 17.97 per 100 000 in 1998–99 to 21.43 in 2002–03. Chart 1.26b depicts the rate of diabetic lower limb amputations. People with diabetes are at risk of developing neuropathy (nerve damage). This is most frequently manifested in ulceration of patients' feet and may lead to lower limb amputation. The chart shows that the rate of lower limb amputations in diabetics in England remained fairly static at around 8.5 per 100 000 population between 1998–99 and 2002–03. In Australia, the diabetic amputation rate in 1995–98 was 13.97 per 100 000 population (Payne, 2000 data not shown).

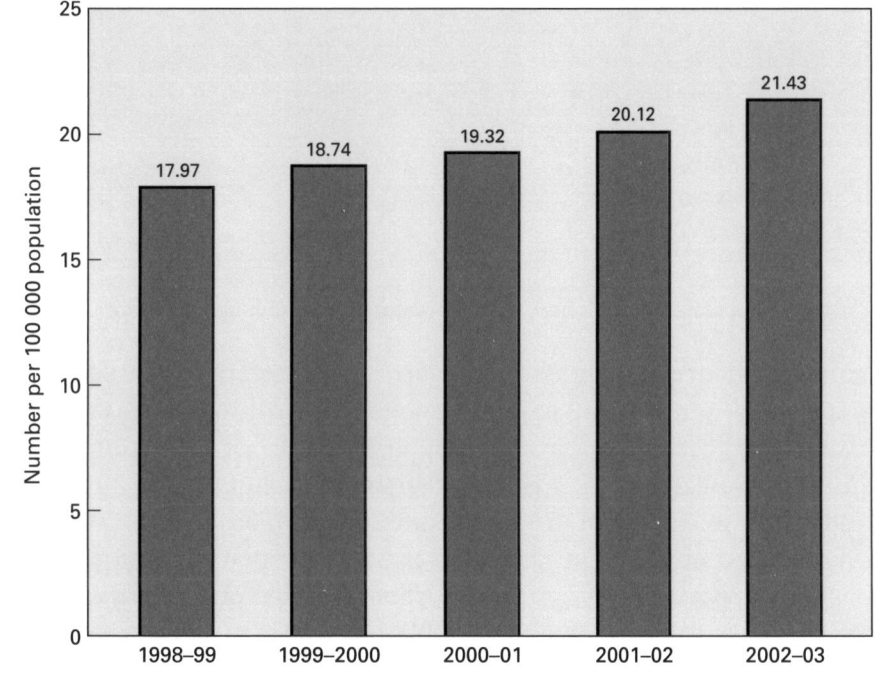

1.26a Episodes of diabetic ketoacidosis and coma, England 1998–99 to 2002–03

Source: Hospital Episode Statistics; NCHOD, 2003 (analysis by Lakhani, Eayres, and Coles).

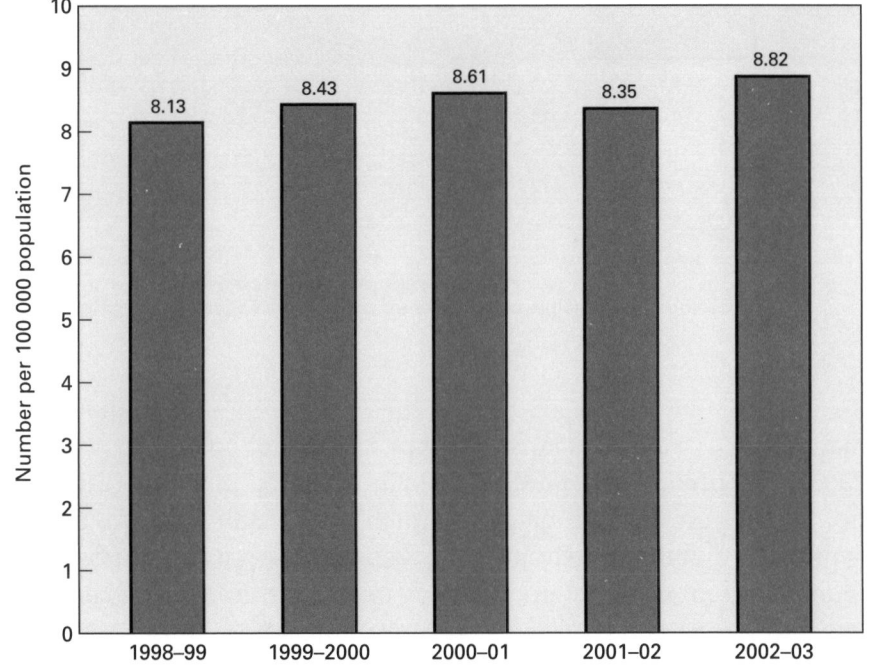

1.26b Lower limb amputations in diabetic patients, England 1998–99 to 2002–03

Source: Hospital Episode Statistics; NCHOD, 2003 (analysis by Lakhani, Eayres, and Coles).

Infectious disease

Infectious diseases account for 41% of the global disease burden and 25% of deaths worldwide (CMO, 2002).

In England, the decline in death and serious illness from infectious disease during the twentieth century was striking.

- In 1901, the death rate from infectious disease was 369 per 100 000 population; by 2000 it had fallen to 9 per 100 000 population.
- In 1953, there were 2832 cases of paralytic poliomyelitis; in 2000, there were none.
- In 1949 there were 371 341 cases of measles, resulting in 290 deaths and more than 400 cases of encephalitis attributed to the disease. In 2000, there were 72 confirmed cases, with 1 death and 4 cases of encephalitis.

Despite this progress, infectious diseases continue to pose significant healthcare problems. In England:

- Infections account for 70 000 deaths per year.

- 40% of people consult their doctor every year because of an infection.
- 150 000 people are hospitalised for infections every year.
- 1 in 11 sexually active women is infected with chlamydia.
- The number of people diagnosed with HIV increased by 40% between 1999 and 2003 to around 29 000 cases.
- 5000 deaths per year are attributed to healthcare-associated infections.
- 100 000 cases of food poisoning occur each year.

(CMO, 2002)

We present data on vaccinations and antibiotic usage. Vaccinations are one of the most cost-effective disease prevention strategies in public health; they are widely accepted as a reliable measure reflecting quality of primary care and public health policy. We also present an analysis of variation in antibiotic prescribing rates in general practice, because inappropriate overuse of antibiotics remains a serious concern and is also a well-accepted quality indicator.

Chart 1.27 Influenza vaccinations (for people ≥ 65 years)

See also Chart 6.10

40

The Quest for Quality in the NHS: a chartbook on quality of care in the UK

Between 10% and 15% of the population may develop influenza in any year. For the majority of people, it is an unpleasant but self-limiting illness. However, for those in high-risk groups (aged 65 and over, or with underlying respiratory or heart disease, diabetes or impaired immunity), influenza is much more serious, and it results in a considerable number of deaths each year. Incidence rates vary but even in years with relatively low incidence rates, 3000 to 4000 deaths in England are attributed to influenza. In epidemic years, mortality rates are much higher. For example, 13 000 deaths were attributed to influenza in 1993 and 29 000 in 1989–90 (DH, 2005). Influenza vaccines are highly effective at preventing illness and reducing hospital admissions among high-risk groups. A national target of 70% uptake of vaccination for people aged ≥ 65 years has been set. Using data from patient surveys conducted in 2004, Chart 1.27a shows that 74% of UK respondents ≥ 65 years of age indicated that they had been vaccinated. Within the UK (Chart 1.27b), the proportion of respondents indicating that they had been vaccinated ranged from 62% in Wales to 82% in Scotland.

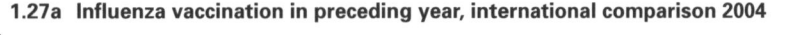

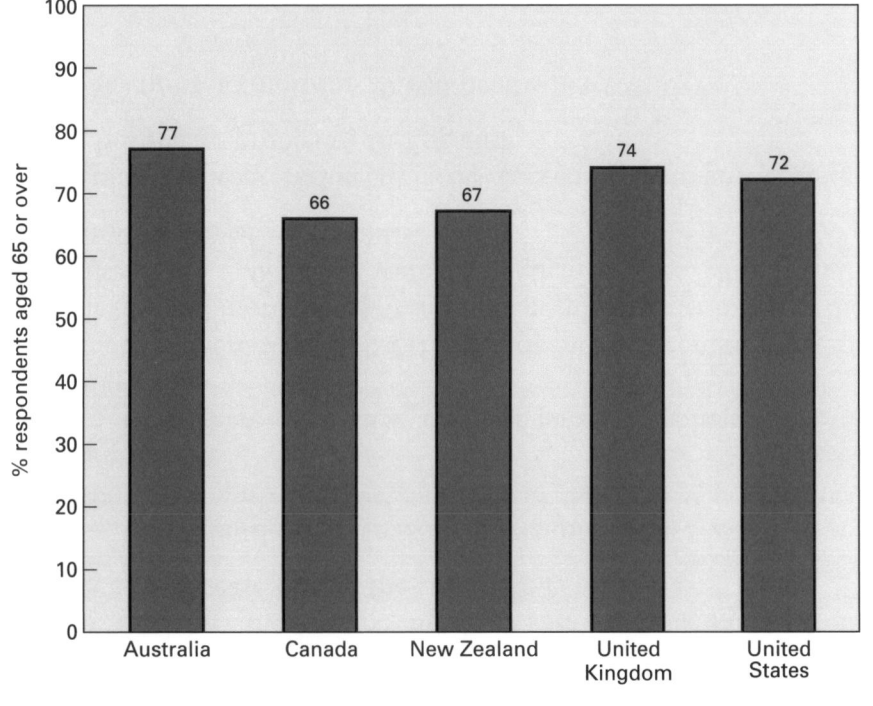

1.27a Influenza vaccination in preceding year, international comparison 2004

Source: Commonwealth Fund, 2004a.

1.27b Influenza vaccination in preceding year, UK countries 2004

Source: Commonwealth Fund, 2004b.

Chart 1.28 Childhood vaccinations by age two

The World Health Organization recommends immunity levels of around 95% to prevent outbreaks of disease (HPA, 2001). Chart 1.28a shows that, across the UK, coverage rates for most childhood vaccinations have been high. However, Chart 1.28b illustrates the exception that has occurred with measles, mumps and rubella (MMR) vaccination rates. In recent years, speculation that the MMR vaccine might be linked to autism and Crohn's disease has affected uptake. Despite repeated, unequivocal and evidence-based assurances that MMR is safe, public scepticism remains a potent force. This chart illustrates and serves as a reminder that patient (and parent) compliance can be an important factor in efforts to improve healthcare quality. In England, MMR vaccination rates have fallen from a high of 91.5% in 1996 to 79.9% in 2003.

1.28a Diphtheria, tetanus, polio and pertussis vaccination coverage at 2 years of age, UK countries 2000–04

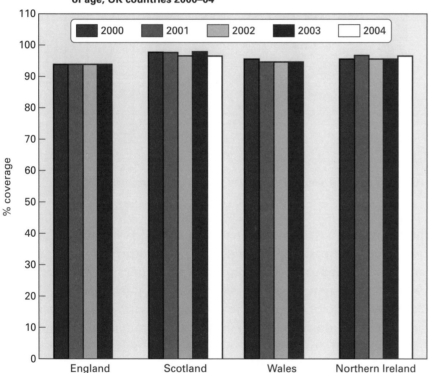

Source: Health Protection Agency.

1.28b MMR vaccination coverage at 2 years of age, UK countries 1993–2004

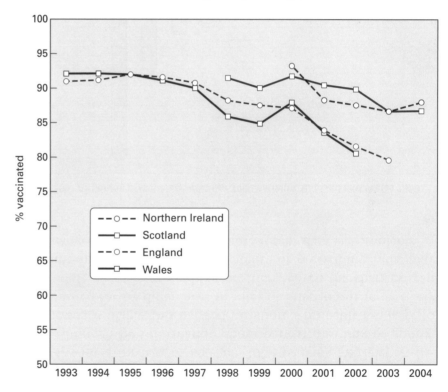

Source: Health Protection Agency.

The Quest for Quality in the NHS: a chartbook on quality of care in the UK

Chart 1.29 Antibiotic prescribing patterns

The Quest for Quality in the NHS: a chartbook on quality of care in the UK

Antibiotics are used to treat bacterial infections and, when used appropriately, are highly effective. However, concerns that antibiotics are used inappropriately for viral infections, such as colds and influenza, are longstanding. Overuse increases the likelihood that antibacterial resistance (e.g. MRSA) will develop. Chart 1.29a illustrates a time series of the rate of liquid antibiotic prescribing in Scotland between 1996 and 2003. Because children are usually dispensed antibiotics in liquid form (and few other patients are), the amount of liquid antibiotics dispensed can be used as a proxy for prescribing rates in children. The chart shows that, over the period of seven years, liquid antibiotic prescribing rates fell by one-third.

Chart 1.29b shows that, in 1998, prescribing rates for antibiotics in 210 general practices in England and Wales varied more than five-fold, ranging from 300 to nearly 1597 prescriptions per 1000 patients, with a median of 660 per 1000 patients (Wrigley *et al.*, 2002). Although no information about patient case mix or appropriateness is available, this marked variation is probably too large to be accounted for by differences in rates of infection; it more likely reflects differences in prescribing practices. Given the changes seen over time in Chart 1.29a, the variability of prescribing rates may have changed since 1998, but no more recent data was available.

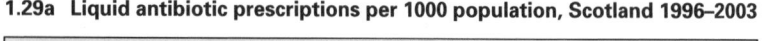

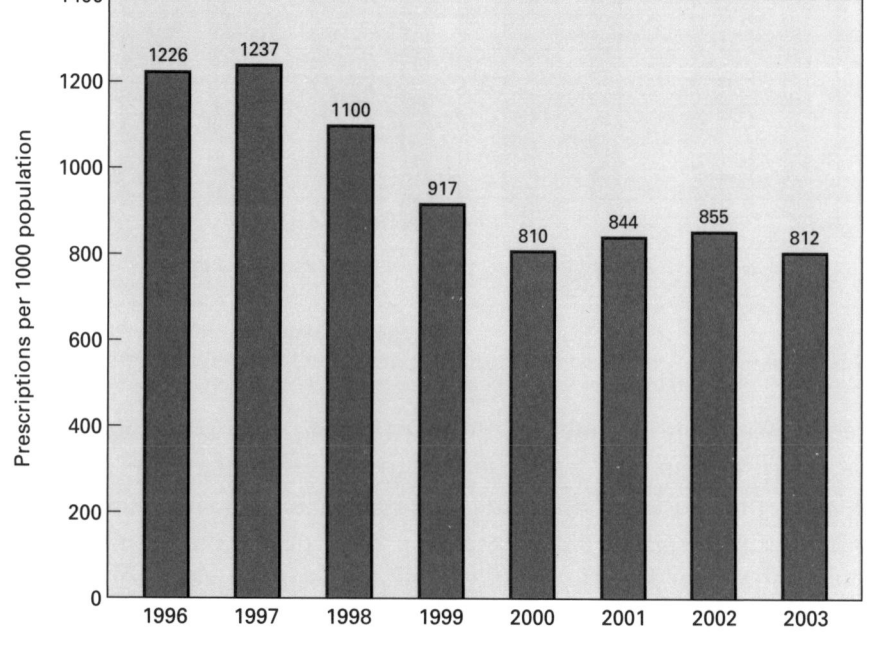

1.29a Liquid antibiotic prescriptions per 1000 population, Scotland 1996–2003

1.29b Antibiotic prescribing rates per 1000 patients, England and Wales 1998

Source: QIS Scotland Health Indicators Report, 2004.

Source: Wrigley *et al.*, 2002.

At any one time around one in six people of working age have a mental health problem, most often anxiety or depression. One person in 250 will have a psychotic illness such as schizophrenia or bipolar affective disorder (manic depression). Most people with mental health problems are cared for by their GP and the primary care team. Generally, for every 100 individuals that consult their GP with a mental health problem, nine will be referred to specialist services for assessment and advice, or for treatment (DH, 1999b).

People with severe mental illness form a small proportion of those with mental health problems but have very high rates of psychological and physical morbidity. The World Health Organization asserts that mental illness represents 10% of the burden of disease in low and middle income countries and 23% in high income countries (WHO, 1999b).

Other estimates suggest that mental illness accounts for about 1.4% of all deaths and 28% of years lived with disability. In 1990, five of the ten leading causes of disability were psychiatric conditions: unipolar depression, alcohol misuse, bipolar affective disorder, schizophrenia and obsessive-compulsive disorder (Murray and Lopez, 1996). People with severe mental illness are also socially excluded, finding it difficult to sustain social and family networks, access education systems and obtain and sustain employment (DH, 1999b).

In a pooled analysis of 20 studies of 36 000 people, mortality among people with schizophrenia was found to be 1.6 times that of the general population; the risk of suicide nine times higher; and the risk of death from other violent incidents more than two times higher (Harris and Barraclough, 1998).

Each suicide represents an individual tragedy and can be devastating for families and friends. In addition to the considerable burdens in personal and family suffering, mental illness costs around £32 billion in England each year. This includes nearly £12 billion in lost employment and approaching £8 billion in benefits payments (Patel and Knapp, 1998).

1 Effectiveness

Suicide

Saving Lives: our healthier nation (DH, 1999a) set a specific target to reduce suicide by one-fifth by 2010. The likelihood of a person committing suicide depends on several factors including both mental and physical illness; stressful life events such as bereavement, separation and divorce, or unemployment; and access to the means of suicide. Suicide accounts for 400 000 years of life lost before the age of 75 years. It is associated with poverty and adverse social circumstances, and studies have demonstrated the correlation between poor housing, low income and mental ill health (Charlton *et al.*, 1994).

Although the overall rate of suicide is falling – by more than 12% since 1982 – more than 4000 deaths from suicide in England still occur each year (ONS, 2003). Risk factors for suicide are quite varied.

- Men are three times more likely than women to commit suicide. Suicide is the leading cause of death among 15–24 year old men and the second most common cause of death among people under 35 years of age.
- Men in unskilled occupations are four times more likely to commit suicide than are those in professional work.
- Among women living in England, those born in India and East Africa have a 40% higher suicide rate than those born in England and Wales.
- Certain occupational groups such as doctors, nurses, pharmacists, veterinarians and farmers are at higher risk, partly because of ease of access to drugs and other means of suicide.

- More than one in ten people with severe mental illness kill themselves.
- Risks are higher for individuals with depression, and those who have suffered a major loss.
- People who have previously harmed themselves, or individuals who misuse drugs or alcohol are at relatively high risk of suicide.
- Suicide rates in prison are high (DH, 1999b).

The National Service Framework for Mental Health (DH, 1999b) asserts that local health and social care communities should prevent suicides by:

- promoting mental health for all, working with individuals and communities
- delivering high quality primary mental healthcare
- ensuring that anyone with a mental health problem can contact local services via the primary care team, a helpline or an A&E department
- ensuring that individuals with severe and enduring mental illness have a care plan that meets their specific needs, including access to services round the clock
- providing safe hospital accommodation for individuals who need it
- enabling individuals caring for someone with severe mental illness to receive the support that they need to continue to care.

Chart 1.30 Suicide rates

The World Health Organization estimates that mental illness represents 23% of the burden of disease in developed economies (WHO, 1999b). Suicide represents the ultimate failure of both the health system and society to help an individual in need of medical and psychosocial care and community support. This chart shows that the suicide rate in England and Wales in 2000 (6.0 per 100 000 people of all ages; 3.3 in those aged 15–19 years; 8.4 in those aged 20–29 years) was low in comparison to the rate in other nations.

Source: Commonwealth Fund, 2004a.

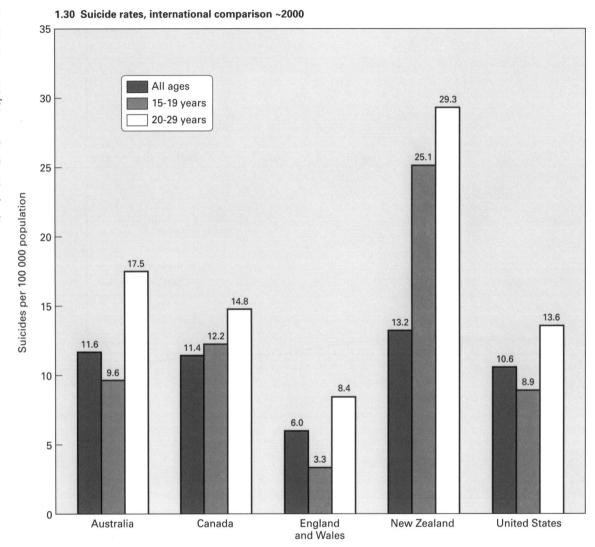

1.30 Suicide rates, international comparison ~2000

Legend:
- All ages
- 15–19 years
- 20–29 years

Y-axis: Suicides per 100 000 population

Country	All ages	15–19 years	20–29 years
Australia	11.6	9.6	17.5
Canada	11.4	12.2	14.8
England and Wales	6.0	3.3	8.4
New Zealand	13.2	25.1	29.3
United States	10.6	8.9	13.6

Chart 1.31 Suicide rates: UK countries time series

The Quest for Quality in the NHS: a chartbook on quality of care in the UK

One in four people who committed suicide, or about 1000 people each year, were in contact with specialist mental health services in the year before their death. Of these, 16% (one in 25 of all suicides) were inpatients at the time of their death, and 24% (one in 16 overall) had been discharged from hospital within the previous three months (Appleby, 1999). Although many individuals were not fully compliant with treatment when discharged, suicide must raise questions about the quality of health and social care. Chart 1.31 provides comparative data for the countries of the UK on suicide rates in people over 14 years of age. It shows, first, that suicide rates have been fairly static since 1997 and, second, that the rate in Scotland (at 21 per 100 000 population) is almost double that of the other countries of the UK. This chart is based on figures for suicides and undetermined deaths (which include 'open verdicts'), which is a more inclusive category than that used for Chart 1.30.

Source: ONS.

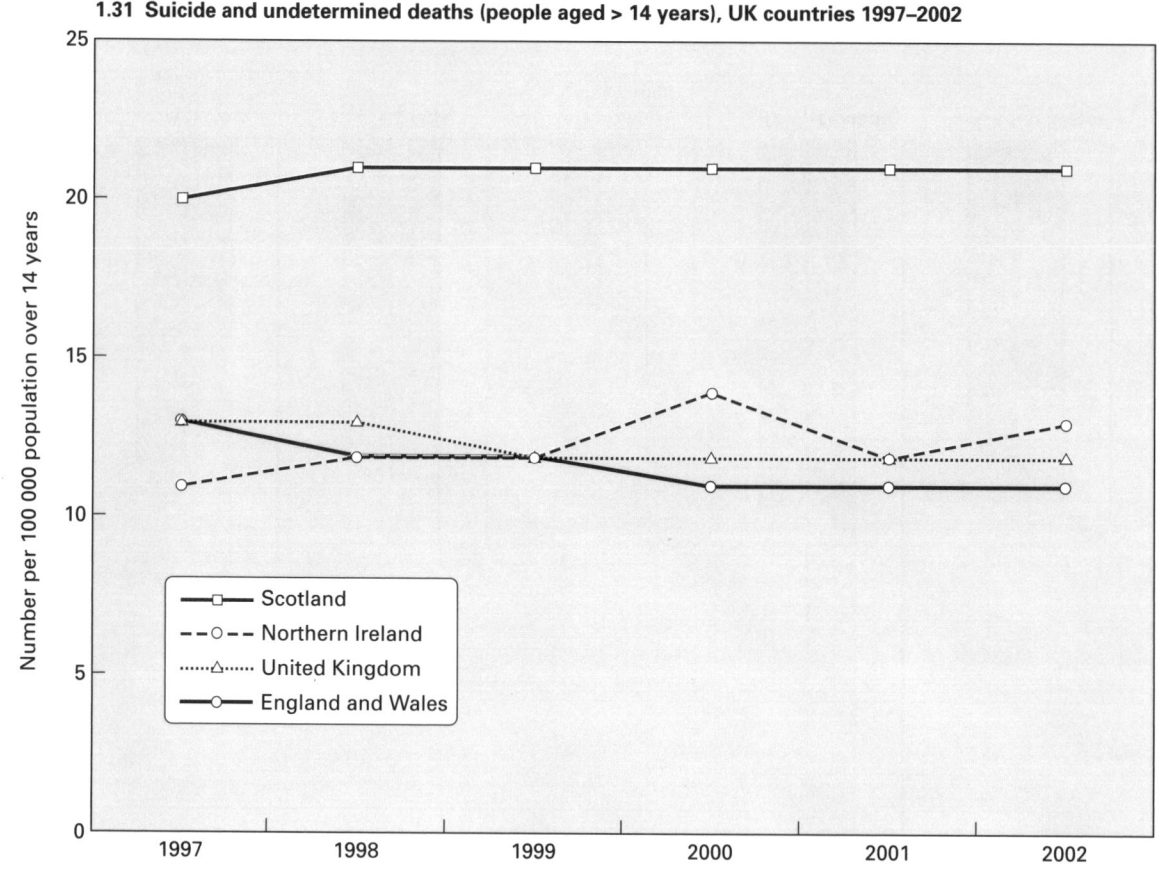

1.31 Suicide and undetermined deaths (people aged > 14 years), UK countries 1997–2002

Number per 100 000 population over 14 years

Legend:
— Scotland
– –o– – Northern Ireland
·····△····· United Kingdom
—o— England and Wales

Chart 1.32 Emergency psychiatric readmissions

The National Service Framework for Mental Health states that each person with severe mental illness should receive the range of mental health services they need. Crises should be anticipated and prevented where possible through prompt and effective help with timely access to an appropriate and safe mental health facility or hospital bed. A high level of emergency psychiatric readmissions suggests that patients were discharged prematurely or that the level of mental health support provided in the community was inadequate, or both. This chart shows the rate of emergency readmissions in England. Until 2001–02 data was collected on emergency readmissions within 90 days of hospital discharge; from 2002 onward, the definition changed to within 28 days of discharge. The reason for this change was that, with the longer period, the likelihood that disease exacerbation prompted readmission was significant; the shorter period gives more information on whether premature discharge is a problem.

Source: Social Services Performance Assessment Framework, 2003.

Note: * within 28 days of discharge.

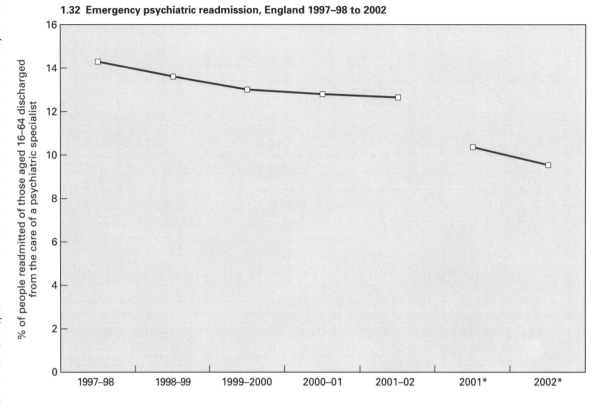

1.32 Emergency psychiatric readmission, England 1997–98 to 2002

The Quest for Quality in the NHS: a chartbook on quality of care in the UK

47

Surgery

Surgery is a large and diverse field. The Hospital Episode Statistics (HES) database in England contains codes for more than 1200 different surgical procedures. In England around 25 000 operations are carried out every day; more than 6.5 million per year (DH, 2000b). In Scotland, there are about 300 000 surgical admissions each year (SASM, 2003). Each episode involves a multidisciplinary team and multiple constituent processes including nursing, technical, clinical and administrative tasks.

In a field so complex, developing meaningful global measures of quality is extremely difficult. Data tends to be collected in specialised fields. We present data commonly accepted as measuring the quality of care in surgical interventions: deaths within 30 days of selected operations; emergency readmissions following pelvic and abdominal surgery; lower limb anthroplasties and caesarean section rates.

Chart 1.33 Surgical outcomes

This pair of charts presents data on two types of surgical outcomes: mortality and emergency readmissions. Both include a range of procedures that account for about one-half of all 'non-minor' elective procedures carried out in Scottish hospitals (for details, *see* Technical Appendix). The procedures represent a wide spectrum of elective surgical activity, in terms of both frequency of the procedures and level of risk expected to accompany the procedures.

Chart 1.33a shows that around three in every 1000 patients died within 30 days of their operation. Some deaths following surgery may be considered unavoidable and others preventable; the data presented here does not allow for any judgements to be made about the level of avoidable deaths. Chart 1.33b shows the rate of emergency readmissions following two major types of operations. Both charts show little change over time.

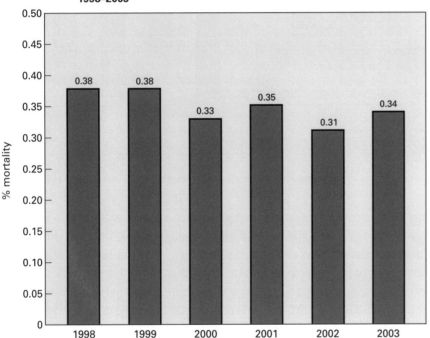

1.33a Mortality within 30 days of selected planned operations, Scotland 1998–2003

Source: Quality Improvement Scotland.

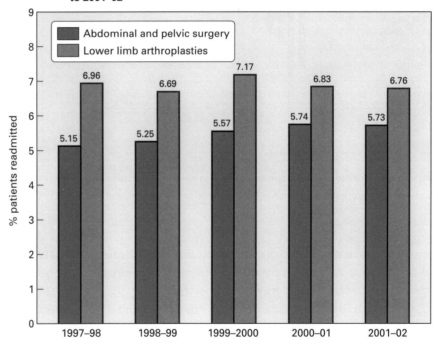

1.33b Emergency readmissions within 28 days of discharge, Scotland 1997–98 to 2001–02

Source: Quality Improvement Scotland.

The Quest for Quality in the NHS: a chartbook on quality of care in the UK

Chart 1.34 Caesarean section rates

The Quest for Quality in the NHS: a chartbook on quality of care in the UK

The public health community has been concerned for many years about the increasing rate of caesarean sections in childbirth. Some estimates call for national caesarean rates to be between 5% and 15% of births (WHO, 1999a). A figure falling below 5% is thought to indicate that a substantial proportion of women do not have access to surgical obstetric care and are at risk. A rate higher than 15% indicates potential overutilisation of the procedure for other than life-saving reasons, incurring unnecessary risk associated with any major surgical operation. The charts illustrate two perspectives of caesarean section rates. Chart 1.34a shows an international comparison of caesarean section rates. Rates across the countries of the UK ranged from 19.3% in Scotland to 24.2% in Wales; all were outside the recommended limits. The UK results are in line with those of the US and Australia but are higher than a number of European comparators. Chart 1.34b shows the variation in rates of caesarean sections across NHS Trusts in England. The percentage of deliveries that were caesarean sections ranged from 6% to 34%; moreover, 15% of NHS Trusts of England had a caesarean section rate of 23%. Further information is needed to analyse how much of the variation within England was a result of differences in actual medical need.

1.34a Caesarean section rates, international comparison, 2000

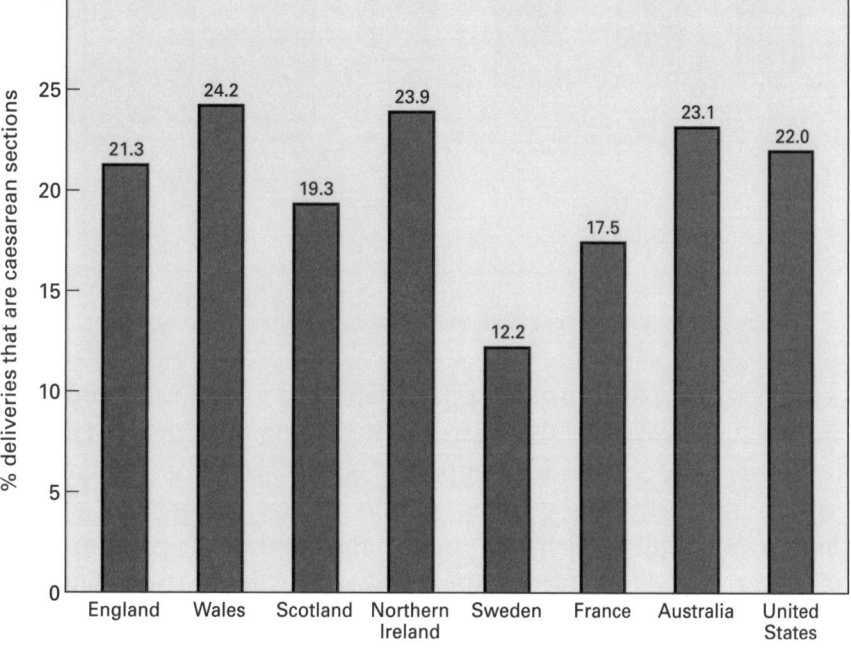

Source: RCOG (Thomas *et al.* 2001); OECD Health Data, 2004.

1.34b Histogram of percentage of deliveries performed by caesarean section in England by Trust, 2000–03

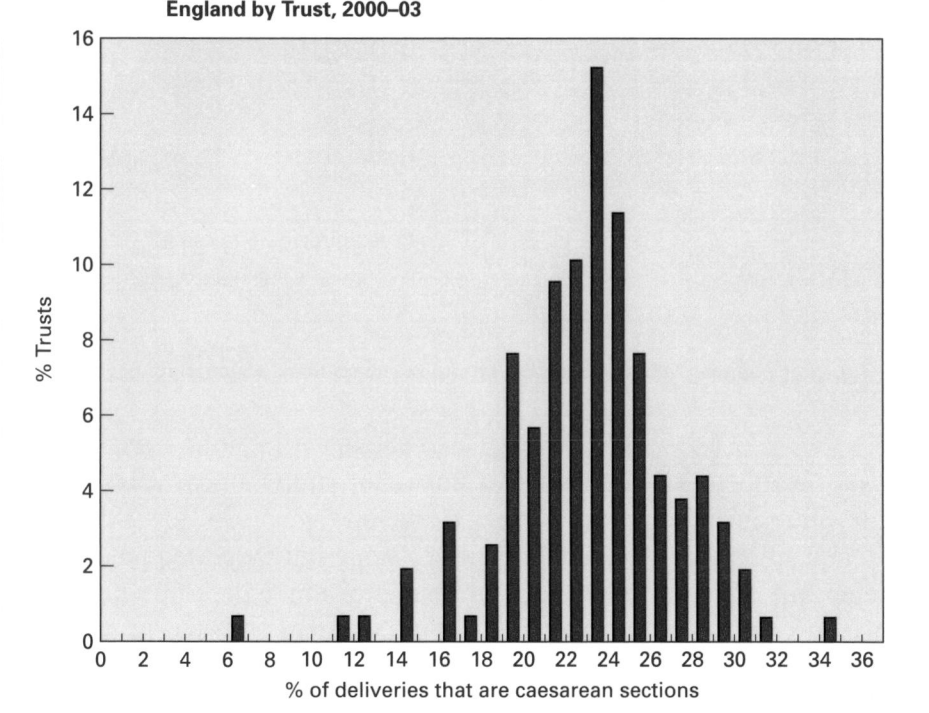

Source: Healthcare Commission (analysis by Raleigh, Irons, Sims).

References

Anbe DT, Armstrong PW, Bates ER *et al.* (2004) ACC/AHA Guidelines for the management of patients with ST-elevation myocardial infarction – Executive Summary. *Circulation.* **110**: 588–636. Available online at: http://circ.ahajournals.org/cgi/content/full/110/5/588 [last accessed 2 February 2005].

Appleby L (1999) *Safer Services: national confidential inquiry into suicide and homicide by people with mental illness.* Department of Health, London. Available online at: www.dh.gov.uk/assetRoot/04/01/45/05/04014505.pdf [last accessed 6 February 2005].

Boersma E, Mass AC, Deckers JW *et al.* (1996) Early thrombolytic treatment in acute myocardial infarction: reappraisal of the golden hour. *Lancet.* **348**(9030): 771–5.

CEEU (2003) *How Hospitals Manage Heart Attacks: Second Public Report of the Myocardial Infarction National Audit Project (MINAP).* Royal College of Physicians, London. Available online at: www.rcplondon.ac.uk/pubs/books/minap/HowHospitalsManageHeartAttacksJune2003.pdf [last accessed 2 February 2005].

CEEU (2004) *How the NHS Manages Heart Attacks: Third Public Report of the Myocardial Infarction National Audit Project (MINAP).* Royal College of Physicians, London. Available online at: www.rcplondon.ac.uk/pubs/books/minap04/HowHospitalsManageHeartAttacksJune2004.pdf [last accessed 2 February 2005].

Charlton J, Kelly S, Dunnell K *et al.* (1994) *The Prevention of Suicide.* HMSO, London.

CMO (2002) *Getting Ahead of the Curve: a strategy for combating infectious diseases.* Chief Medical Officer, Department of Health, London. Available online at: www.publications.doh.gov.uk/cmo/idstrategy/idstrategy2002.pdf [last accessed 2 February 2005].

Commonwealth Fund (2004a) *First Report and Recommendations of the Commonwealth Fund's International Working Group on Quality Indicators.* Commonwealth Fund, New York. Available online at: www.cmwf.org/publications/publications_show.htm?doc_id=227628 [last accessed 2 February 2005].

Commonwealth Fund (2004b) *International Health Policy Survey of Adults' Experiences with Primary Care.* Commonwealth Fund, New York.

DCCT (1993) The effect of intensive treatment of diabetes on the development and progression of long-term complications in insulin-dependent diabetes mellitus. The Diabetes Control and Complications Trial Research Group. *NEJM.* **329**: 977–86.

Department of Health (1999a) *Saving Lives: our healthier nation.* The Stationery Office, London. Available online at: www.archive.official-documents.co.uk/document/cm43/4386/4386.htm [last accessed 6 February 2005].

Department of Health (1999b) *Mental Health National Service Framework.* Department of Health, London. Available online at: www.dh.gov.uk/assetRoot/04/07/72/09/04077209.pdf [last accessed 6 February 2005].

Department of Health (2000a) *National Service Framework for Coronary Heart Disease.* Department of Health, London. Available online at: www.dh.gov.uk/assetRoot/04/04/90/70/04049070.pdf [last accessed 6 February 2005].

Department of Health (2000b) *The NHS Plan: a plan for investment, a plan for reform.* The Stationery Office, London. Available online at: www.dh.gov.uk/assetRoot/04/05/57/83/04055783.pdf [last accessed 2 February 2005].

Department of Health (2001) *National Service Framework for Diabetes.* Department of Health, London. Available online at: www.dh.gov.uk/assetRoot/04/05/89/38/04058938.pdf [last accessed 2 February 2005].

Department of Health (2003) *Social Services Performance Assessment Framework 2002–2003.* Department of Health, London.

Department of Health (2004a) Reid announces new national screening programme to tackle bowel cancer. Press release 2004/0383. Available online at: www.dh.gov.uk/PublicationsAndStatistics/PressReleases/PressReleasesNotices/fs/en?CONTENT_ID=4092376&chk=F1jw5w [last accessed 2 February 2005].

Department of Health (2004b) *Chief Executive's Report to the NHS: Statistical Supplement December 2004.* Department of Health, London. Available online at: www.dh.gov.uk/assetRoot/04/09/75/40/04097540.pdf [last accessed 2 February 2005].

Department of Health (2005) *Summary of Flu Immunisation Policy.* Available online at: www.dh.gov.uk/PolicyAndGuidance/HealthAndSocialCareTopics/Flu/FluGeneralInformation/FluGeneral/fs/en?CONTENT_ID=4001688&chk=BbJebs [last accessed 2 February 2005].

DHSSPS (2004) *Health and Social Care: comparative data for Northern Ireland and other countries.* Department of Health, Social Services and Public Safety, Belfast. Available online at: www.dhsspsni.gov.uk/publications/2004/COMPARATIVE_DATA_12MAY04.pdf [last accessed 2 February 2005].

Downs JR, Clearfield M, Weis S *et al.* (1998) Primary prevention of acute coronary events with lovastatin in men and women with average cholesterol levels: results of AFCAPS/TexCAPS. *JAMA.* **279**: 1615–22.

Giuffrida A, Gravelle H and Roland M (1999) Measuring quality of care with routine data: avoiding confusion between performance indicators and health outcomes. *BMJ.* **319**(7202): 94–8.

Hardcastle JD, Chamberlain JO, Robinson MH *et al.* (1996) Randomised controlled trial of faecal-occult-blood screening for colorectal cancer. *Lancet.* **348**(9040): 1472–77.

Harris EC and Barraclough B (1998) Excess mortality of mental disorder. *Br J Psychiatry.* **173**: 11–53.

Heart Protection Study Collaborative Group (2002) MRC/BHF Heart protection study of cholesterol lowering with simvastatin in 20 536 high-risk individuals: a randomised placebo-controlled trial. *Lancet.* **360**(9326): 7–22.

Heart Protection Study Collaborative Group (2004) Effects of cholesterol-lowering with simvastatin in stroke and other major vascular events in 20 536 people with cerebrovascular disease or other high risk conditions. *Lancet.* **363** (9411): 757–67.

Hemingway H, Crook AM, Feder G *et al.* (2001) Underuse of coronary revascularisation procedures in patients considered appropriate candidates for revascularisation. *NEJM.* **344**(9): 645–54.

HPA (2001) *Vaccine uptake data.* Health Protection Agency, London. Available online at: www.hpa.org.uk/hpa/news/phls_archive/infections_news/2001/010928.htm [last accessed 3 February 2005].

HPA (online) *Vaccination coverage.* Health Protection Agency, London. Available at: www.hpa.org.uk/infections/topics_az/vaccination/vac_coverage.htm [last accessed 6 February 2005].

Hurtado MP, Swift EK and Corrigan JM (eds) (2001) *Envisioning the National Health Care Quality Report.* Institute of Medicine, Washington, DC.

International Agency for Research on Cancer (2002) *IARC Handbooks on Cancer Prevention: breast cancer screening.* Vol. 7. International Agency for Research on Cancer, Lyon, France.

ISD Scotland (2004) *Scottish Health Statistics: Cancer* [Online]. Available at: www.isdscotland.org/isd/info3.jsp?pContentID=338&p_applic=CCC&p_service=Content.show& [last accessed 2 February 2005].

Korda RJ and Butler JRG (2004) *The Impact of Health Care on Mortality: time trends in avoidable mortality in Australia 1968–2001.* NCEPH Working Paper No. 49. National Centre for Epidemiology and Population Health, The Australian National University. Available at: http://nceph.anu.edu.au/Publications/Working_Papers/WP49.pdf [last accessed 2 February 2005]

Lipid Research Clinics Program (1984) The Lipid Research Clinics Coronary Primary Prevention Trial results, I: reduction in incidence of coronary heart disease. *JAMA.* **251**: 351–64.

Marso SP (ed.) (2003) *The Handbook of Diabetes Mellitus and Cardiovascular Disease.* Remedica Publishing, London.

Medline-plus Encyclopaedia (2005) *Diabetic Ketoacidosis.* Available online at: www.nlm.nih.gov/medlineplus/ency/article/000320.htm [last accessed 2 February 2005].

Miettinen TA, Pyorala K, Olsson AG *et al.* (1997) Cholesterol-lowering therapy in women and elderly patients with myocardial infarction or angina pectoris: findings from the Scandinavian Simvastatin Survival Study (4S). *Circulation.* **96**(12): 4211–18.

Murray C and Lopez A (1996) *The Global Burden of Disease.* Harvard University Press, Harvard, CT.

National Paediatric Diabetes Audit (2004) *Results from the Audit Year 2002.* Diabetes UK. Available online at: www.diabetes.org.uk/audit/downloads/PaediatricAuditReport.pdf [last accessed 2 February 2005].

NCHOD (2003) *Compendium of Clinical and Health Indicators 2003.* National Centre for Health Outcomes Development, Oxford.

NHS Breast Screening Programme (2004) *Changing Lives: annual review.* NHS Cancer Screening Programme, Sheffield. Available online at: www.cancerscreening.nhs.uk/breastscreen/publications/nhsbsp-annualreview2004.pdf [last accessed 2 February 2005].

NHS Cancer Screening Programme (2005) *English Colorectal Cancer Screening Pilot.* Available online at: www.cancerscreening.nhs.uk/colorectal/#how [last accessed 2 February 2005].

Nolte E and McKee M (2004) *Does Healthcare Save Lives? Avoidable mortality revisited.* The Nuffield Trust, London.

OECD (2004) *OECD Health Data 2004.* Organisation for Economic Co-operation and Development, Paris.

OECD Health Project (2004) *Towards High-Performing Health Systems.* Organisation for Economic Cooperation and Development, Paris.

ONS (2003) *Mortality Statistics.* Office for National Statistics, London. Available online at: www.statistics.gov.uk/STATBASE/Product.asp?vlnk=618 [last accessed 6 February 2005].

ONS (2004a) *Annual Abstract of Statistics, 2004 Edition.* Office for National Statistics, London.

ONS (2004b) *Cancer Statistics Registrations: registrations of cancer diagnosed in 2001, England.* Office for National Statistics, London. Available online at: www.statistics.gov.uk/downloads/theme_health/MB1_32/MB1_32.pdf [last accessed 2 February 2005].

ONS (2004c) *Cancer.* Available online at: www.statistics.gov.uk/CCI/nugget.asp?ID=915&Pos=2&ColRank=2&Rank=224 [last accessed 2 February 2005].

ONS (2004d) *Childhood Cancer.* Office for National Statistics. Available online at: www.statistics.gov.uk/CCI/nugget.asp?ID=854&Pos=&ColRank=1&Rank=374 [last accessed 6 February 2005].

ONS (2004e) *Mortality: circulatory diseases – leading cause group* [Online]. Available at: www.statistics.gov.uk/CCI/nugget.asp?ID=919&Pos=6&ColRank=2&Rank=224 [last accessed 6 February 2005].

Patel A and Knapp M (1998) Costs of mental illness in England. *PSSRU Mental Health Research Review.* **5**: 4–10.

Payne CB (2000) Diabetes-related lower-limb amputations. *Medical Journal of Australia.* **173**(7): 352–4.

Pignone M, Rich M, Teutsch SM, Berg AO and Lohr KN (2002) Screening for colorectal cancer in adults at average risk: A summary of the evidence for the US Preventive Services Task Force. *Annals of Internal Medicine.* **137**: 132–141.

RCOG (2001) *National Sentinel Caesarean Section Audit.* Royal College of Obstetricians and Gynaecologists, London. Available online at: www.rcog.org.uk/resources/public/pdf/nscs_audit.pdf [last accessed 6 February 2005].

SASM (2003) *Scottish Audit of Surgical Mortality Summary Report.* Available online at: www.sasm.org.uk/Reports/2003Report/Summary_Annual_Report_final_2003_data.pdf [last accessed 6 February 2005].

Scandinavian Simvastatin Survival Study Group (1994) Randomised trial of cholesterol lowering in 4444 patients with coronary heart disease. *Lancet.* **344**(8934): 1383–9.

Scottish Cancer Registry (2002) *Cancer in Scotland.* ISD, NHSScotland, Edinburgh. Available online at: www.isdscotland.org/isd/files/Cancer_in_Scotland_Summary_m.pdf [last accessed 2 February 2005].

Serruys PW, de Feyter P, Macaya C *et al.* (2002) Fluvastatin for prevention of cardiac events following successful first percutaneous coronary intervention: a randomized controlled trial. *JAMA.* **287**(24): 3215–22.

Shepherd J, Cobb SM, Ford I *et al.* (1995) Prevention of coronary heart disease with Pravastatin in men with hypercholesterolemia. *NEJM.* **333**: 1301–8.

Stroke Association (2004) *Facts and Figures About Stroke* [Online]. Available at: www.stroke.org.uk/media_centre/facts_and_figures/index.html [last accessed 6 February 2005].

Summerfield C and Babb P (eds) (2004) *Social Trends 34: a portrait of British society.* Office for National Statistics, London. Available online at: www.statistics.gov.uk/downloads/theme_social/Social_Trends34/Social_Trends34.pdf [last accessed 2 February 2005].

Thomas J, Paranjothy S and the Royal College of Obstetricians and Gynaecologists Clinical Effectiveness Support Unit (2001) *National Sentinel Caesarean Section Audit Report.* RCOG Press, London.

UKPDS (1998) Tight blood pressure control and risk of macrovascular and microvascular complications in type 2 diabetes: UK Prospective Diabetes Study Group. *BMJ.* **317**: 703–16.

Unal B, Critchley JA and Capewell S (2004) Explaining the decline in coronary heart disease mortality in England and Wales between 1981 and 2000. *Circulation.* **109**(9):1101–7.

Walley T, Folino-Gallo P, Schwabe U and van Ganse E (2004) Variations and increase in use of statins across Europe: data from administrative databases. *BMJ.* **328**(7436): 385–6.

Watkins P, Amiel S, Howell S and Turner E (2003) *Diabetes and its Management* (6e). Blackwell, London.

Watkins PJ (ed.) (2003) *ABC of Diabetes* (5e). BMJ Publishing Group, London.

Weitz J, Koch M, Debus J *et al.* (2005) Colorectal cancer. *Lancet.* **365**: 153–65.

WHO (1999a) *Indicators to Monitor Maternal Health Goals* [Online]. Available at: www.who.int/reproductive-health/publications/MSM_94_14/MSM_94_14_chapter3.en.html [last accessed 2 February 2005].

WHO (1999b) *The World Health Report 1999: making a difference.* WHO, Geneva. Available online at: www.who.int/whr/1999/en/ [last accessed 6 February 2005].

Wolfe C (2002) *The Incidence, Natural History, Resource Use and Outcomes of Stroke.* Department of Health, London. Available online at: www.dh.gov.uk/PolicyAndGuidance/ResearchAndDevelopment/ResearchAndDevelopmentAZ/CardiovascularDiseaseAndStroke/CardiovascularDiseaseAndStrokeArticle/fs/en?CONTENT_ID=4001897&chk=8uIeVM. and www.dh.gov.uk/PolicyAndGuidance/ResearchAndDevelopment/ResearchAndDevelopmentAZ/CardiovascularDiseaseAndStroke/CardiovascularDiseaseAndStrokeArticle/fs/en?CONTENT_ID=4001899&chk=ZDLGdE [last accessed 6 February 2005].

Wrigley T, Tinto A and Majeed A (2002) Age and sex-specific antibiotic prescribing patterns in general practice in England and Wales, 1994 to 1998. *Health Statistics Quarterly.* **14**: 14–20. Available online at: www.statistics.gov.uk/downloads/theme_health/HSQ14_v4.pdf [last accessed 6 February 2005].

1 Effectiveness

The issue of access to healthcare is a significant health policy concern in many countries around the world. Barriers to access are many and varied. They include long waits for service, inconvenience of location or hours of service, the cost of insurance coverage, lack of personal or public transport, and cultural or language differences between patients and health professionals. Poor access has potentially serious consequences, including deterioration in individuals' health status and subsequent extra costs for health systems.

In countries with no public health insurance, costs and afford-ability are the primary barriers to access. Waiting times, in contrast, tend to be most problematic in countries that combine public health insurance and constraints on capacity. Hence the overriding concerns regarding access to care in the publicly funded NHS are with waits and queues. This chapter accordingly focuses on those issues. However, healthcare systems always juggle trade-offs between equity of provision and costs and queuing. This trade-off is illustrated by data from an international patient survey that showed that 39% of UK respondents indicated that waiting times were one of the biggest problems facing their healthcare system compared to 3% of US respondents. Conversely, only 6% of UK respondents indicated that high costs were problematic, compared with 48% of US respondents (Commonwealth Fund, 2002). Further data on the role of cost disincentives appears in Chapter 6; for example Chart 6.8 illustrates that relatively few people in the UK fail to obtain care for health problems because of concerns about their ability to pay.

Problems with excessive waiting times are thought to be rooted in the dramatic increase in the demand for health services that has occurred in recent decades. In many countries, supply has struggled to keep pace with demand. This imbalance between supply and demand has been most marked in the case of non-urgent surgical procedures such as cataract removal and hip replacement. In some respects the situation is a case of healthcare systems being the victims of their success; increased demand is a result of improvements in a broad spectrum of medical, surgical and mental health services and technologies. In publicly funded systems such as the NHS, optimum waiting times for elective admissions may not be zero. It is cost-effective to maintain short queues of elective patients because the adverse health consequences of short delays are small and because of the efficiency gains that accrue from operating at high capacity (Hurst and Siciliani, 2003). Balancing supply and demand is a continuing challenge for healthcare systems in attempting to optim-ise efficiency while maximising effectiveness and patient responsive-ness.

Consistently rated as the foremost concern in public opinion surveys (Jowell *et al.*, 2000), improving access to reliable and timely health services has been a central policy theme in the UK for decades. England has in recent years embarked on a concerted effort to address waiting list problems, largely through supply-side interventions such as setting maximum waiting time targets, increas-ing system capacity and designing incentives for institutional and individual healthcare providers to increase access and throughput. As Charts 2.3 and 2.4 show, this policy has met with considerable success. Nevertheless, several service areas continue to be plagued by problems with access and timeliness; and there are concerns that recent increases in supply may fuel yet more demand.

The charts in this chapter focus on three key areas of access that have been most problematic for the NHS: waiting for hospital admission; waiting for primary care; and waiting for treatment for specific conditions.

The Quest for Quality in the NHS: a chartbook on quality of care in the UK

Waiting for hospital care

Waiting for hospital care encompasses waiting for elective surgery, waiting for outpatient appointments, and receiving timely care in Accident and Emergency (A&E).

Waiting times for elective surgery are a significant health policy concern in many healthcare systems. No international consensus exists on what represents 'excessive' waiting, but in recent years several countries have set targets of either three months or six months for maximum waiting times. A recent OECD project found that waiting times are a serious health policy issue in Australia, Canada, Denmark, Finland, Ireland, Italy, the Netherlands, New Zealand, Norway, Spain, Sweden and the United Kingdom. The study found that excessive waiting times are associated with:

- low numbers, or availability, of doctors
- low availability of acute care beds and
- salaried (rather than fee for service) remuneration for specialists.

Further, the study found evidence to suggest that activity-based funding (i.e. where funding is based on levels of activity rather than on fixed budgets) for hospitals may help reduce waiting times (Siciliani and Hurst, 2003). These findings highlight the close association between the quality domains of access and system capacity. Chapter 3 explores many of the underlying capacity-based determinants of excessive waiting lists.

With respect to elective surgery, waiting list figures currently cover the period from when a patient is added to the waiting list until his or her operation. Although this is standard practice across many OECD countries, it is somewhat misleading, as the reported waiting time may represent as little as one-third of the full period that patients wait from their initial general practitioner appointment. This is set to change, at least in England, where the Health Secretary has pledged that by the end of 2008, the entire waiting time will be measured.

Waiting list statistics are closely watched in the UK and serious consequences befall those organisations with poor results. For those reasons, there is a risk that waiting list data is subject to 'gaming'. Because of this concern, both the Audit Commission and the National Audit Office have undertaken studies of inpatient waiting lists and found:

Inappropriate Adjustments to NHS Waiting Lists (NAO, 2001)

- nine NHS Trusts inappropriately adjusted their waiting lists
- of these, three Trusts adjusted their waiting lists inappropriately for three years or more, affecting nearly 6000 patient records

Waiting List Accuracy (Audit Commission, 2003)

- auditors carried out 'spot checks' at 41 Trusts in 2002
- there was evidence of deliberate misreporting of waiting list information at three Trusts
- in a further 19 Trusts, auditors found evidence of reporting errors in at least one waiting list indicator
- in three Trusts, the spot checks revealed no significant problems.

Chart 2.1 Waiting for elective surgery

Waiting times for elective surgery is a common policy concern across the world. However, little comparative data is available (Hurst and Siciliani, 2003). Chart 2.1a draws on two international patient surveys conducted in 1998 and 2001 and shows the percentages of respondents who waited more than four months for elective surgery in the two years preceding the surveys. The UK had the highest percentages in both time periods. Chart 2.1b illustrates median waiting time data for hip replacements, cataract operations and coronary artery bypass grafts (CABG). Elective surgery waits in England, for the year 2000, were far longer than those in comparator countries. However, marked improvements in England have occurred since the time frame of these charts, as shown in Charts 2.3 and 2.4.

2.1a Patients waiting > 4 months for elective surgery, international comparison 1998 and 2001

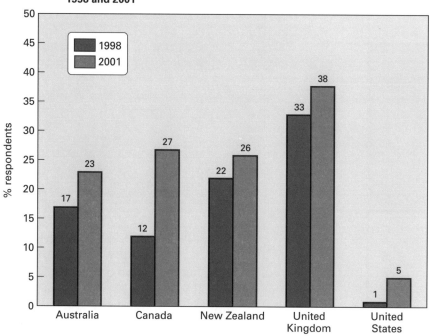

Source: Commonwealth Fund 1998; 2001.

2.1b Median waits for elective surgery, international comparison 2000

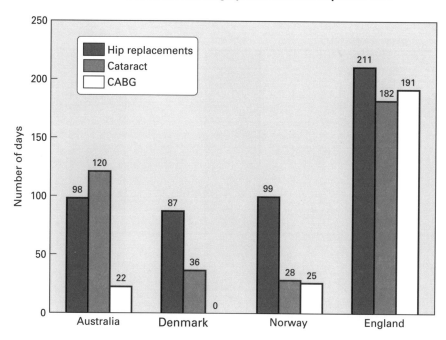

Source: Siciliani and Hurst, 2003.

The Quest for Quality in the NHS: a chartbook on quality of care in the UK

2 Access

The Quest for Quality in the NHS: a chartbook on quality of care in the UK

Chart 2.2 Proportion of population waiting for inpatient admission

This chart provides some context for understanding the scale of waiting lists for hospital admission in the UK. The data, for September 2004, shows the number of people on the inpatient waiting lists in each country of the UK per 1000 population. Per capita, England has the lowest number of people on the waiting lists and Northern Ireland, the highest. Eliminating waits entirely, however, may neither be possible nor desirable.

Source: DH, StatsWales, ISD Scotland, DHSSPS (*see* Technical Appendix for details).

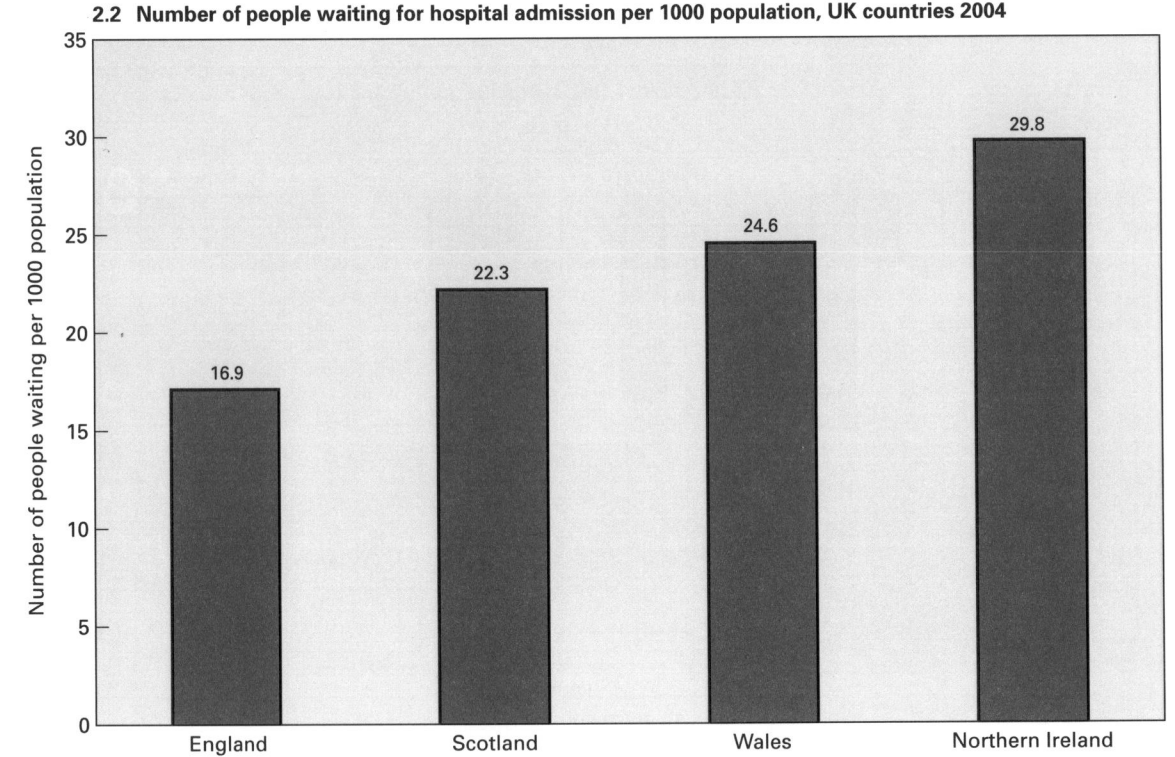

2.2 Number of people waiting for hospital admission per 1000 population, UK countries 2004

Chart 2.3 Excessive waits: intra-UK comparison

In September 2004, the percentage of UK patients on the inpatient waiting list that had been waiting more than six months ranged from 7% in Scotland to 36% in Wales (no data was available for Northern Ireland). The percentages of patients that had been waiting more than 12 months ranged from 0% in England and Scotland to 13% in Northern Ireland. In recent years, England's Department of Health has made a concerted effort to reduce waiting lists, particularly excessively long waits of more than 12 months. The chart illustrates the changes that have occurred in England since 1999: the percentage of patients on the waiting list waiting longer than 12 months fell from 5% to zero and the percentage of patients waiting longer than six months from 21% to 9%.*

Sources: DH, ISD Scotland, StatsWales, DHSSPS (*see* Technical Appendix for details)

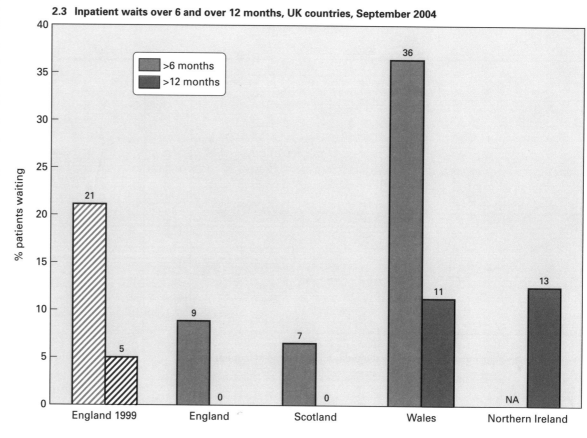

2.3 Inpatient waits over 6 and over 12 months, UK countries, September 2004

Legend:
- >6 months
- >12 months

y-axis: % patients waiting

England 1999: 21, 5
England: 9, 0
Scotland: 7, 0
Wales: 36, 11
Northern Ireland: NA, 13

The Quest for Quality in the NHS: a chartbook on quality of care in the UK

* Scotland figures are for those patients without an Availability Status Code (ASC); *see* Technical Appendix for details.

Chart 2.4 Numbers of patients waiting for hospital admission and median length of waits

The Quest for Quality in the NHS: a chartbook on quality of care in the UK

The number of people waiting an excessively long time for admission into hospital in England has decreased markedly. Chart 2.4a shows that the number of English patients who had been waiting more than six months for hospital admission fell from 275 621 in 1999 to 75 050 in 2004. More than 90% of patients on the waiting list in September 2004 had been waiting less than six months (*see* Chart 2.3). Since 2003 there has been no quarter when more than 100 patients had been waiting longer than 12 months. In 2000, the NHS Plan pledged that, by the end of 2005, the maximum wait for inpatient treatment would be six months; progress has been good, but this remains a challenging target. Although the size of the waiting list is of great interest, an indication of the length of wait is sometimes more relevant, especially to patients. Chart 2.4b depicts the median time that patients on the waiting list (at the end of each financial year) had been waiting. This indicator also shows considerable, although less dramatic, improvement from a peak of 14.2 weeks in 1998 to 10.2 weeks in 2004.

2.4a Number of patients waiting 6–11 months and > 12 months, England 1999–2000 to 2004–05

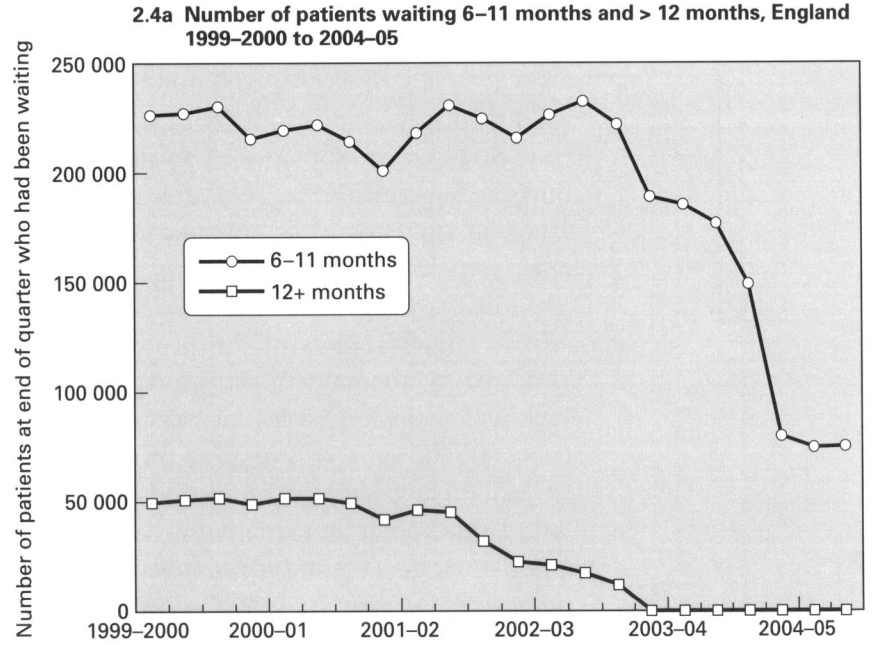

Source: DH.

2.4b Median waiting time for inpatient admission, England 1997–2004

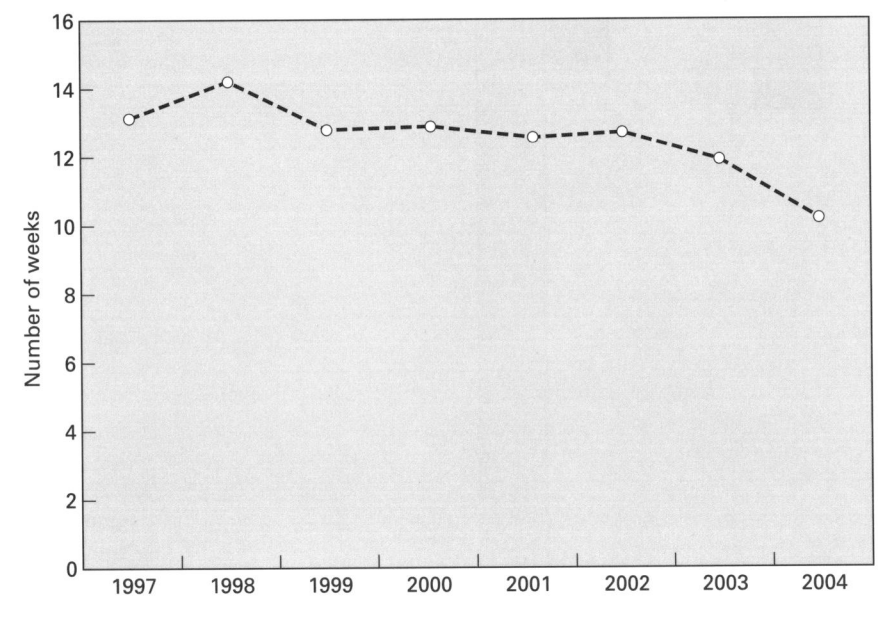

Source: DH.

Chart 2.5 Cancelled operations and rescheduling

The cancellation of operations at short notice is distressing and inconvenient for patients and their families. The NHS Plan (DH, 2000b) pledged that, from 2002, when a patient's operation is cancelled, the hospital must offer another binding appointment rescheduling the surgery for within 28 days or fund the patient's treatment at the time and hospital of the patient's choice (either public or private). This measure is important because it acts as a disincentive to the artificial reduction of waiting lists by offering a date for operation, subsequently cancelling it for non-clinical reasons, and, in so doing, 'resetting' the waiting clock. The number of last-minute cancellations has made no significant sustained improvement over the past six years. The number of patients who did not have their operations rescheduled within 28 days following a cancellation has fallen from a peak of 5437 in 2001 to 1410 in September 2004.

Source: DH.

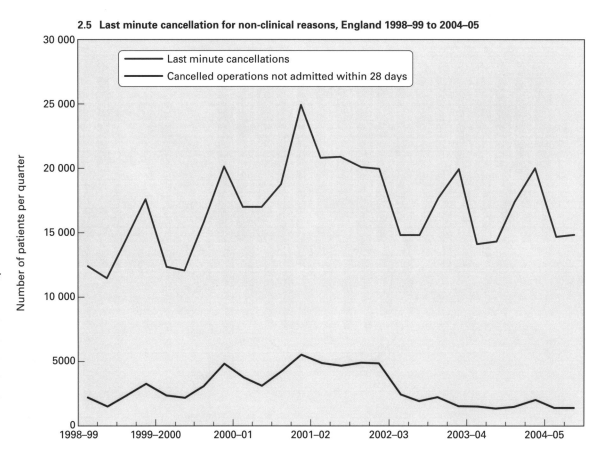

2.5 **Last minute cancellation for non-clinical reasons, England 1998–99 to 2004–05**

Legend:
- Last minute cancellations
- Cancelled operations not admitted within 28 days

Y-axis: Number of patients per quarter

The Quest for Quality in the NHS: a chartbook on quality of care in the UK

Chart 2.6 Delayed discharges and transfers

Reducing unnecessary days in hospital is an important factor in ameliorating the problem of waiting lists. Delayed discharge or 'bed blocking' has different definitions. In England, it refers to the situation when a patient's medical condition no longer requires inpatient hospital care but the patient remains in an acute hospital bed, waiting for assessment or for arrangements for support at home or other suitable intermediate care. Chart 2.6a shows a steady decrease in the number of delayed discharges in English hospitals from 7065 in September 2001 to 2742 in September 2004.

In Scotland, delayed discharge statistics include patients who are clinically ready, and are waiting, for transfer to the next stage of care (including further inpatient episode, patient's home, care home, etc.). Chart 2.6b depicts Scottish data and shows that while there has been a decrease in the number of delayed transfers, in October 2004 there were 1908 patients affected, 1109 of which had been ready for transfer for over six weeks. Further (and not charted) there were 80 patients who had been delayed for a year or more.

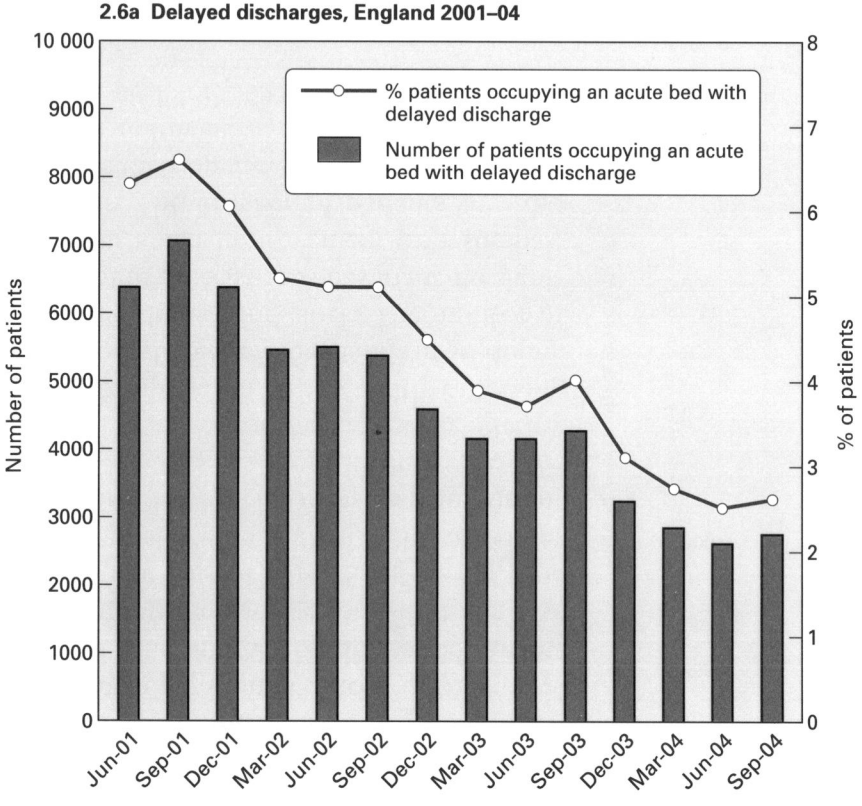

2.6a Delayed discharges, England 2001–04

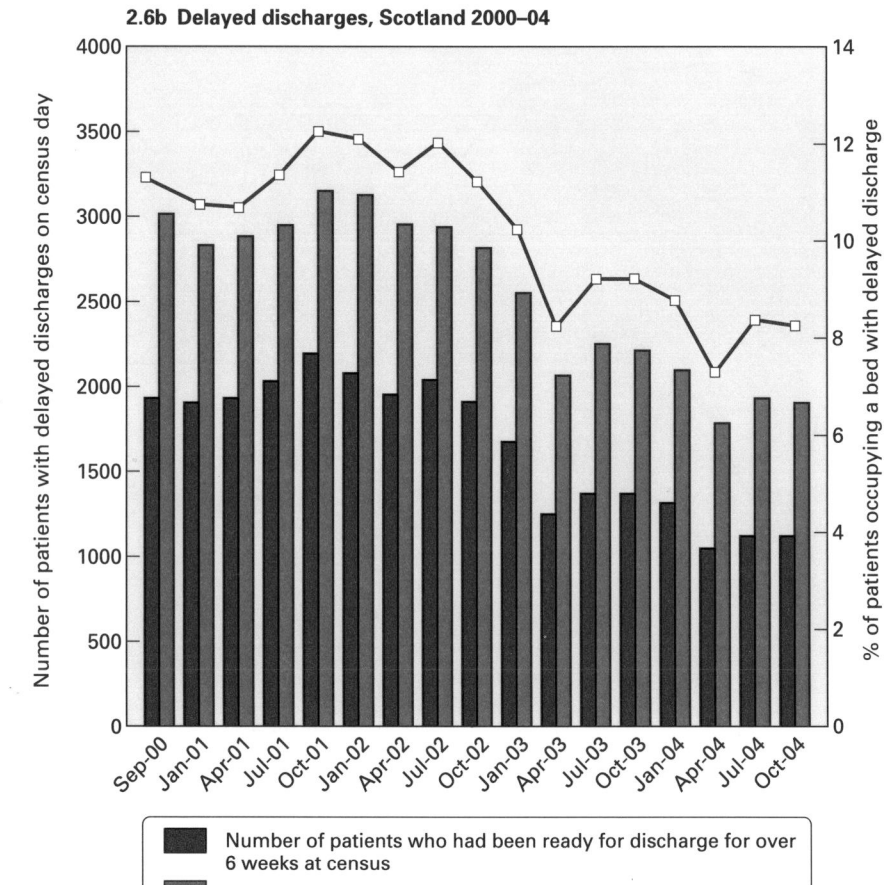

2.6b Delayed discharges, Scotland 2000–04

Number of patients who had been ready for discharge for over 6 weeks at census

Total number of patients with delayed discharges

Patients ready for discharge as a percentage of occupied beds

Sources: DH, SAFFR, ISD Scotland (*see* Technical Appendix for details).

Note: In Scotland there is an agreed six-week period beyond a 'clinically ready for discharge date' during which all assessment and follow-on arrangements are put in place.

Sources: DH, SAFFR, ISD Scotland (*see* Technical Appendix for details).

Chart 2.7 Outpatient waits

Data on waiting lists for outpatient appointments is collected and presented in two ways. Chart 2.7a is based on completed waits, i.e. of all outpatients seen in a particular time period (e.g. quarter or year), the percentage who had waited over 13 weeks. It shows that the percentage of patients who waited over 13 weeks for an outpatient appointment between 1999–2000 and 2004–05 fell in England (by 7.8%) but rose in Northern Ireland (by 7.9%) and in Scotland (by 8.1%). Chart 2.7b is based on waiting lists on a particular day, i.e. of all patients on the waiting list at the end of the month/quarter, the percentage who had been waiting over 13 weeks. It shows that between 2000–01 and 2003–04 the percentage of patients waiting over 13 weeks increased by 5.2% in Wales and 6.9% in Northern

Ireland. We have presented the Northern Ireland data in both charts to underline how different methods of presenting waiting list data can depict different aspects of performance. The completed waits give a fuller picture of activity as they include patients who are seen quickly within reporting periods. The 'length of wait to date' figures focus on the waiting list itself. Further complexity is added by the use of different definitions across comparator countries, e.g. the Auditor General for Wales (2005) highlighted that Wales counts a broader range of patients in their outpatient waiting statistics and estimated that the Welsh waiting list is 20–30% larger than it would be if the definitions used in England were applied.

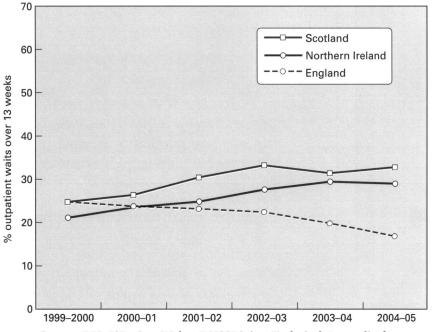

2.7a Outpatient waits > 13 weeks (completed waits), England, Scotland and Northern Ireland, 1999–2000 to 2004–05

Source: DH, ISD, StatsWales, DHSSPS (*see* Technical Appendix for details).

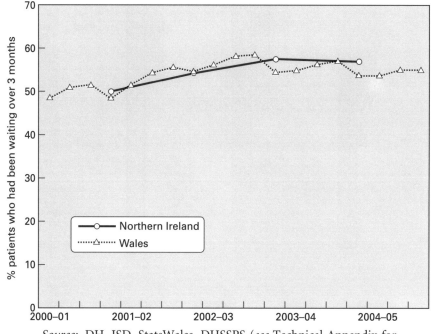

2.7b Outpatient waits > 13 weeks (length of wait to date at census), Wales and Northern Ireland, 2000–01 to 2004–05

Source: DH, ISD, StatsWales, DHSSPS (*see* Technical Appendix for details).
* 2004–05 data based on three quarters only.

Chart 2.8 Waiting in Accident and Emergency (A&E)

The Quest for Quality in the NHS: a chartbook on quality of care in the UK

The 2004 Commonwealth Fund International Health Policy Survey asked respondents: *The last time you went to the hospital emergency room, how long did you wait before being treated?* Of all UK respondents, 82% indicated that they were treated in less than four hours, a figure broadly in line with comparator countries. Official data from the Department of Health indicates that 94% of patients in England wait less than four hours from arrival to admission, transfer or discharge.

Source: Commonwealth Fund, 2004.

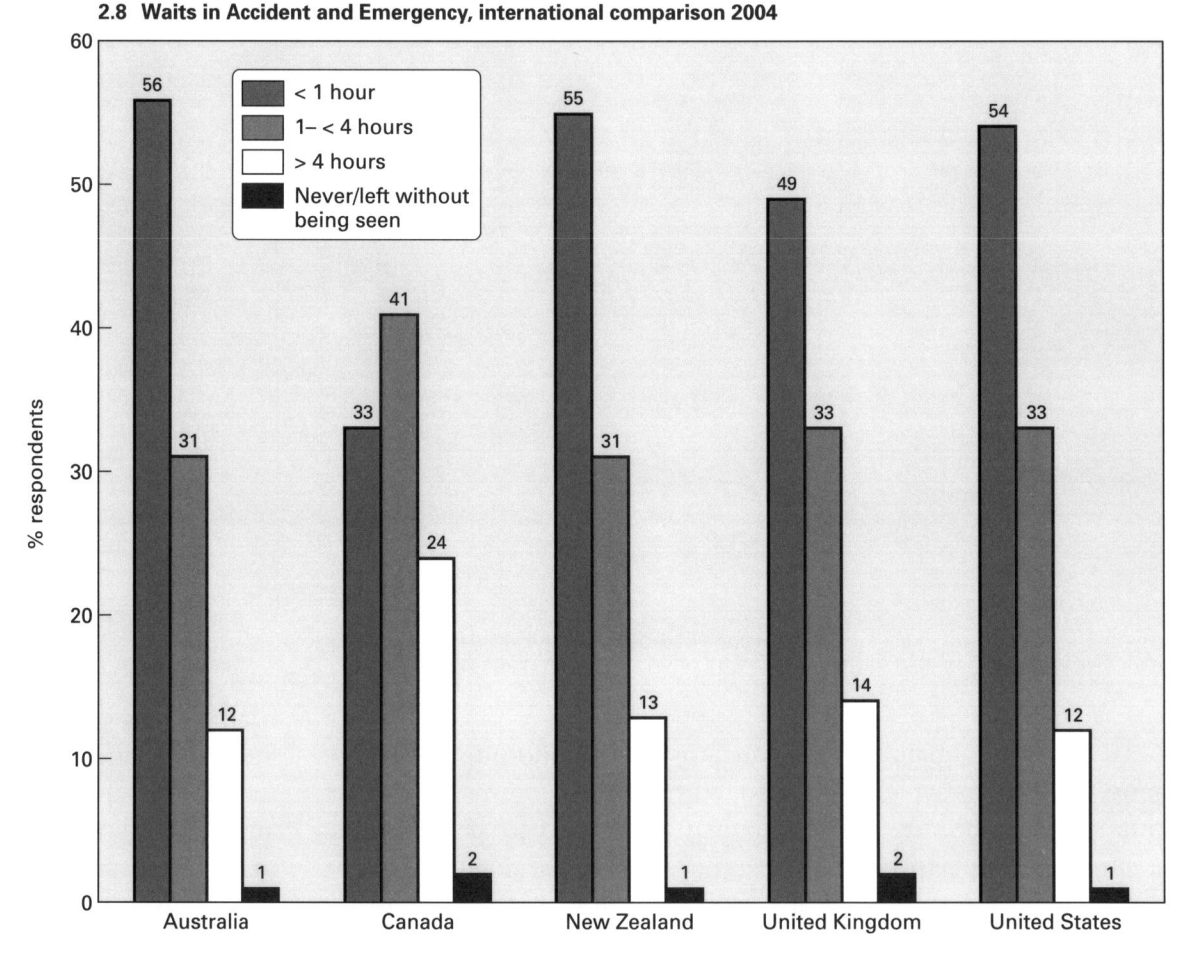

2.8 Waits in Accident and Emergency, international comparison 2004

Legend:
- < 1 hour
- 1– < 4 hours
- > 4 hours
- Never/left without being seen

% respondents

Country	< 1 hour	1– < 4 hours	> 4 hours	Never/left without being seen
Australia	56	31	12	1
Canada	33	41	24	2
New Zealand	55	31	13	1
United Kingdom	49	33	14	2
United States	54	33	12	1

Waiting for primary care

Primary care is the cornerstone of healthcare in the UK. It represents the first point of contact for health services, provides a comprehensive range of services underpinned by continuity of care, acts as coordinator and, increasingly, purchaser of specialist services, and plays a central role in efforts to improve population health (Starfield, 1994).

The Department of Health has asserted that: 'The future of the NHS rests on the strength of its primary care services. Nine out of ten NHS patients are seen in primary care, while it remains the gateway to secondary care and has a key role in helping people stay at home and out of hospital' (DH, 2001: p. 2). However, primary care, like the rest of the health service, suffered decades of underinvestment. In return for extra funding, the Government (through the NHS Confederation) negotiated a new GP contract in 2003 with explicit quality requirements, and swifter access for patients.

Waiting times for primary care are much shorter than those for secondary care but nevertheless have been a serious and widespread concern. In England, the NHS Plan (DH, 2000b) set a target that by 2004 all patients will be able to see a primary care professional within 24 hours and a GP within 48 hours. In Scotland, *Our National Health: a plan for action, a plan for change* (Scottish Executive, 2000) pledged that patients should get access to an appropriate member of the primary care team in no more than 48 hours.

The Quest for Quality in the NHS: a chartbook on quality of care in the UK

Chart 2.9 Waits for primary care: international survey data

The Quest for Quality in the NHS: a chartbook on quality of care in the UK

The 2004 Commonwealth Fund International Health Policy Survey focused on primary care. It was supplemented by an enlarged sample of respondents within the four countries of the UK. This chart illustrates the responses in both samples to the survey question: *Last time you were sick or needed medical attention, how quickly could you* *get an appointment to see a doctor?* New Zealand and Australian respondents received the most prompt attention in primary care. The UK outperformed both the US and Canada. Within the UK, 60% of English respondents were seen on the same or next day, compared to 45% in Scotland.

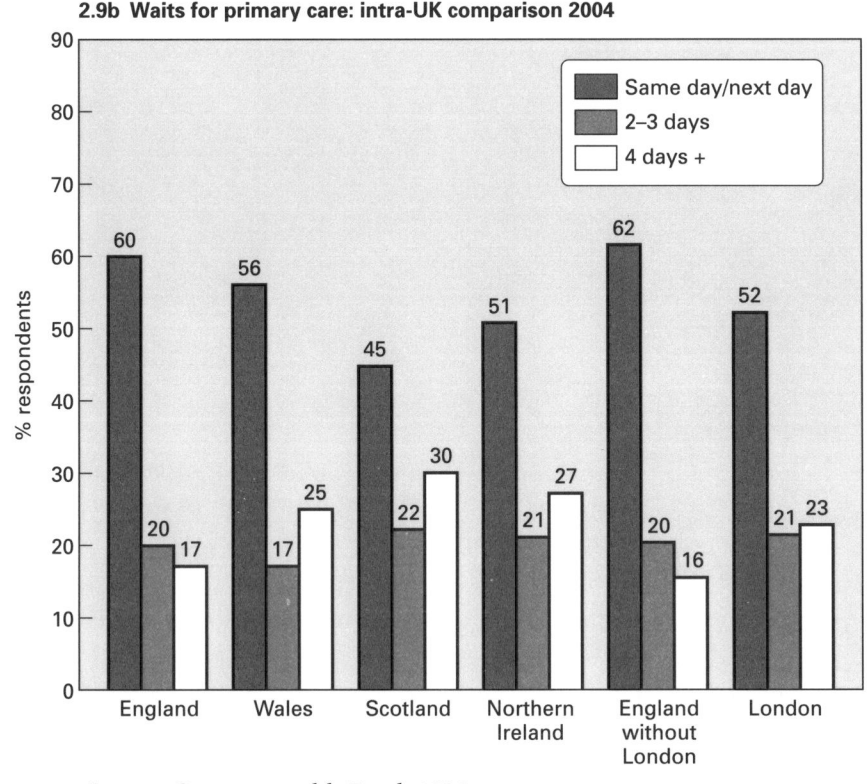

2.9a Waits for primary care: international comparison 2004

Legend:
- Same day/next day
- 2–3 days
- 4 days +

% respondents

	Australia	Canada	New Zealand	United Kingdom	United States
Same day/next day	75	42	84	59	51
2–3 days	14	19	9	20	18
4 days +	9	31	4	19	26

Source: Commonwealth Fund, 2004.

2.9b Waits for primary care: intra-UK comparison 2004

Legend:
- Same day/next day
- 2–3 days
- 4 days +

% respondents

	England	Wales	Scotland	Northern Ireland	England without London	London
Same day/next day	60	56	45	51	62	52
2–3 days	20	17	22	21	20	21
4 days +	17	25	30	27	16	23

Source: Commonwealth Fund, 2004.

Chart 2.10 Waits for primary care appointments

The Healthcare Commission undertakes large patient surveys in England, focusing on different patient subpopulations. In 2003 and 2004, surveys of primary care trusts were undertaken. This chart shows the responses to the questions: *Did you have to wait for a [primary care] appointment?* in 2003 and *The last time you saw a doctor from your GP surgery did you have to wait for an appointment?* in 2004. Almost one-quarter of respondents, in both surveys, waited longer than two days for an appointment. This result differs markedly from official data, which reports that in November 2004, 99.2% patients were offered an appointment with a GP within two working days, and 99.3% offered an appointment with a primary care professional within one working day (DH, 2004).

Source: Healthcare Commission/nhssurveys.org.

Note: Pre-planned appointment refers to non-urgent routine appointment spaced at regular intervals.

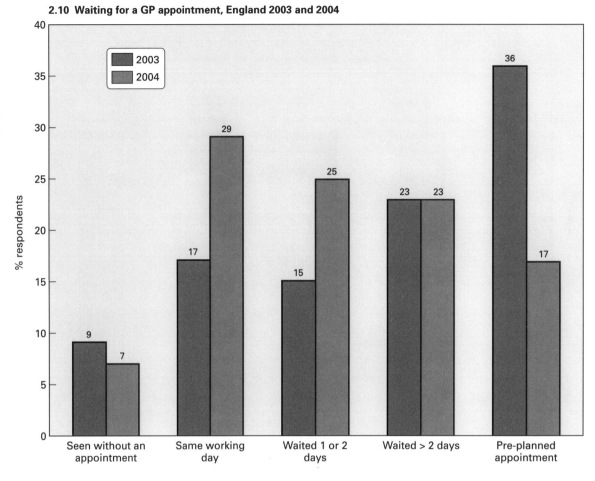

2.10 Waiting for a GP appointment, England 2003 and 2004

The Quest for Quality in the NHS: a chartbook on quality of care in the UK

Chart 2.11 Using Accident and Emergency (A&E) for primary care

This chart illustrates the responses to the following question from the 2004 Commonwealth Fund International Health Policy Survey: *The last time you went to the hospital emergency room, was it for a condition that you thought could have been treated by your regular doctor had he or she been available?* A high rate of positive responses would suggest that access to primary care is problematic. The UK had the best performance of all countries studied; only about one in five respondents who had been to A&E indicated that their visit would have been unnecessary if appropriate primary care had been available. About half of the American and Canadian respondents indicated that this was the case.

Source: Commonwealth Fund, 2004.

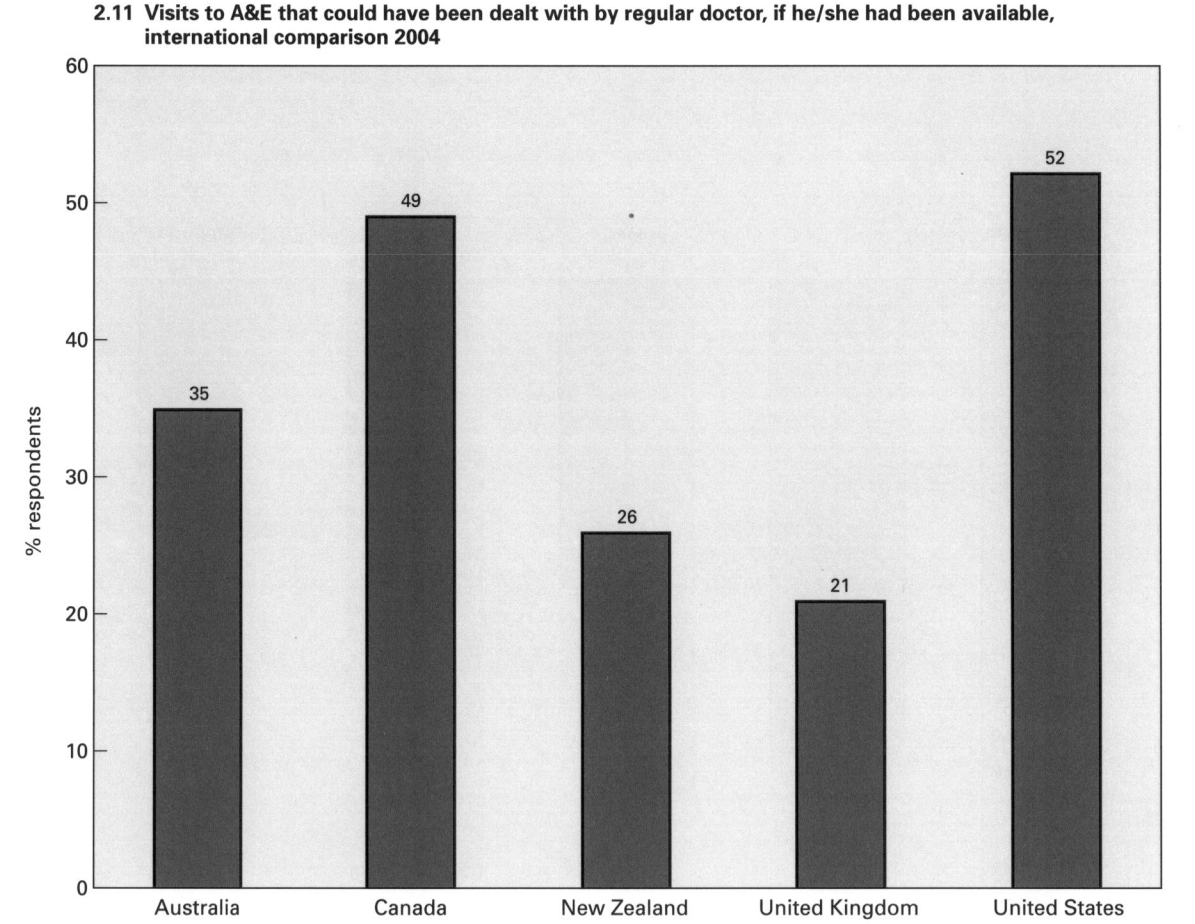

2.11 Visits to A&E that could have been dealt with by regular doctor, if he/she had been available, international comparison 2004

Waiting for specific treatments

The drive to improve access to care in the UK has drawn on a range of interventions. These have included additional investment, setting standards, adding facilities, establishing targets, measuring performance and introducing new contracts for physicians.

In particular, a great deal of work has been done on establishing national standards of care and minimum service level requirements for specific disease and patient groups across the UK. In England and Wales the delineation of appropriate and effective care pathways and discussion of requisite resources has culminated in the production of National Service Frameworks (NSFs). Each NSF is grounded in the research evidence base and developed with the assistance of an external reference group, bringing together health professionals, service users and carers, health service managers, partner agencies and other advocates. Many of the NSFs contain standards that define maximum waiting times for diagnostic procedures and treatment. These have been used as targets to galvanise efforts and resources towards key processes in patient care. In Scotland the development and dissemination of evidence-based guidelines is a well-established feature of the healthcare system. In recent times, such guidelines have been complemented by specific commitments from the Scottish Executive to improve access to key procedures. In this section, we focus on aspects of two major clinical areas: coronary heart disease and cancer. The coronary heart disease data emanates from Scotland where reducing waits for revascularisation procedures has been an important goal. The cancer data is drawn from England where The Cancer Plan (DH, 2000a) was the inaugural NSF in an iterative programme of development and dissemination. Targets for times between initial presentation of the patient in primary care, diagnosis and the start of treatment have accompanied the NSF.

In both cases, as of December 2004, timely access to care in the particular areas highlighted by policy documents was approaching 100%.

Chart 2.12 Coronary heart disease waits

See Coronary heart disease pp19–32

The Quest for Quality in the NHS: a chartbook on quality of care in the UK

The Scottish Executive has made two key commitments regarding waiting times in coronary heart disease:

1 by December 2004, the maximum wait for angiography will be eight weeks from the time of seeing a specialist
2 by June 2004, the maximum wait for surgery (cardiac revascularisation) will be 18 weeks from the time of angiography (Scottish Executive, 2000).

This chart shows that, in September 2004, 88.3% of patients were waiting less than the target time of eight weeks for angiography, and 100% of patients waited less than the target 18 weeks for revascularisation surgery. The percentage of revascularisations performed within 12 weeks is also shown (93% in September 2004).

Source: ISD Scotland.

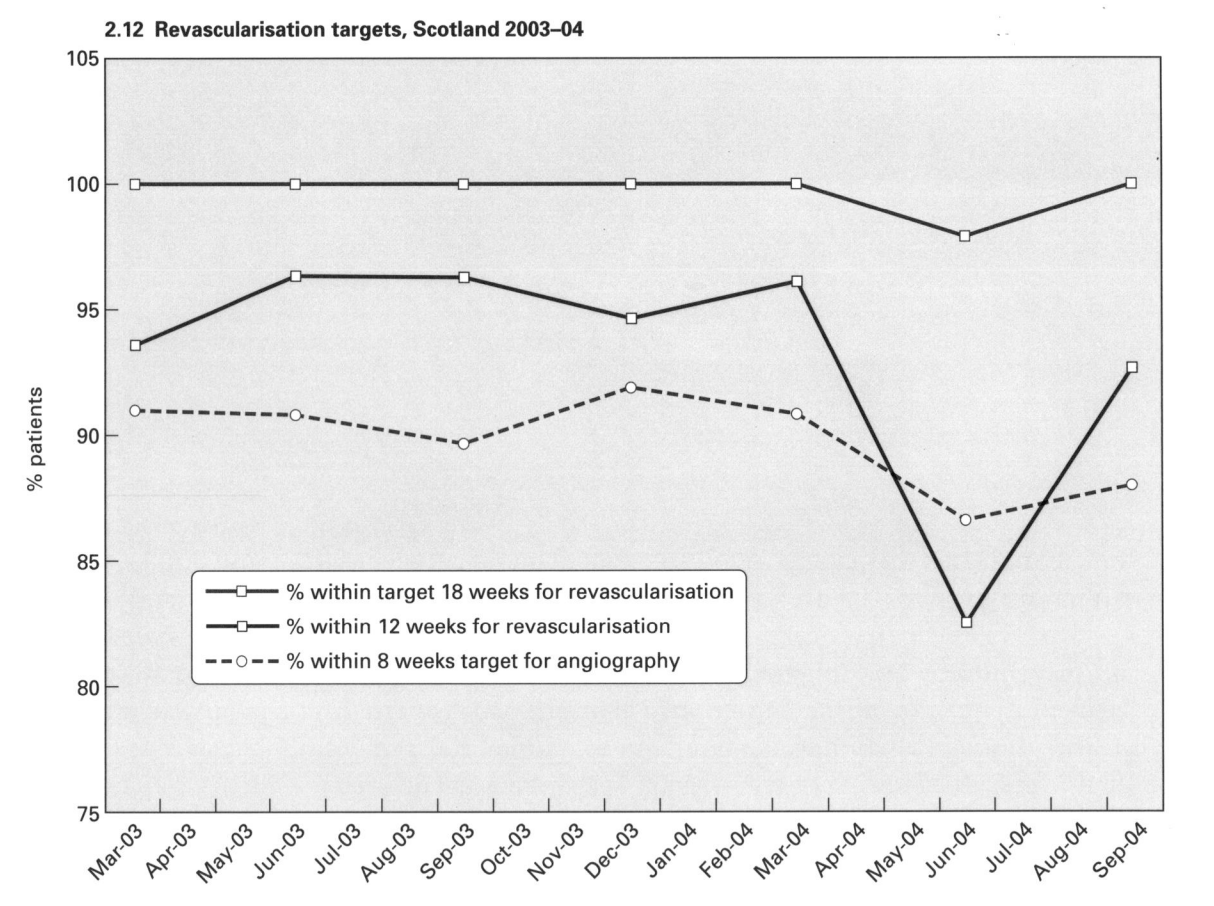

2.12 Revascularisation targets, Scotland 2003–04

% patients

Legend:
— □ — % within target 18 weeks for revascularisation
— □ — % within 12 weeks for revascularisation
- - ○ - - % within 8 weeks target for angiography

Chart 2.13 Cancer waits

In 1997, *The New NHS: modern, dependable* (DH, 1997) made a commitment that by 2000, all patients referred urgently to cancer specialists would be seen within two weeks. Additional objectives were articulated in The Cancer Plan (DH, 2000a) including: a maximum one-month wait from diagnosis to treatment for breast cancer and a maximum two-month wait from urgent GP referral to treatment for breast cancer. The chart illustrates data for September 2004. On all three indicators, the level of compliance was high: 99.5% of patients referred urgently to cancer specialists were seen within two weeks; 97.5% of breast cancer patients waited less than a month between diagnosis and commencing treatment; and 96.5% of breast cancer patient waited less than two months from urgent GP referral to treatment.

Source: DH.

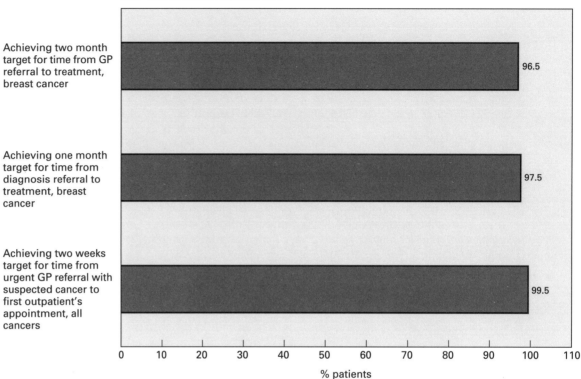

2.13 Cancer waits, England 2004

Achieving two month target for time from GP referral to treatment, breast cancer — 96.5

Achieving one month target for time from diagnosis referral to treatment, breast cancer — 97.5

Achieving two weeks target for time from urgent GP referral with suspected cancer to first outpatient's appointment, all cancers — 99.5

% patients

The Quest for Quality in the NHS: a chartbook on quality of care in the UK

References

The Quest for Quality in the NHS: a chartbook on quality of care in the UK

Audit Commission (2003) *Waiting List Accuracy: assessing the accuracy of waiting list information in NHS hospitals in England*. CW Print, Loughton, Essex.

Auditor General for Wales (2005) *NHS Waiting Times in Wales*. Auditor General for Wales, Cardiff. Available online at: www.agw.wales.gov.uk/notices/2004/agw2004_11pn.htm [last accessed 13 February 2005].

Commonwealth Fund (1998) *1998 International Health Policy Survey*. Commonwealth Fund, New York.

Commonwealth Fund (2001) *2001 International Health Policy Survey*. Commonwealth Fund, New York.

Commonwealth Fund (2002) *International Health Policy Survey of Adults with Health Problems*. Commonwealth Fund, New York.

Commonwealth Fund (2004) *International Health Policy Survey of Adults' Experiences with Primary Care*. Commonwealth Fund, New York.

Department of Health (1997) *The New NHS: modern, dependable: a national framework for assessing performance*. Stationery Office, London. Available online at www.archive.official-documents.co.uk/document/doh/newnhs/newnhs.htm [last accessed 31 January 2005].

Department of Health (2000a) *The NHS Cancer Plan: a plan for investment, a plan for reform*. Stationery Office, London. Available online at: www.dh.gov.uk/assetRoot/04/01/45/13/04014513.pdf [last accessed 31 January 2005].

Department of Health (2000b) *The NHS Plan: a plan for investment, a plan for reform*. The Stationery Office, London. Available online at: www.dh.gov.uk/assetRoot/04/05/57/83/04055783.pdf [last accessed 31 January 2005].

Department of Health (2001) *Primary Care, General Practice and the NHS Plan: information for GPs, nurses, other health professionals and staff working in primary care in England*. The Stationery Office, London. Available online at: www.dh.gov.uk/assetRoot/04/08/27/00/04082700.pdf [last accessed 31 January 2005].

Department of Health (2004) *Chief Executive's Report to the NHS, December 2004: statistical supplement*. DH, London. Available online at: www.dh.gov.uk/assetRoot/04/09/75/40/04097540.pdf [last accessed 31 January 2005].

Department of Health Cancer Waiting Times Statistics [Online]. Available at: www.performance.doh.gov.uk/cancerwaits/ [last accessed 31 January 2005].

Department of Health Hospital Activity Statistics: Cancelled Operations Data Files [Online]. Available at: www.performance.doh.gov.uk/hospitalactivity/data_requests/cancelled_operations.htm [last accessed 31 January 2005].

Department of Health Hospital Waiting Times/List Statistics [Online]. Available at: www.performance.doh.gov.uk/waitingtimes/index.htm [last accessed 31 January 2005].

Hurst J and Siciliani L (2003) *Tackling Excessive Waiting Times for Elective Surgery: a comparison of policies in twelve OECD countries*. OECD Working Papers No. 6. OECD, Paris. Available online at: www.oecd.org/dataoecd/24/32/5162353.pdf [last accessed 31 January 2005].

Jowell R, Curtice J, Park A *et al.* (eds) (2000) *British Social Attitudes: the 17th report: focusing on diversity*. Sage, London.

National Audit Office (2001) *Inappropriate Adjustments to NHS Waiting Lists: report by the comptroller and auditor general*. The Stationery Office, London.

Scottish Executive (2000) *Our National Health: a plan for action, a plan for change*. Scottish Executive, Edinburgh. Available online at: www.scotland.gov.uk/library3/health/onh-00.asp [last accessed 31 January 2005].

Siciliani L and Hurst J (2003) *Explaining Waiting Times Variations for Elective Surgery Across OECD Countries*. OECD Working Papers No. 7. OECD, Paris. Available online at: www.oecd.org/dataoecd/31/10/17256025.pdf [last accessed 31 January 2005].

Starfield B (1994) Is primary care essential? *Lancet*. **22 Oct**: 1129–33.

3 Capacity

In 1997, health spending per capita in the UK was lower than in almost all comparator countries. Australia, Sweden and the Netherlands spent 20% to 30% more than the UK; France and Germany spent 41% and 57% more, respectively; and the US spent 157% more on health per person (OECD, 2004).

At the turn of the twenty-first century, sustained underinvestment in the NHS was widely acknowledged to have taken its toll. Buildings were poorly maintained; hospitals were understaffed; primary care was overstretched; and waits for diagnostic and treatment services were unacceptably long.

> The NHS has suffered from decades of under investment . . . UK spending on healthcare has consistently lagged behind other developed countries. Since 1960, OECD countries have on average increased health spending per capita by 5.5% in real terms compared with only 3.6% in the UK. Between 1979–97 the average annual increase in Government spending on health was even less – just 2.9% . . . As a consequence the NHS has been left with insufficient capacity to provide services the public expect. England has too few hospital beds per head of population compared with most other health systems. The NHS lacks sufficient doctors, nurses and other skilled staff . . . The backlog of maintenance in the NHS now stands at £3.1 billion.
>
> DH, 2000b: p31

In response to these concerns, in April 2002 the UK government announced a 7.4% increase in expenditure in real terms each fiscal year between 2003–04 and 2007–08. This will translate into an increase in the percentage of gross domestic product (GDP) spent on healthcare from 7.7% in 2003 to 9.4% in 2008 (Robinson, 2002). The comprehensive and influential Wanless review which was commissioned by HM Treasury (Wanless, 2002) argued that over the next 20 years, the UK will need substantially to increase that figure further, from 7.7% of GDP in 2002–03 to a level between 10.6% and 12.5% of GDP in 2022–23 (depending on level of public engagement, efficiency of services and technological development).

The Wanless review emphasised that success in the quest for quality in healthcare does not depend solely on adequate resourcing; it also depends on the prudent and efficient use of resources. It asserted that maximising the use of resources requires:

- use of national standards for clinical care
- an integrated information and communication technology (ICT) system
- appropriate incentives and targets
- a balance between national and local priorities; health and social care; primary and secondary care; treatment and prevention
- rigorous independent audit of healthcare spending to ensure efficiency and effectiveness
- greater public engagement both in individuals' own health and in the healthcare system as a whole.

The capacity charts included in this chapter display data on some of the areas of shortage that have compromised the performance of the NHS in recent years. Most show some improvement as a response to the infusion of more funding.

The Quest for Quality in the NHS: a chartbook on quality of care in the UK

Chart 3.1 Spending on health

In 1980, the UK was a comparatively low spender on health, although the overall variation between the countries shown in terms of per capita spending was quite small. The announcement of increased funding for health in the UK in 2000 was beginning to have an impact on the 2002 figures. Chart 3.1a shows per capita spending in $US PPP (purchasing power parity) in the UK increased by 17% between 2000 and 2002 compared to a 16% increase in the US, 13% increase in France and 7% increase in Germany. Chart 3.1b shows that increases in spending as a percentage of GDP have been less dramatic, with increases between 2000 and 2002 of 0.3% in Germany, 0.4% in France and the UK, 0.8% in Sweden and 1.5% in the US.

3.1a Average spend on health per capita ($US PPP), international comparison 1980–2002

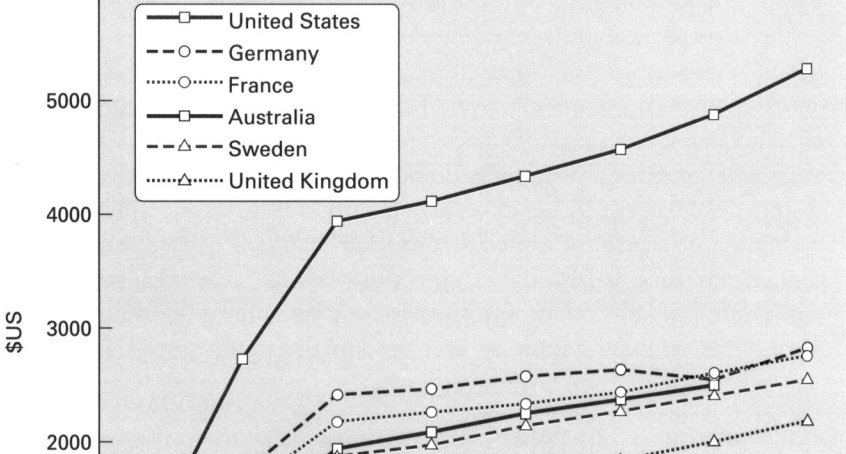

Source: OECD Health Data, 2004.

3.1b Total expenditure on health as % GDP, international comparison 1980–2002

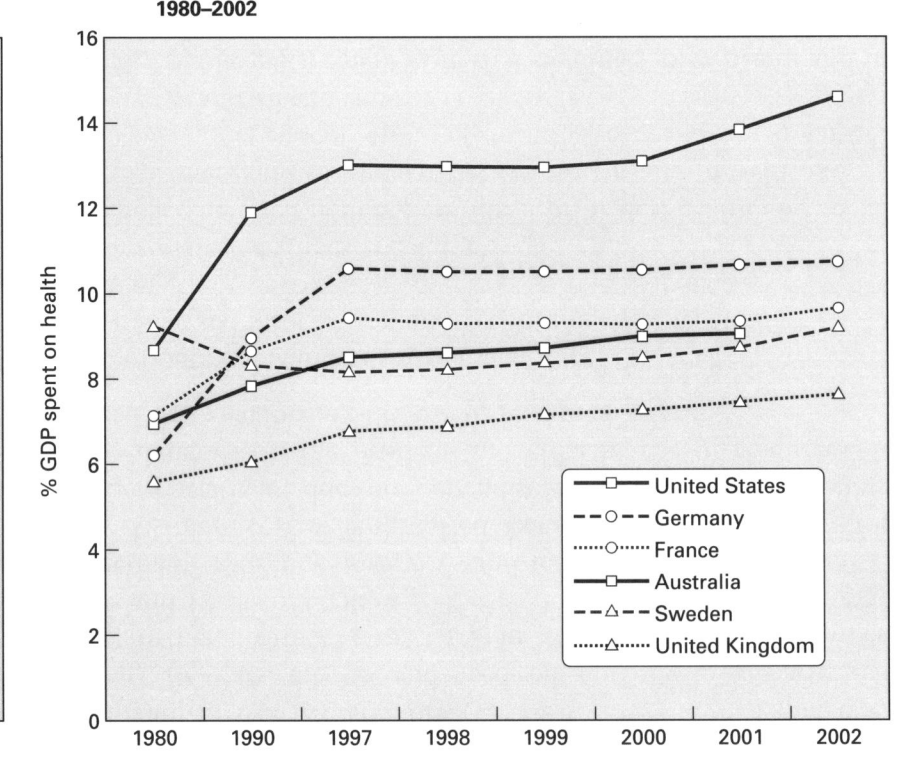

Source: OECD Health Data, 2004.

Chart 3.2 Practising physicians per 1000 population

The *NHS Plan* (DH, 2000b: p50) identified shortages in staff as the biggest constraint facing the NHS and made a series of commitments to increase staff numbers in England by 2004: 7500 more consultants; 2000 more GPs; 20 000 more nurses (for progress against these targets *see* Charts 3.3, 3.4 and 3.5). This chart, which displays figures for head counts of practising physicians per 1000 population (where physician is used as a generic term for doctor), provides some context for interpreting the progress made against those targets. The number of practising physicians per 1000 population increased between 1995 and 2002 in the UK, but figures are still below those of comparator countries, particularly France and Germany.

Source: OECD Health Data, 2004.

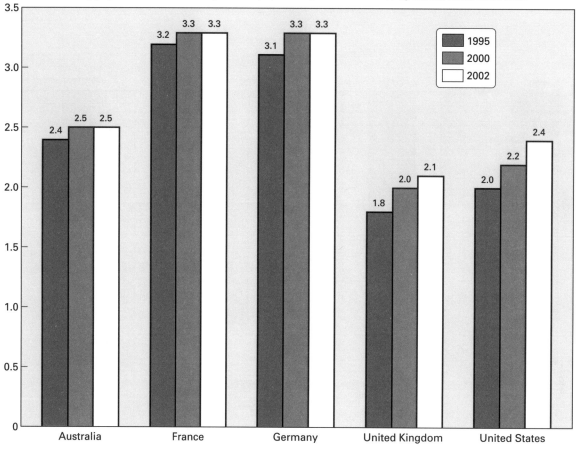

3.2 Practising physicians (head count) per 1000 population, international comparison, 1995, 2000, 2002

The Quest for Quality in the NHS: a chartbook on quality of care in the UK

75

Chart 3.3 Staffing: number of consultants

This chart provides two perspectives on numbers of consultants (i.e. specialists) working in the NHS. Chart 3.3a illustrates the extent of variation in the number of consultants per 1000 population between the countries of the UK. In 2003 the figures ranged from 0.49 in Wales to 0.65 in Scotland (wte – whole-time equivalent – where 1 wte equals a full-time post). Chart 3.3b looks more closely at figures just for England; between 2000 and 2004 the number of consultants increased by about 25%. The target set in *The NHS Plan* (2000) for a net increase of 7500 consultants (headcount) by 2004 was not met.

3.3a Number of consultants per 1000 population, UK countries 2003 (wte)

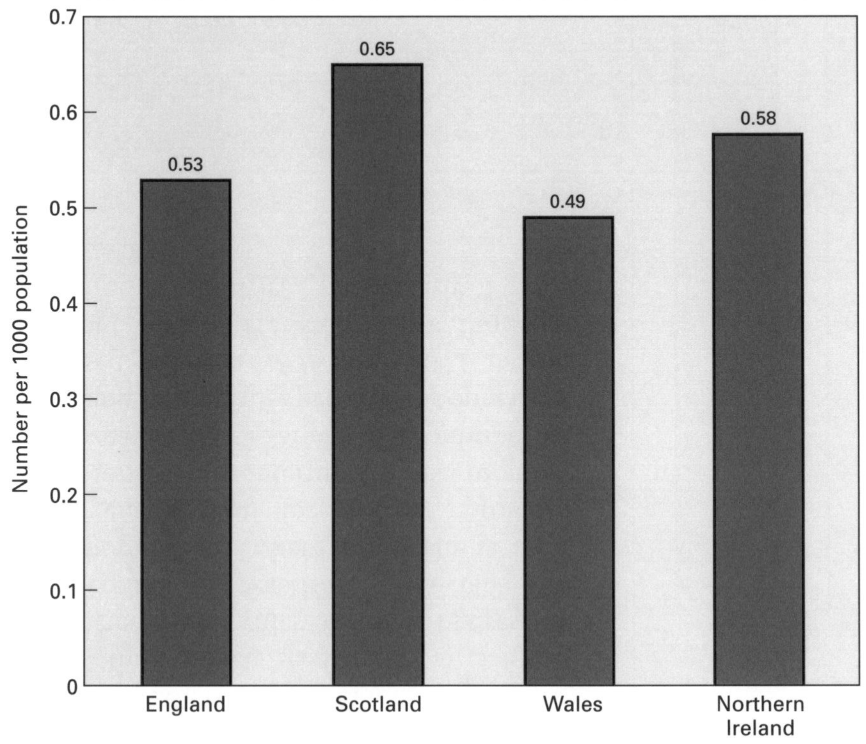

Number per 1000 population

- England: 0.53
- Scotland: 0.65
- Wales: 0.49
- Northern Ireland: 0.58

Sources: DH, NHS Wales, ISD, DHSSPSNI.

3.3b Consultant numbers, England 2000–04

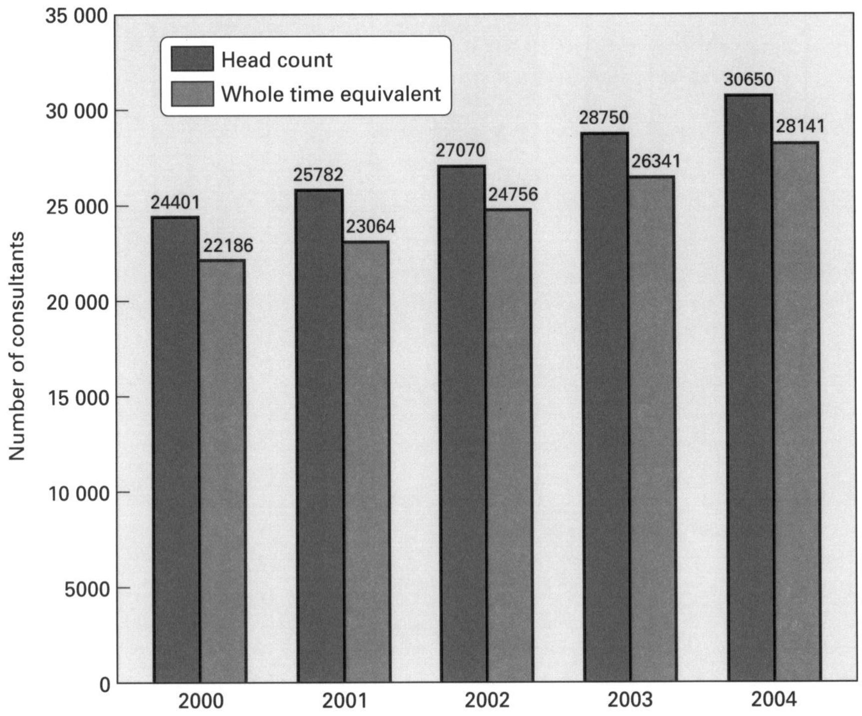

Number of consultants

Legend:
- Head count
- Whole time equivalent

Year	Head count	Whole time equivalent
2000	24401	22186
2001	25782	23064
2002	27070	24756
2003	28750	26341
2004	30650	28141

Source: DH.

Chart 3.4 Staffing: number of general practitioners

This chart provides two perspectives on general practitioner (GP) numbers. Chart 3.4a illustrates the extent of variation in the number of GPs per 1000 population between the countries of the UK. The data is for unrestricted principals and equivalents (UPEs) (*see* Technical Appendix for details). In 2003, the number of GPs ranged from 0.53 in England to 0.70 in Scotland. Chart 3.4b gives just England's figures on three categories of GP: all practitioners, unrestricted principals and NHS Plan group (*see* Technical Appendix for details). Between 2000 and June 2004 the whole-time equivalent (wte, where 1 wte is equivalent to a full-time post) of All Practitioners (excluding GP retainers) increased from 28 154 to 30 576, an increase of 2422 (9%). Within this group of 'all practitioners', the wte of UPEs increased by 483 (2%). The NHS Plan target of 2000 additional GPs does not pertain to either of these groups however. The target is based on headcount rather than wte figures, and is a subset of 'all practitioners' which excludes retainers and registrars. Between 2000 and June 2004, NHS Plan group numbers increased from 28 593 to 31 215, an increase of 2622 (9%).

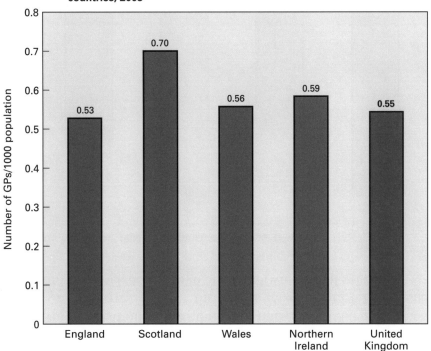

3.4a Number of whole-time equivalent GPs (UPEs) per 1000 population UK countries, 2003

Sources: DH, NHS Wales, ISD Scotland, DHSSPSNI.

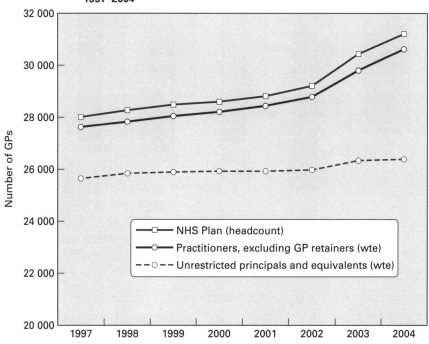

3.4b Number of GPs in England (all practitioners, UPEs, NHS Plan group), 1997–2004

Note: Data is from September each year (except 2004 which is from June).

The Quest for Quality in the NHS: a chartbook on quality of care in the UK

The Quest for Quality in the NHS: a chartbook on quality of care in the UK

Chart 3.5 Staffing: number of nurses

As with the charts pertaining to numbers of doctors, these charts provide two perspectives on numbers of nurses. Chart 3.5a illustrates the extent of variation in the number of nurses per 1000 population across UK countries. In 2003 the figures ranged from 6.1 per 1000 population in England to 7.6 in Scotland (wte – whole-time equiva-

lent – where 1 wte equals a full-time post). Chart 3.5b displays data for England, and shows that between 2000 and 2004 the number of nurses (wte) rose by 48 453 (an 18% increase). The target set in *The NHS Plan* (2000) for 20 000 additional nurses by 2004 was exceeded.

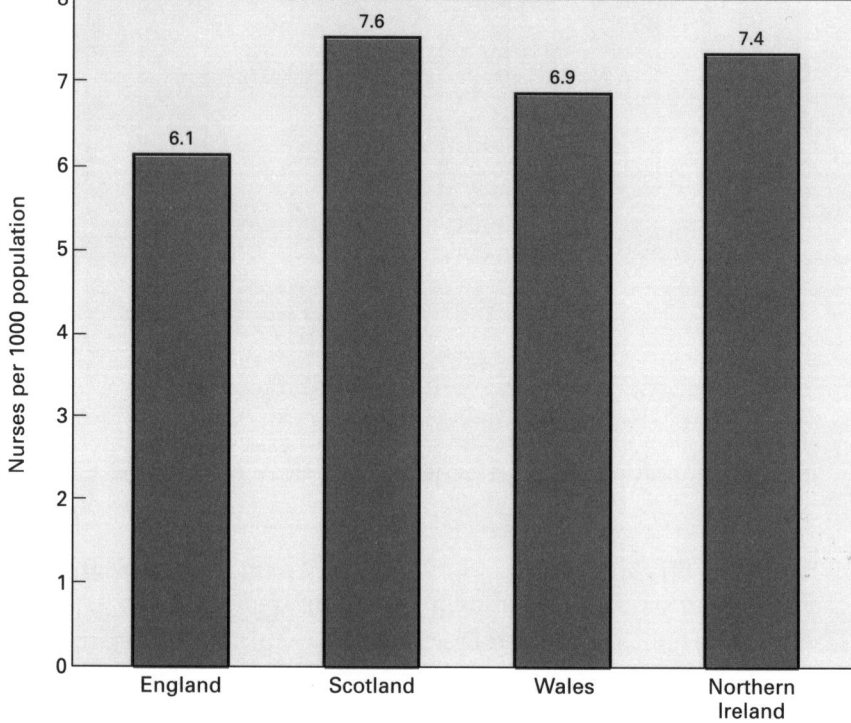

3.5a Nurses per 1000 population (wte), UK countries 2003

Sources: DH, NHS Wales, ISD Scotland, DHSSPSNI.

3.5b Qualified nursing staff, England 2000–04

Source: DH.

Chart 3.6 Staffing: number of dentists

Dentistry is a critical area of deficient capacity in the UK. In 2001, compared to similar countries, the UK had fewer dentists per capita. Less than 50% of the population are currently registered with an NHS dentist. This may reflect a deliberate choice on the part of patients to pay for dentistry services or, much more likely, the low availability of dentists willing to work within the NHS. In some areas of the UK, no dentists will accept adult NHS patients, effectively discriminating against those with low incomes (Boulos and Picton-Phillips, 2004).

Sources: ONS, OECD Health Data 2004.

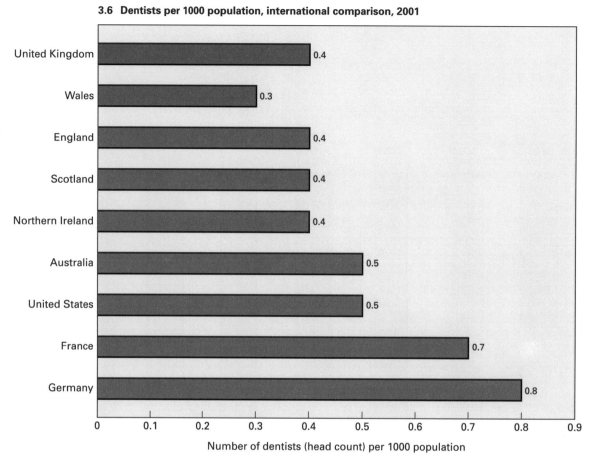

3.6 Dentists per 1000 population, international comparison, 2001

Number of dentists (head count) per 1000 population

The Quest for Quality in the NHS: a chartbook on quality of care in the UK

79

Chart 3.7 Number of beds per 1000 population

The Quest for Quality in the NHS: a chartbook on quality of care in the UK

The number of hospital beds has been declining since the 1960s, largely as a result of medical advances, shorter hospital stays, the development of day surgery, and the growth of 'care in the community' for older people and those with mental illnesses (DH, 2000c). All of the UK countries have fewer beds per 1000 population than the EU average. There is a wide variation within the UK with numbers of beds ranging from 3.7 per 1000 in England to 5.9 per 1000 in Scotland.

Sources: Eurostat; DH, ISD Scotland, NHS Wales, DHSSPSNI.

3.7 Beds per 1000 population, international comparison 2003–04

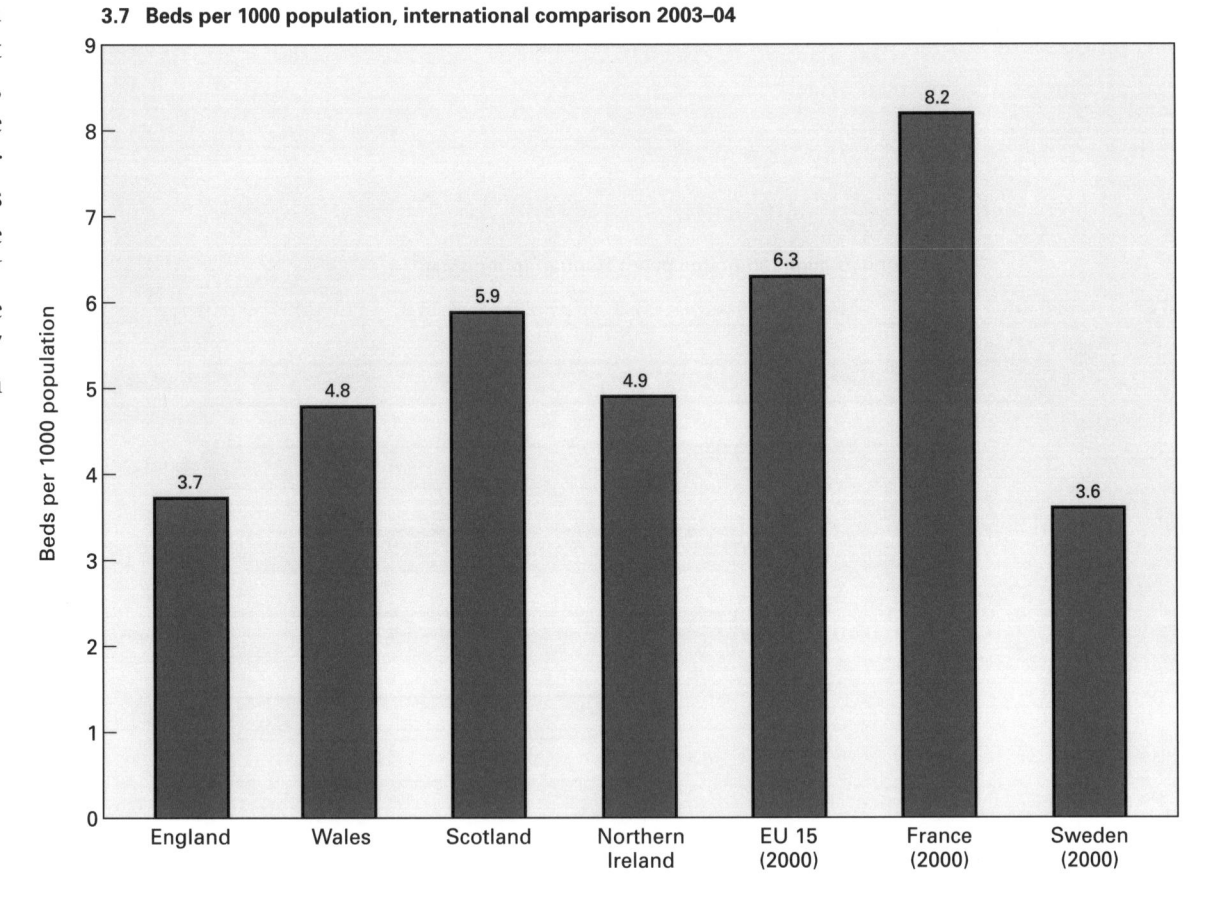

Chart 3.8 Critical care beds

Critical care beds include both Intensive Care Unit (ICU) beds and beds on high dependency units (HDUs) which provide an intermediate level of care for patients not well enough to go on to general wards. Critical care is very labour-intensive; a typical six-bed ICU unit is staffed by several consultants and an average of 30 to 50 nurses (Intensive Care Society, 2002). International comparisons have shown that the UK allocates about 2.6% of its beds to critical care, a relatively low proportion compared to other European countries; Denmark, with 4.1%, has the highest allocation (DH, 2000a). Resource constraints, high demand for beds and subsequent early transfer to general wards have been shown to have serious consequences for outcomes and patient mortality (Smith *et al.*, 1999). Chart 3.8a displays data comparing the number of ICU beds in UK countries, ranging from 2.4 per 100 000 population in Northern Ireland to 4.5 per 100 000 in Wales. *The NHS Plan* (DH, 2000b) set a target to increase critical care beds in England by 30% by 2003. Chart 3.8b shows that this was achieved. The most recent data available for England indicates that the number of critical care beds per 100 000 population in July 2004 was 6.33; the corresponding figure for ICU beds was 3.50.

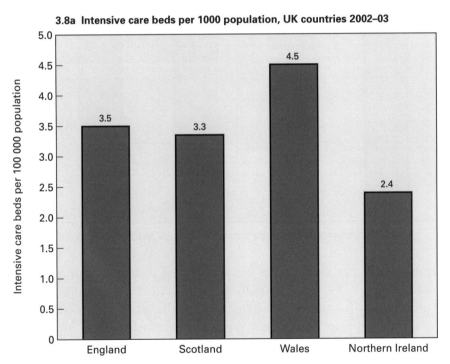

3.8a Intensive care beds per 1000 population, UK countries 2002–03

Sources: DH; StatsWales, ISD Scotland; DHSSPS (*see* Technical Appendix for details).

Note: NI data from 2000.

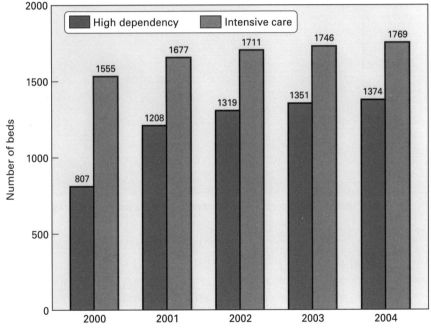

3.8b Critical care beds, England 2000–04

Source: DH.

The Quest for Quality in the NHS: a chartbook on quality of care in the UK

Chart 3.9 Imaging equipment

Problems with availability and timeliness of imaging and radiographic services represent one of the major bottlenecks hampering efforts to reduce waiting lists for inpatient and outpatient care in the NHS. In comparison with similar countries, the UK has low numbers of imaging equipment such as computed tomography (CT) scanners and magnetic resonance imaging (MRI) units. Further, the Society of Radiographers (SOR) have stated that long waiting times for scans and cancer treatment are likely to continue for at least three years because of staff shortages (Society Guardian, 2004). Chart 3.9a shows that, in 2001, Germany and the US had more than double the number (per million population) of CT scanners than the UK had. Chart 3.9b shows that the UK also had a lower number of MRI units (per million population) than comparator countries except France.

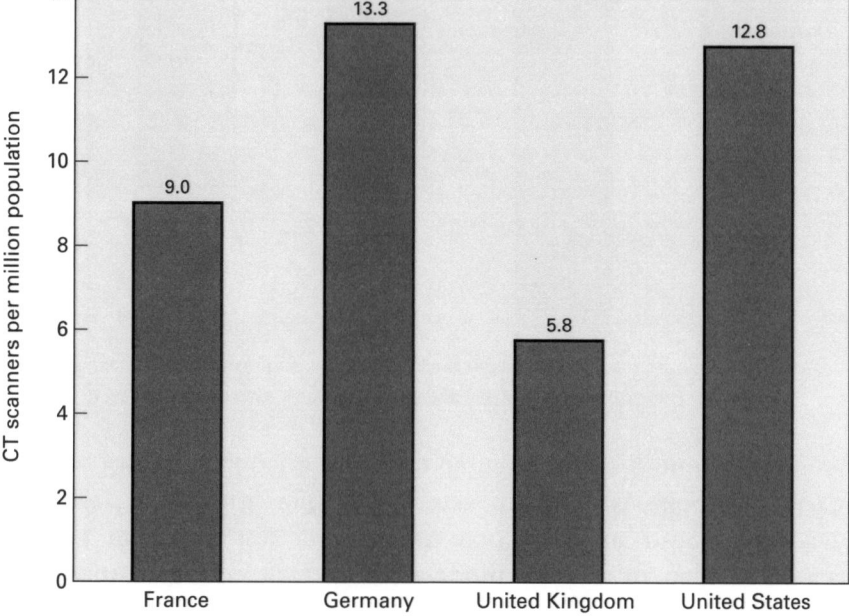

3.9a CT scanners per million population, international comparison, 2001–02

Source: OECD Health Data 2004.

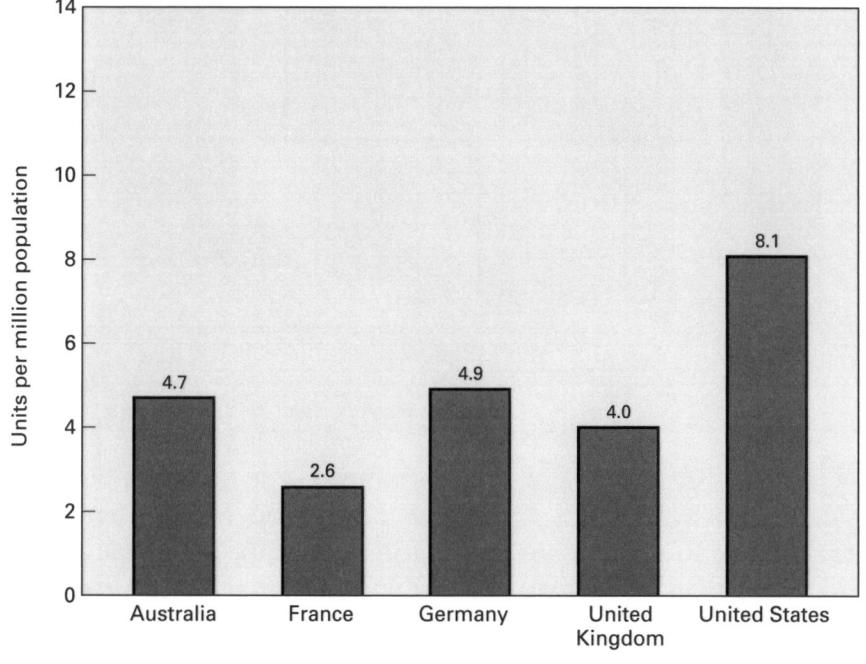

3.9b MRI units per million population, international comparison, 2000

Source: OECD Health Data 2004.

Chart 3.10 Percutaneous coronary interventions

See Revascularisation p27

Rates of revascularisation in the UK are lower than in comparator countries (*see* Chart 1.19), leading to concerns about insufficient capacity. Percutaneous coronary interventions (PCI) are a type of revascularisation used to treat coronary heart disease, and includes percutaneous transluminal coronary angioplasty (PTCA) and other new techniques capable of relieving coronary narrowing such as rotational atherectomy, directional atherectomy, extraction atherectomy, laser angioplasty, implantation of intracoronary stents, and other catheter devices for treating coronary atherosclerosis (Smith *et al.*, 2001). The British Cardiovascular Intervention Society (BCIS, 2004) conducts an annual audit of PCIs. The 2003 audit reported a 17% increase in PCI activity between 2002 and 2003. PCI rates for the UK increased by 122% between 1997 and 2003. Within the UK, rates of PCI per million population in 2003 varied from 592 in Wales to 1044 in Northern Ireland. As a reference point, in 2001 the PCI rate in the US was approximately 1700 per million population (Smith *et al.*, 2001).

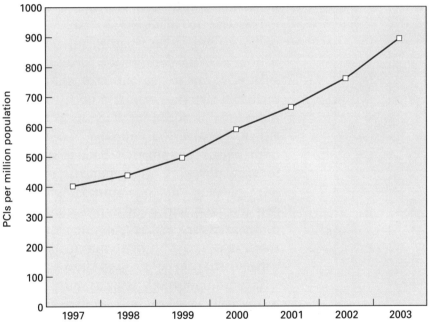

3.10a PCI rates per million population, UK countries 1997–2003

Source: BCIS Audit, 2004.

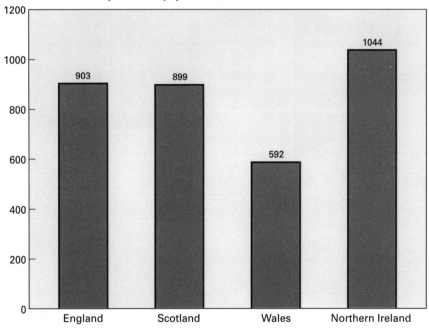

3.10b PCI rates per million population, UK countries 2003

Source: BCIS Audit, 2004.

The Quest for Quality in the NHS: a chartbook on quality of care in the UK

Chart 3.11 Stroke units

See Stroke pp33–4

The Quest for Quality in the NHS: a chartbook on quality of care in the UK

There is strong evidence to suggest that stroke patients who receive inpatient care on a specialised stroke unit are more likely to survive, to be more independent, and to be living at home one year after their stroke (Stroke Unit Trialists' Collaboration, 2001). In 1998, only 48% of NHS Trusts had a stroke team/unit (CEEU, 2002). The chart shows that in 2004, stroke care capacity in Wales remained around that level but had improved considerably in England and Northern Ireland, with 82% and 85% of hospitals having a dedicated stroke unit, respectively. Despite an increase in the number of stroke units, problems with capacity persist; on a typical weekday, estimates are that just over one-half of stroke patients are on a stroke unit. Moreover, even though provision for stroke care is improving in hospitals, the development of services in the community has been much slower; in 2004, only 25% of sites had a specialist stroke community team to provide support to rehabilitating patients (data not shown).

Sources: CEEU, 2004; Royal College of Physicians.

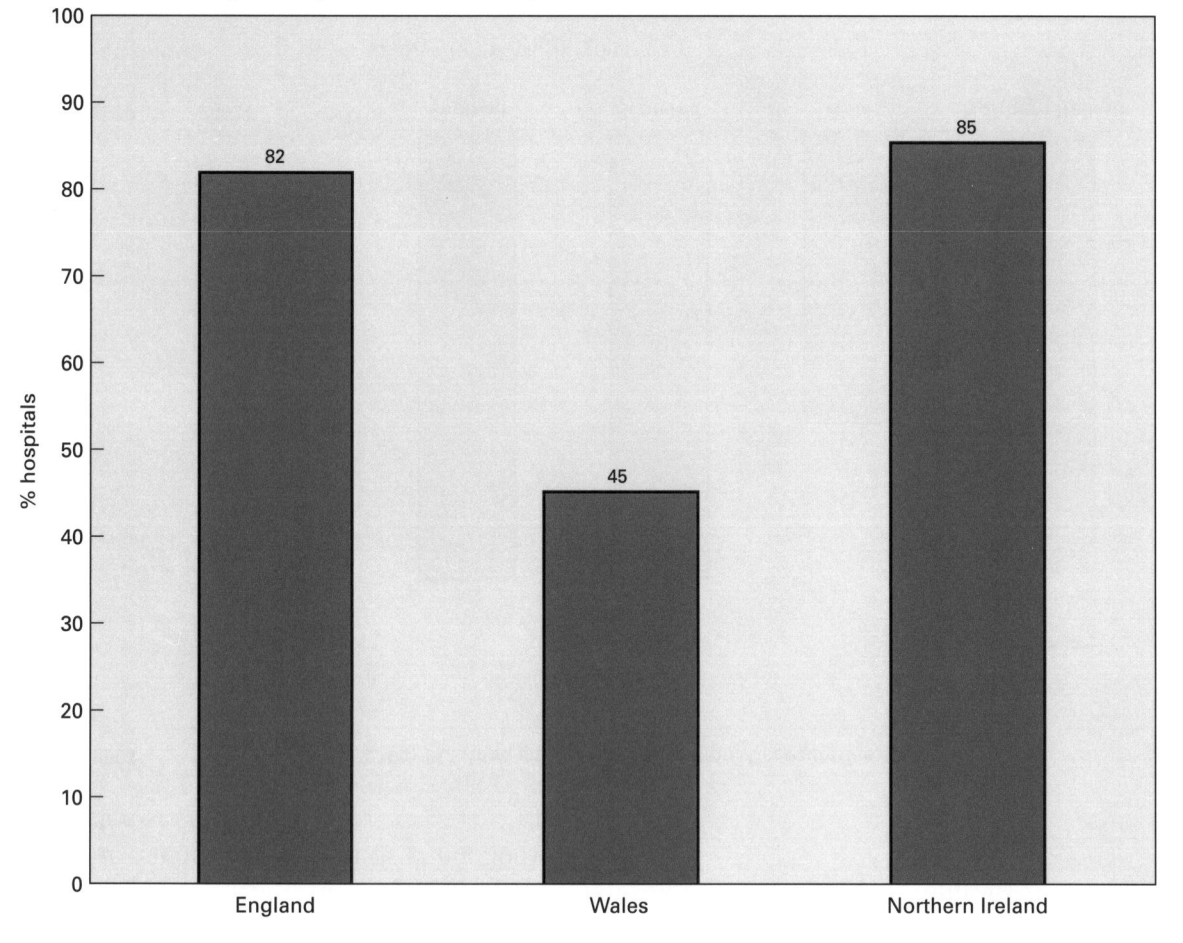

3.11 Percentage of hospitals with stroke unit, UK countries 2004

Chart 3.12 Acute stroke units: facilities audit

See Stroke pp33–4

Effective early management of stroke can reduce mortality and morbidity and lower unnecessary use of scarce health and social services resources (Royal College of Physicians, 2004). Of the 256 stroke units in England, Wales and Northern Ireland, 88 are acute units that admit patients immediately after they have suffered a stroke but usually discharge patients within seven days. Acute stroke units generally provide an intensive model of care with continuous monitoring and high nurse staffing levels. The characteristics depicted in the chart are all regarded as beneficial in acute stroke care. The chart shows that their availability is far from universal.

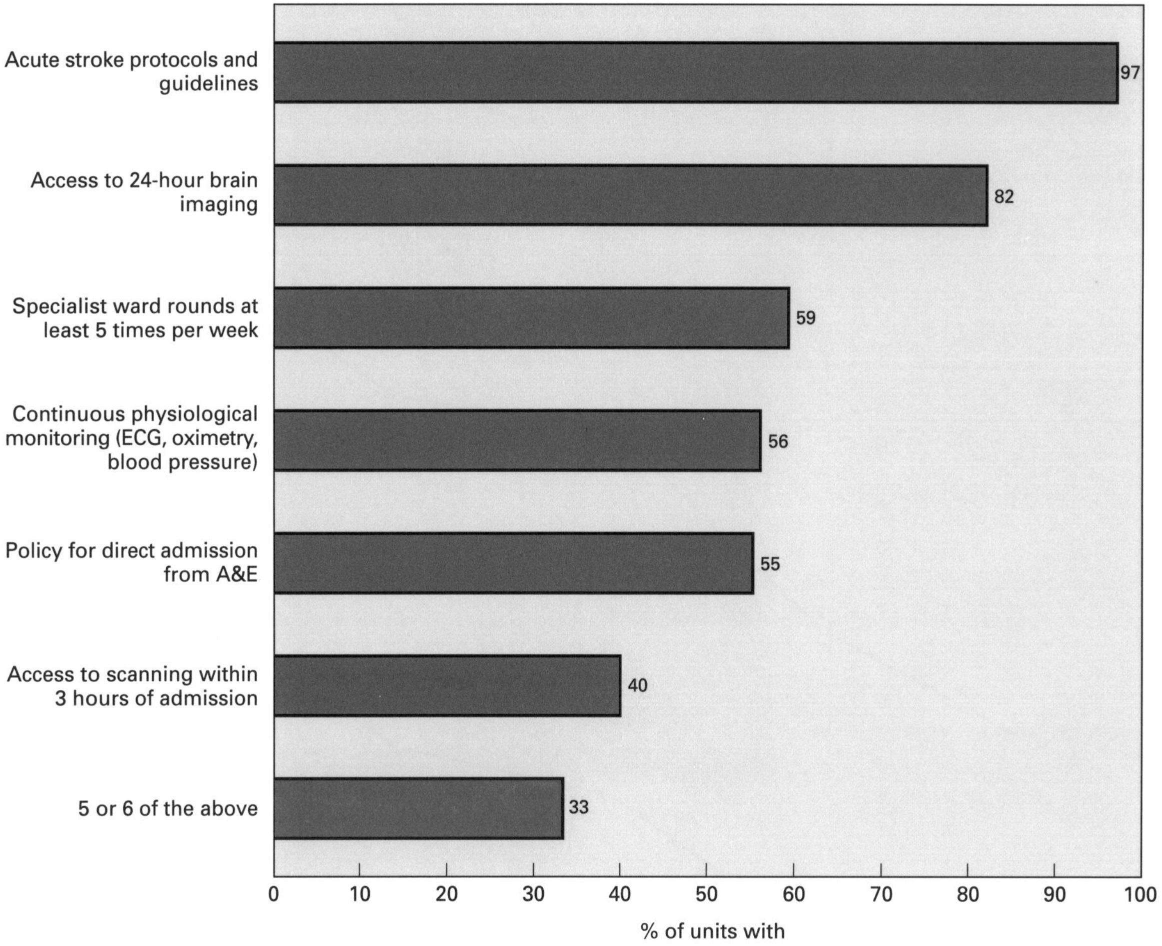

Source: CEEU, 2004; Royal College of Physicians.

3.12 Acute stroke unit facilities: England, Wales and Northern Ireland, 2004

Facility	% of units with
Acute stroke protocols and guidelines	97
Access to 24-hour brain imaging	82
Specialist ward rounds at least 5 times per week	59
Continuous physiological monitoring (ECG, oximetry, blood pressure)	56
Policy for direct admission from A&E	55
Access to scanning within 3 hours of admission	40
5 or 6 of the above	33

% of units with

85

Chart 3.13 Mental health services teams

See Mental health overview p43

The Quest for Quality in the NHS: a chartbook on quality of care in the UK

Innovative approaches to mental health services provision have been enthusiastically pursued in recent years. *Assertive outreach teams* provide intensive support for severely mentally ill people who are difficult to engage in more traditional services. Care and support is offered in their homes or some other community setting, at times suited to them. The NHS Plan target for 220 teams by December 2003 was met.

Crisis resolution teams provide 24-hour intensive support for people in mental health crises in their own homes. They aim to provide prompt and effective home treatment, including medication, to prevent hospital admissions and support family and other carers. The NHS Plan pledged 335 teams by December 2004. *Early intervention teams* aim to help people between 14 and 35 years of age who either show symptoms of psychosis for the first time or are in the first three years of a psychotic illness. They focus on prevention, early detection and more effective treatment at the beginning of illness. The NHS Plan pledged the formation of 50 teams by 2003. Progress was made in increasing numbers of both crisis resolution and early intervention teams, but the ambitious Government-set targets were not fully met.

Source: Annual Service Mapping Exercise, University of Durham, 2004.

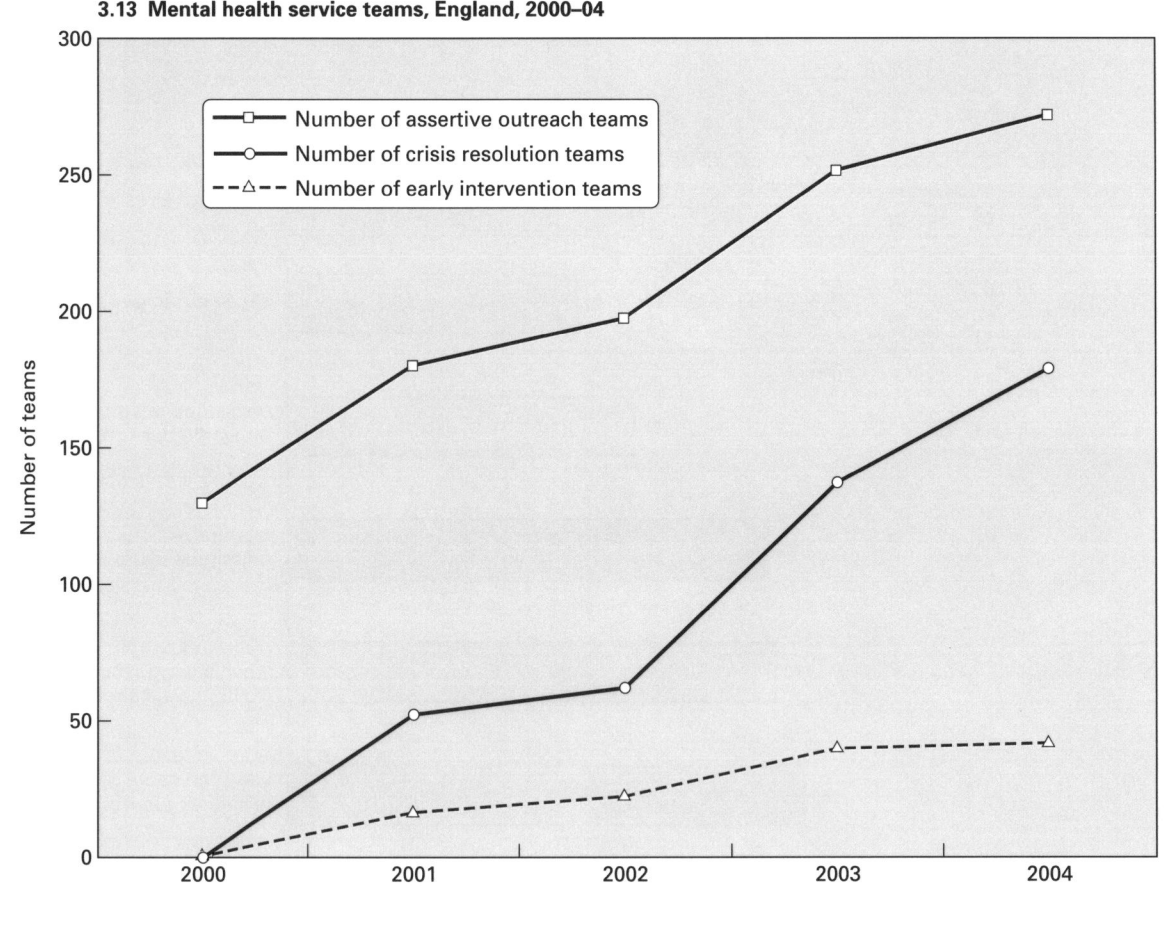

3.13 Mental health service teams, England, 2000–04

Number of teams

— □ — Number of assertive outreach teams
— ○ — Number of crisis resolution teams
- - △ - - Number of early intervention teams

References

Annual Service Mapping Exercise, University of Durham. Data drawn from: Department of Health (2004) *Chief Executive's Report to the NHS*. Department of Health, London. Available online at: www.dh.gov.uk/assetRoot/04/09/75/40/04097540.pdf [last accessed 31 January 2005].

BCIS (2004) *BCIS Audit Data 2003*. British Cardiovascular Intervention Society. Available online at: www.bcis.org.uk/cgi-bin/item.cgi?id=218&d=1&h=28&f=29&dateformat=%o%20%B%20%Y [last accessed 31 January 2005].

Boulos MNK and Picton-Phillips G (2004) Is NHS Dentistry in crisis? 'Traffic light' maps of dentists distribution in England and Wales. *International Journal of Health Geographics*. 3: 10.

CEEU (2002) *Summary Report of the National Sentinel Stroke Audit 2001/02*. Clinical Evaluation and Effectiveness Unit, Royal College of Physicians, London. Available online at: www.rcplondon.ac.uk/pubs/strokeaudit01-02.pdf [last accessed 31 January 2005].

CEEU (2004) *National Sentinel Stroke Audit*. Clinical Evaluation and Effectiveness Unit, Royal College of Physicians, London. Available online at: www.rcplondon.ac.uk/pubs/books/strokeaudit/strokeaudit2004.pdf [last accessed 31 January 2005].

Department of Health (2000a) *Comprehensive Critical Care: a review of adult critical care services*. Department of Health, London. Available online at: www.dh.gov.uk/assetRoot/04/08/28/72/04082872.pdf [last accessed 31 January 2005].

Department of Health (2000b) *The NHS Plan: a plan for investment, a plan for reform*. The Stationery Office, London. Available online at: www.dh.gov.uk/assetRoot/04/05/57/83/04055783.pdf [last accessed 31 January 2005].

Department of Health (2000c) *Shaping the Future NHS: long term planning for hospitals and related services*. Consultation document on the findings of the National Beds Inquiry. Department of Health, London. Available online at: www.dh.gov.uk/assetRoot/04/02/04/69/04020469.pdf [last accessed 31 January 2005].

Department of Health (2004) *Average daily number of available and occupied beds by sector, England, 2003–04* [Online]. Available at: www.performance.doh.gov.uk/hospitalactivity/data_requests/download/beds_open_overnight/bed_04_summary.xls [last accessed 31 January 2005.].

Department of Health (2004) *Hospital Activity Statistics* [Online]. Available at: www.performance.doh.gov.uk/hospitalactivity/data_requests/critical_care_beds.htm [last accessed 31 January 2005.].

Department of Health, Social Services and Public Safety (2004) *Hospital Statistics 1 April 2003–31 March 2004 Volume 1: Programme of Care* [Online]. Available at: www.dhsspsni.gov.uk/publications/2004/poc-contents.pdf [last accessed 31 January 2005].

Intensive Care Society (2002) *Critical Insight: an Intensive Care Society introduction to UK adult critical care services*. Available online at: www.ics.ac.uk/press/CRITICAL%20INSIGHT%20FINAL.pdf.

ISD Scotland (2004) *National Statistics Release: Inpatient Facilities – by Specialty* [Online]. Available at: www.isdscotland.org/isd/files/Annual_trends_in_available_beds_March_2004_NovRelease.xls [last accessed 31 January 2005].

National Assembly for Wales (2004) *NHS Beds, 2003–04* [Online]. Available at: www.wales.gov.uk/keypubstatisticsforwalesheadline/content/health/2004/hdw20040908-e.htm [last accessed 31 January 2005].

Organisation for Economic Co-operation and Development (2004) *OECD Health Data 2004*. OECD, Paris.

Robinson R (2002) Gold for the NHS: good news that raises questions on consistency and sustainability *BMJ*. 324: 987–8.

Royal College of Physicians (2004) *National Clinical Guidelines for Stroke* (2e). Royal College of Physicians, London.

Smith L, Orts CM, O'Neil I *et al.* (1999) TISS and mortality after discharge from intensive care. *Intensive Care Medicine*. 25 (10): 1061–5.

Smith SC, Dove JT, Jacobs AK *et al.* (2001) ACC/AHA Guidelines for percutaneous coronary intervention. Executive summary. *Circulation*. 103: 3019.

SocietyGuardian [Online] (2004) Radiographers warn of staffing crisis. 28 September. Available at: http://society.guardian.co.uk/NHSstaff/story/0,7991,1314629,00.html [last accessed 31 January 2005].

Stroke Unit Trialists' Collaboration (2001) Organised inpatient (stroke unit) care for stroke. *The Cochrane Database of Systematic Reviews*. 3. Art. No.: CD000197. DOI: 10.1002/14651858.CD000197. Available online at: www.cochrane.org/cochrane/revabstr/AB000197.htm [last accessed 31 January 2005].

Wanless D (2002) *Securing our Future Health: taking a long-term view*. The Public Inquiry Unit, HM Treasury, London.

Safety is a fundamental attribute of healthcare quality. It encompasses avoidance of medical error and elimination of unnecessary risk of harm to patients. Safety has in recent years commanded considerable attention internationally (Brennan *et al.*, 1991; Wilson *et al.* 1995; Davis *et al.* 2002; Baker *et al.*, 2004), with key publications released on both sides of the Atlantic including the Institute of Medicine report, *To Err is Human* (Kohn *et al.*, 2000) in the United States and *An Organisation with a Memory* (DH, 2000) in the United Kingdom.

An Organisation with a Memory articulated four key safety targets for England:

- by 2001, reduce to zero the number of patients dying or being paralysed by maladministered spinal injections
- by March 2002, reduce to zero the number of suicides by mental health patients as a result of hanging from non-collapsible bed or shower curtain rails
- by the end of 2005, reduce by 25% the number of instances of harm in the field of obstetrics and gynaecology that result in litigation
- by the end of 2005, reduce by 40% the number of serious errors in the use of prescribed drugs.

Highlighting the critical importance that safety issues are now accorded, the World Health Organization (WHO) in 2004 established a world alliance for patient safety (www.who.int/patientsafety). The alliance seeks to be a forum to coordinate and capitalise on different countries' efforts to improve safety and to establish standardised terminology, common methods of measurement, and compatible reporting of adverse events. Similarly, the OECD has recently published a set of 21 indicators for patient safety, based on consensus recommendations of an international expert panel. Those indicators are:

Healthcare-Associated Infections (also referred to as Hospital-Acquired Infections (HAI)

- ventilator pneumonia
- wound infection
- infection due to medical care
- decubitus ulcer

Sentinel events

- transfusion reaction
- wrong blood type
- wrong-site surgery
- foreign body left in during procedure
- medical equipment related adverse event
- medication errors

Operative and postoperative complications

- complication of anaesthesia
- postoperative hip fracture
- postoperative pulmonary embolism or deep vein thrombosis
- postoperative sepsis
- technical difficulty with procedure

Obstetrics

- birth trauma – injury to neonate
- obstetric trauma – vaginal delivery
- obstetric trauma – caesarean delivery
- problems with childbirth

Other care-related adverse events

- patient falls
- in-hospital hip fracture or fall

Source: Millar *et al.*, 2004

The Quest for Quality in the NHS: a chartbook on quality of care in the UK

The Quest for Quality in the NHS: a chartbook on quality of care in the UK

Currently, such a comprehensive set of indicators is largely aspirational in the UK. Compared with other domains of quality, safety is marked by a relative insufficiency in the amount of data readily available. The paucity of publicly reported safety data is often attributed to concerns that incident reporting may allow an individual and/or organisation to be identified, resulting in reprisals. Such concerns are seen to be an impediment both to transparency and to learning in a constructive and blame-free process. There are, however, a number of ways to address 'reporting reticence', including the promotion of an organisational culture that supports learning from mistakes; the development of easy-to-use internal reporting tools; and the creation of a central repository that collects safety data in confidence, aggregates it and releases it in an anonymised form (Edmondson, 2004).

Providing robust and timely safety data is not merely a measurement issue. Although it is of great interest and helps chart how the NHS performs over time, its particular strength is as a means to secure improved performance in the future. Once detected and reported, patterns of errors may be revealed; once uncovered, patterns of errors may be rectified through professional feedback and education, thus resulting in the correction of unsafe organisational practices or systemic problems.

As a result of 'reporting reticence', the type and source of data must be considered when interpreting information on patient safety. For example, an increase in rates of adverse events may at face value seem to indicate a deterioration in quality. If the data are based on voluntary reporting, however, the increase may reflect a greater propensity to report adverse events (facilitating subsequent analysis and prevention) rather than increased incidence. Similarly, in comparisons across countries or hospitals, higher figures may be a reflection of more accurate reporting or data collection, rather than poorer relative performance.

The concerns about, and subsequent constraints on, public release of data mean that the safety charts are somewhat limited in scope. When system-wide data is not accessible, we make use of individual case studies.

Safety charts focus on four areas:

1 adverse events
2 medication errors
3 healthcare-associated infections
4 patient and professional perceptions about safety issues.

Adverse events

An **adverse event** is defined as 'an event or omission arising during clinical care and causing physical or psychological injury to a patient' (DH, 2000). Not all are the result of error, nor are all of them preventable. Patient injuries resulting from drug therapy are one of the more common types of adverse events that occur in hospitals. Incidence rates of **adverse drug events** (ADEs) in the US have been estimated to occur at a rate of between 2 and 7 per 100 admissions (Classen *et al.*, 1997; Bates *et al.*, 1995; Jha *et al.*, 1998). ADEs can result in a range of physical consequences, from temporary discomfort to death. Thomas *et al.* (1999) estimated that 9.7% of ADEs cause permanent disability. An earlier study estimated that the increased risk of death for a patient who experiences an ADE is nearly twice that of a patient who does not (Classen *et al.*, 1997). The distribution of different types of injuries among patients who suffered ADEs in the US are shown in Figure A (as this is US data it is not contained in the chart set). In a 700-bed hospital in the US, the cost of ADEs was an estimated $2.8 million per year (Bates *et al.*, 1997).

Source: www.ahrq.gov/qual/aderia/aderia.htm#14.

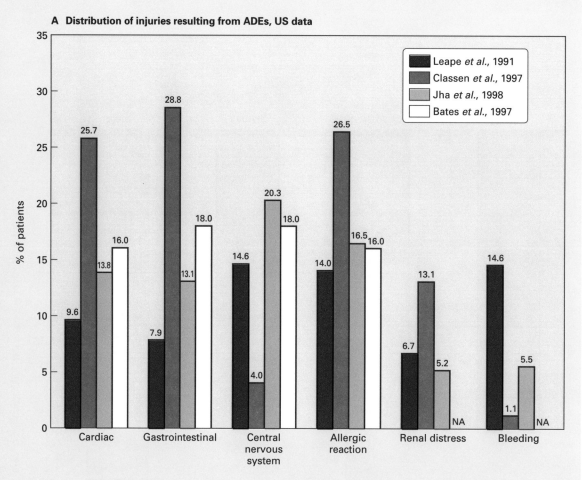

A   Distribution of injuries resulting from ADEs, US data

The Quest for Quality in the NHS: a chartbook on quality of care in the UK

Chart 4.1 Adverse events: routine data source

The Quest for Quality in the NHS: a chartbook on quality of care in the UK

A retrospective review of Hospital Episode Statistics (HES) from 1999–2000 to 2002–03 found, on average, that 2.2% of all episodes (276 514 per year) were coded for an adverse event. Incidence did not change over time. Adverse events were more common in men than women, more frequent in emergency than elective admissions, and more common in elderly patients (data not shown). The researchers acknowledged that adverse events are likely to be underrecorded in HES data; they pointed out that some Trusts report no adverse events, which seems unlikely, thus raising questions about the validity of the reporting.

4.1 Rate of adverse events, England 1999–2000 to 2002–03

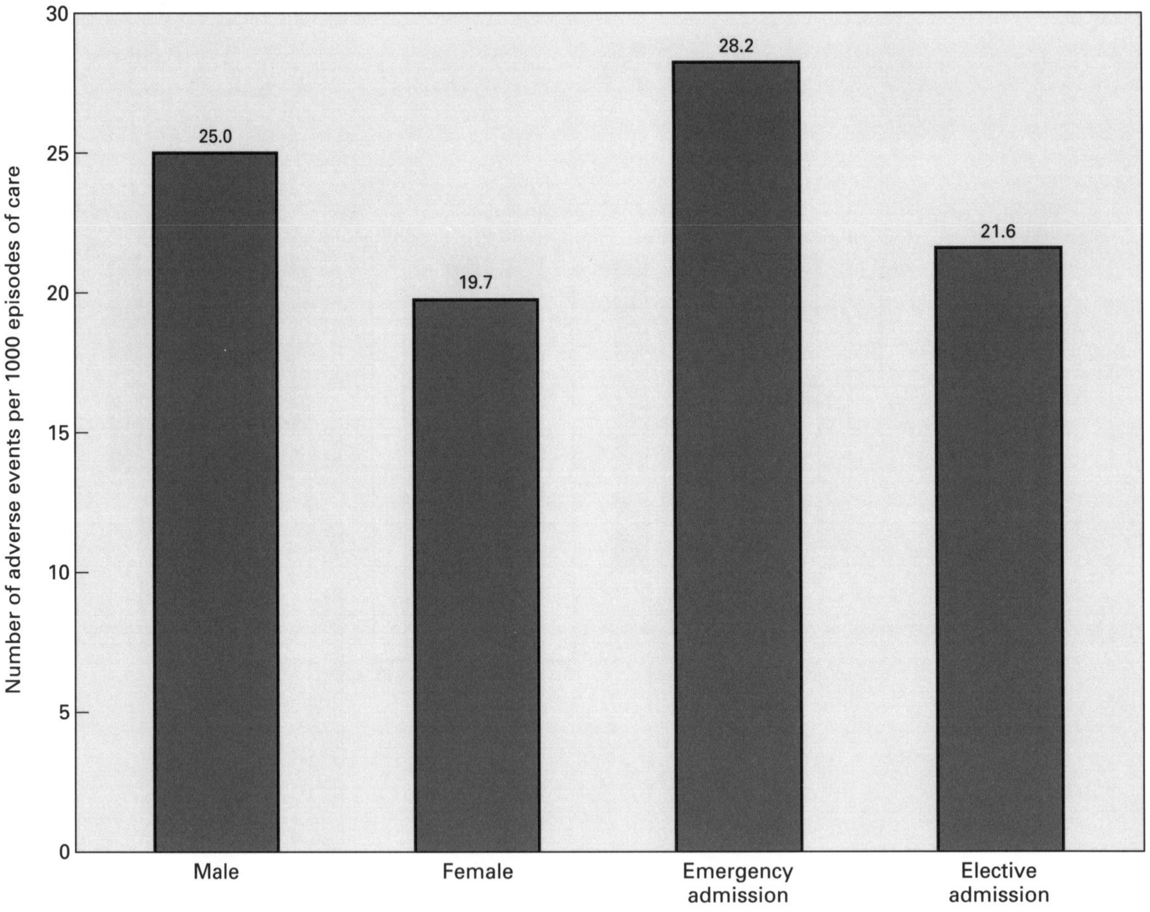

Source: Aylin *et al.*, 2004.

Chart 4.2 Adverse events: case notes review

This chart is based on a retrospective review of 1014 medical and nursing records drawn from two acute hospitals in London. One in 10 patients (10.8%) experienced an adverse event. Of these events, about one-half were judged preventable with ordinary standards of care; reviewers considered that one-third led to moderate or greater disability or death. For the 110 patients who experienced an adverse event, the mean length of stay was increased by 8.5 days at an additional cost of £290 000. Extrapolating these findings to England and Wales suggests that adverse events might occur at a rate in excess of 850 000 per year. The Department of Health estimates that adverse events incur some £2 billion of direct costs in additional bed days per year (Chief Pharmaceutical Officer, 2004).

Source: Vincent *et al.*, 2001.

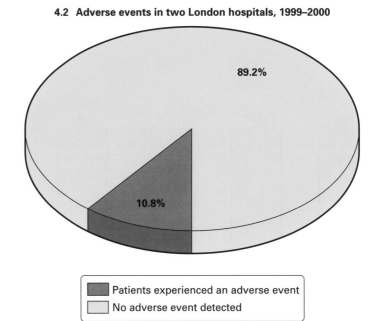

4.2 Adverse events in two London hospitals, 1999–2000

89.2%

10.8%

Patients experienced an adverse event
No adverse event detected

The Quest for Quality in the NHS: a chartbook on quality of care in the UK

Chart 4.3 Adverse events under surgical care

The Quest for Quality in the NHS: a chartbook on quality of care in the UK

The 2003 Scottish Audit of Surgical Mortality reported that 4478 patients died under surgical care, representing 1.5% of the 295 034 total surgical admissions. Of these, 700 cases were recorded as including an adverse event or an area for concern. In 2003, data collection processes changed: between 1998 and 2002, cases with adverse events were recorded according to the categories shown in the chart. In 2003, the category 'made no difference to eventual outcome' was divided into 'areas for consideration but they made no difference to eventual outcome' and 'areas of concern but they made no difference to eventual outcome'. Therefore, the data from 2003 is not strictly comparable to that from earlier years. The increase in levels of reported adverse events in 2003 may reflect more comprehensive reporting.

Source: Scottish Audit of Surgical Mortality 2002; 2003.

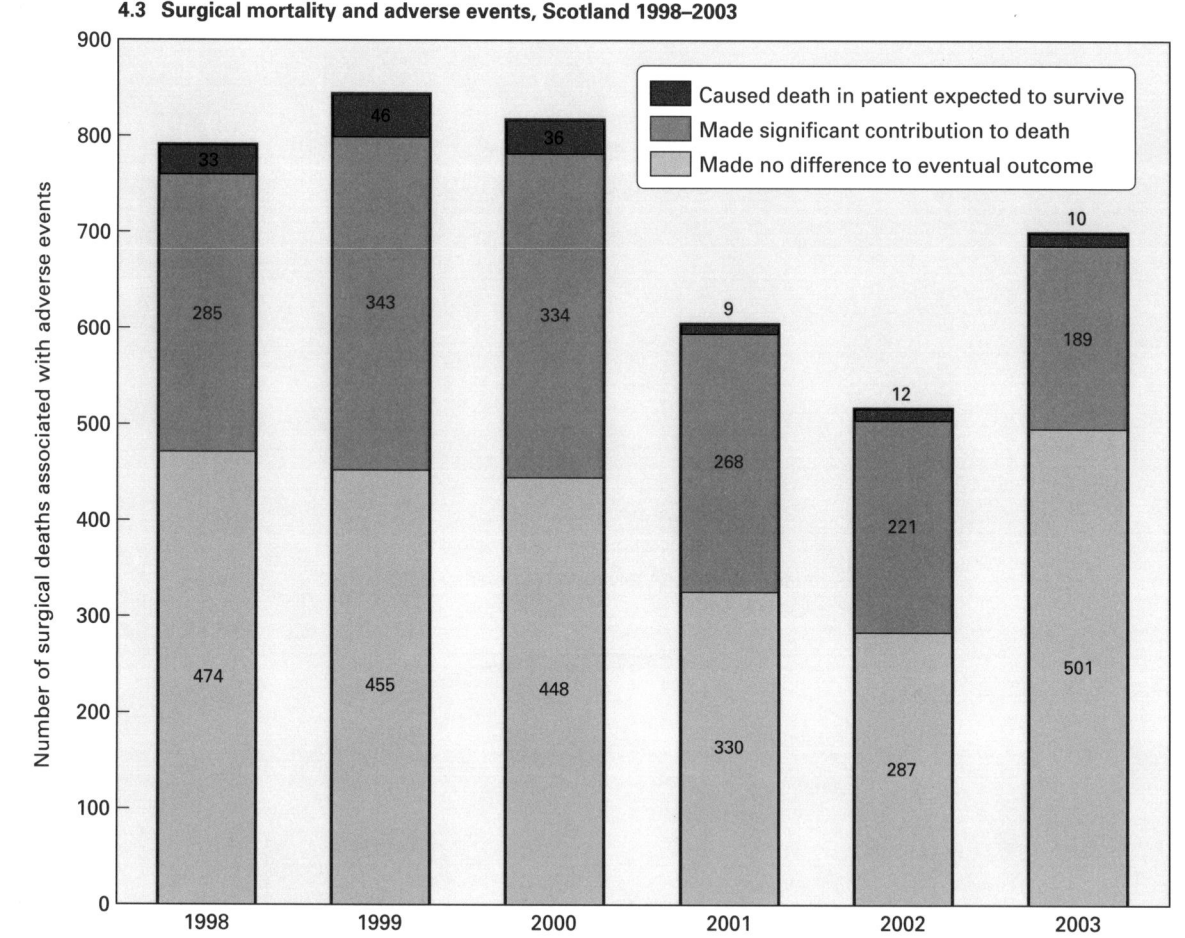

4.3 Surgical mortality and adverse events, Scotland 1998–2003

Legend:
- Caused death in patient expected to survive
- Made significant contribution to death
- Made no difference to eventual outcome

Number of surgical deaths associated with adverse events

Year	Made no difference to eventual outcome	Made significant contribution to death	Caused death in patient expected to survive
1998	474	285	33
1999	455	343	46
2000	448	334	36
2001	330 / 9	268	9
2002	287 / 221	—	12
2003	501	189	10

Medication errors

Medication errors have been defined as 'any preventable event that may cause or lead to inappropriate medication use or patient harm while the medication is in the control of health professional, patient or consumer' (US National Coordinating Council for Medication Error Reporting and Prevention). Medication errors are mistakes or lapses that occur while medicines are prescribed, dispensed or administered. Most do not cause harm to the patient. Medication errors represent 10–20% of all adverse events (Chief Pharmaceutical Officer, 2004). In the US, studies have calculated medication error rates ranging from 3.13 to 62.4 per 1000 medication orders and rates of clinically significant errors ranging from 1.81 to 19.2 per 1000 orders (Lesar *et al.*, 1997; Bobb *et al.*, 2004). Medication errors cost the NHS hospitals an estimated £200–400 million per year (Chief Pharmaceutical Officer, 2004). Research conducted in the US indicates that medication errors occur at different points in the medication process at the following frequencies:

- physician prescribing/ordering: 39–49%
- transcription: 11–12%
- pharmacy dispensing: 11–14%
- medication administration: 26–38% (AHRQ, 2001).

US research has also quantified the percentage of adverse drug events caused by various types of medication error (*see* Figure B).

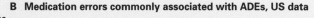

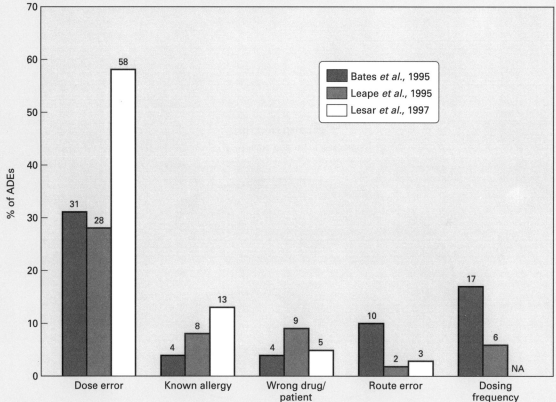

Source: AHRQ.

The Quest for Quality in the NHS: a chartbook on quality of care in the UK

4 Safety

Chart 4.4 Errors in the preparation of intravenous infusions, two UK hospitals

This chart illustrates data collected from 10 wards in two UK hospitals on the incidence and severity of errors in the preparation and administration of intravenous drugs. At least one error occurred in 212 of the 430 intravenous drug doses observed. Of the total observed doses, 3 (1%) were judged to have potentially serious errors, 126 (29%) moderate errors and 83 (19%) minor errors.

Source: Taxis and Barber, 2003.

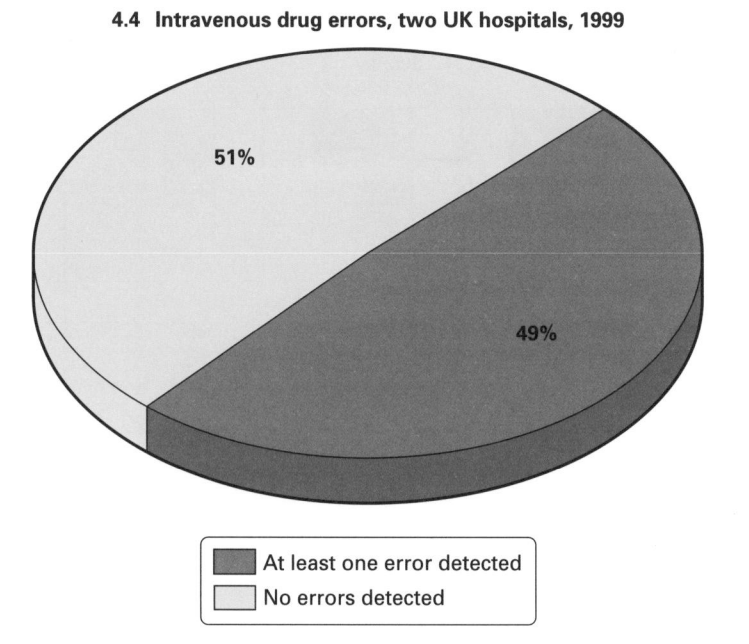

4.4 Intravenous drug errors, two UK hospitals, 1999

51%

49%

At least one error detected
No errors detected

The Quest for Quality in the NHS: a chartbook on quality of care in the UK

Chart 4.5 Errors in the preparation of intravenous acetylcysteine infusions: four UK hospitals

This chart illustrates data derived from direct sampling and analysis of intravenous infusions of acetylcysteine (used to treat paracetamol overdose). The infusion samples were collected in four hospitals in England, Wales and Scotland. Dosages were calculated directly (based on the patient's weight) or read from a published table by a junior doctor and checked by a nurse or pharmacist. The infusions were prepared by nursing staff in three study sites and by pharmacists in the fourth. The concentration of acetylcysteine in infusion bags was independently assayed and compared to the required dose. Just over one-third of infusions were within 10% of the correct dose. Almost two-thirds were within 20% of the correct dose. Concentration of active drug for one in 10 of the infusions was more than 50% different from the correct dose. The study provides no details about the extent to which patients were adversely affected as a result of the medication errors detected. However, significant concerns both in terms of efficacy and potential overdose are warranted if errors of this magnitude are occurring, where either half or double the intended dose is administered to some patients.

Source: Ferner *et al.*, 2001.

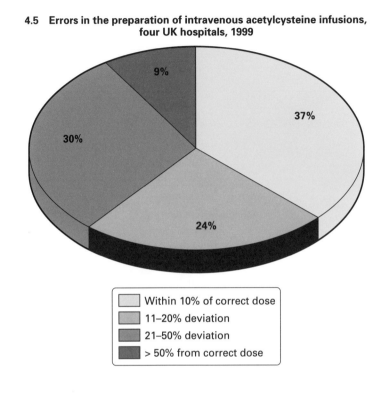

4.5   Errors in the preparation of intravenous acetylcysteine infusions, four UK hospitals, 1999

- Within 10% of correct dose
- 11–20% deviation
- 21–50% deviation
- > 50% from correct dose

The Quest for Quality in the NHS: a chartbook on quality of care in the UK

Chart 4.6 Infusion error incident study: six hospitals in England and Wales

The Quest for Quality in the NHS: a chartbook on quality of care in the UK

Fifteen million infusions (also known as IVs or drips) are given to NHS patients every year. The Medicines and Healthcare Products Regulatory Agency (MHRA) receives more than 700 reports of unsafe incidents with infusion devices (including 10 deaths) every year* (National Patient Safety Agency, 2004). A pilot study conducted by the National Patient Safety Agency (NPSA), across six hospitals in England and Wales, sought to identify root causes of infusion device incidents. The study identified 321 incidents in one year; overinfusion and user error were especially frequent incidents. The study also reported (data not displayed) that, of a total of 6387 infusion devices across the six pilot sites, 1200 (19%) were more than 10 years old, raising concerns about obsolescence.

'Other' causes include prescription error; wrong prescription; wrong patient; incorrect mixing of drugs; and housekeeping.

Source: National Patient Safety Agency, 2004.

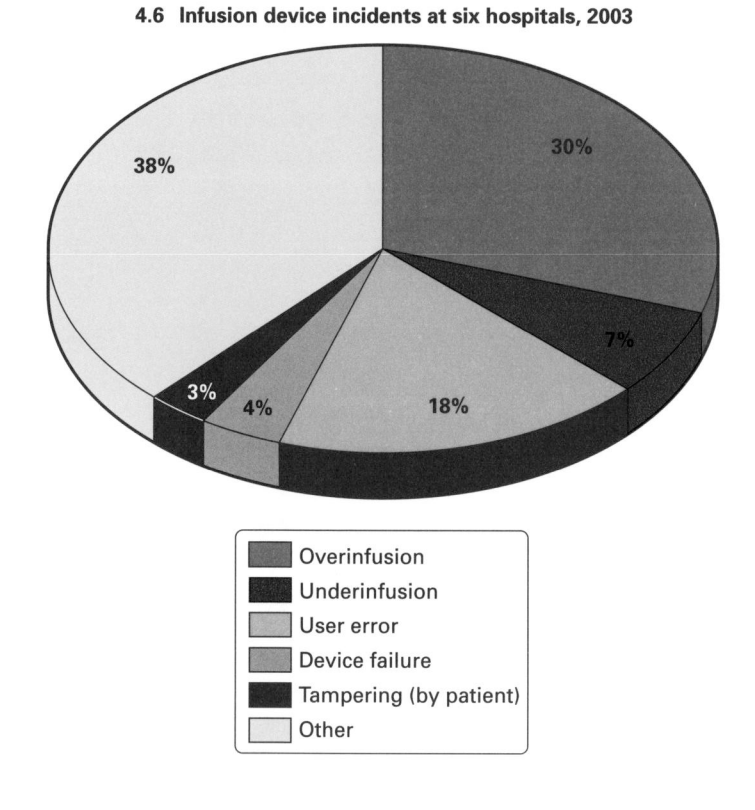

4.6 Infusion device incidents at six hospitals, 2003

- Overinfusion
- Underinfusion
- User error
- Device failure
- Tampering (by patient)
- Other

* http://81.144.177.110/site/media/documents/526_npsa_saferpractice_01.pdf.

Healthcare-associated infections and MRSA

Healthcare-associated infections (HAIs) affect nearly one in 10 NHS hospital patients each year (Chief Medical Officer, 2003). The impact of HAIs is profound. Plowman *et al.* (2001) in a study of a single English hospital found that patients with HAIs had almost a threefold increase in both length of stay and hospital costs. The human impact ranges from increased levels of discomfort or prolonged or permanent disability to at least 5000 patient deaths each year (National Audit Office, 2004). The National Audit Office (2000, 2004) has calculated that HAIs cost the NHS £1 billion per year. An estimated 15% of HAIs could be prevented by better application of good infection control practices (National Audit Office, 2004).

The approximate prevalence of HAIs as a proportion of hospitalised patients in different countries is shown below.

USA	5–10%
Denmark	8%
Australia	6%
France	6–10%
Norway	7%
Netherlands	7%
England	9%
Spain	8%

Source: CMO, 2003.

Surveillance for HAI tends to focus on those infections, particularly bacteraemias, caused by methicillin-resistant *Staphylococcus aureus* (MRSA). *Staph aureus* is a bacterium that colonises or lives harmlessly on the skin of normal, healthy people. It can cause problems when it invades the body, causing an infection. MRSA infections are very problematic because the bacteria's resistance renders them unsusceptible to many antibiotics, making them extremely difficult to treat. Bacteraemia (or blood poisoning) data is used for surveillance because positive results indicate infection, which is clinically significant, rather than colonisation, which is not. In addition, bacteraemia data is not distorted by variation in infection control screening policies, allowing comparison over time and between organisations and countries.

Over the past decade the increase in HAIs has been marked; it has been attributed to:

- more seriously ill patients susceptible to infection
- more invasive procedures
- mixing of patient populations
- high bed occupancy rates
- increasing antimicrobial resistance
- poorer standards of cleanliness and hygiene
- a lack of senior management attention to HAI.

Source: Chief Medical Officer, 2002

International experience has shown that MRSA rates can be controlled. The Netherlands has adopted a policy of screening patients for MRSA and isolating those found to be carrying or infected with the organism. Coupled with the use of single rooms and high healthcare-worker-to-patient ratios, this approach has been highly successful. The proportion of *Staph aureus* bloodstream isolates resistant to methicillin among hospital patients is less than 1% in the Netherlands compared to 41% in the UK.

In November 2004, the Health Secretary in England announced a new target to reduce MRSA bloodstream infections by 50% in hospitals by 2008 (DH Press release 2004/0396). All NHS Trusts will be expected to draw up comprehensive action plans to prevent or isolate MRSA and will be tasked with achieving an annual reduction up to and beyond March 2008.

The Quest for Quality in the NHS: a chartbook on quality of care in the UK

Chart 4.7 Surgical healthcare-associated infections

Healthcare-associated infections (HAIs) cause significant morbidity and mortality. This chart focuses on morbidity for surgical patients, drawing on data from the Nosocomial Infection National Surveillance Service (NINSS) for 168 NHS Trusts in England. Of 107 492 patients on whom an operation was performed from 1997 to 2002, 4% contracted an HAI. Infection rates varied widely depending on the site and type of operation.

4.7 Percentage of surgical patients with surgical site infections, 168 NHS Trusts, England 1997–2002

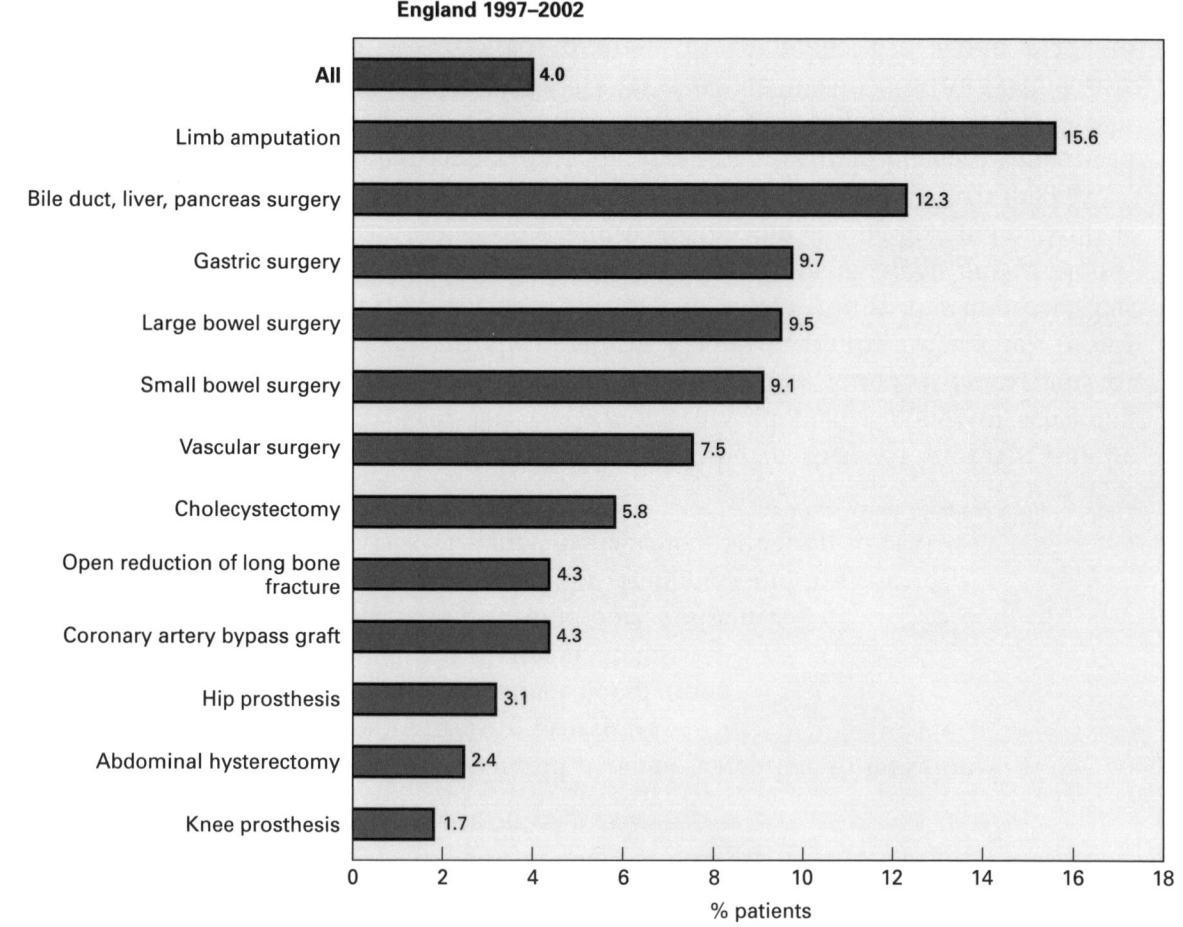

% patients

Source: Health Protection Agency, 2003.

The Quest for Quality in the NHS: a chartbook on quality of care in the UK

Chart 4.8 HAIs as a factor in surgical mortality

Chart 4.7 showed that in 1997–2002 4% of surgical patients in England suffered from a healthcare-associated infection. This chart takes a different view of the HAI problem focusing on mortality. It illustrates the extent to which HAIs were associated with post-surgical deaths in Scotland. It draws on data from the 2003 Scottish Audit of Surgical Mortality. Of 4084 patients who died in hospital under surgical care, 344 (8.4%) had developed an HAI.

Source: SASM, 2003.

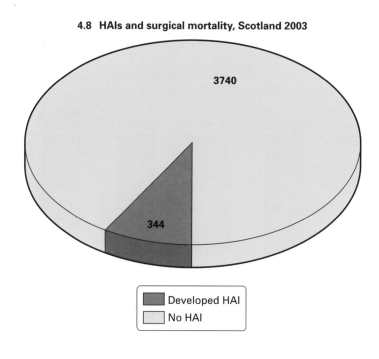

4.8 HAIs and surgical mortality, Scotland 2003

3740

344

Developed HAI

No HAI

The Quest for Quality in the NHS: a chartbook on quality of care in the UK

Chart 4.9 MRSA as a proportion of all *Staphylococcus aureus* bacteraemias

The Quest for Quality in the NHS: a chartbook on quality of care in the UK

The European Antimicrobial Resistance Surveillance System (EARSS) collects, collates and validates data on antimicrobial resistance. This chart is based on EARSS data for the number of methicillin-resistant *Staphylococcus aureus* (MRSA) isolates from blood cultures as a percentage of all *Staph aureus* bacteraemias between 1999 and 2002. These percentages vary widely across Europe; the figure in Greece was 75 times greater than that in the Netherlands, for example. The UK performs relatively poorly in comparison to its European neighbours.

Source: Tiemersma *et al.*, 2004.

4.9 MRSA bacteraemia as a proportion of all *Staphylococcus aureus* bacteraemias, international comparison, 1999–2002

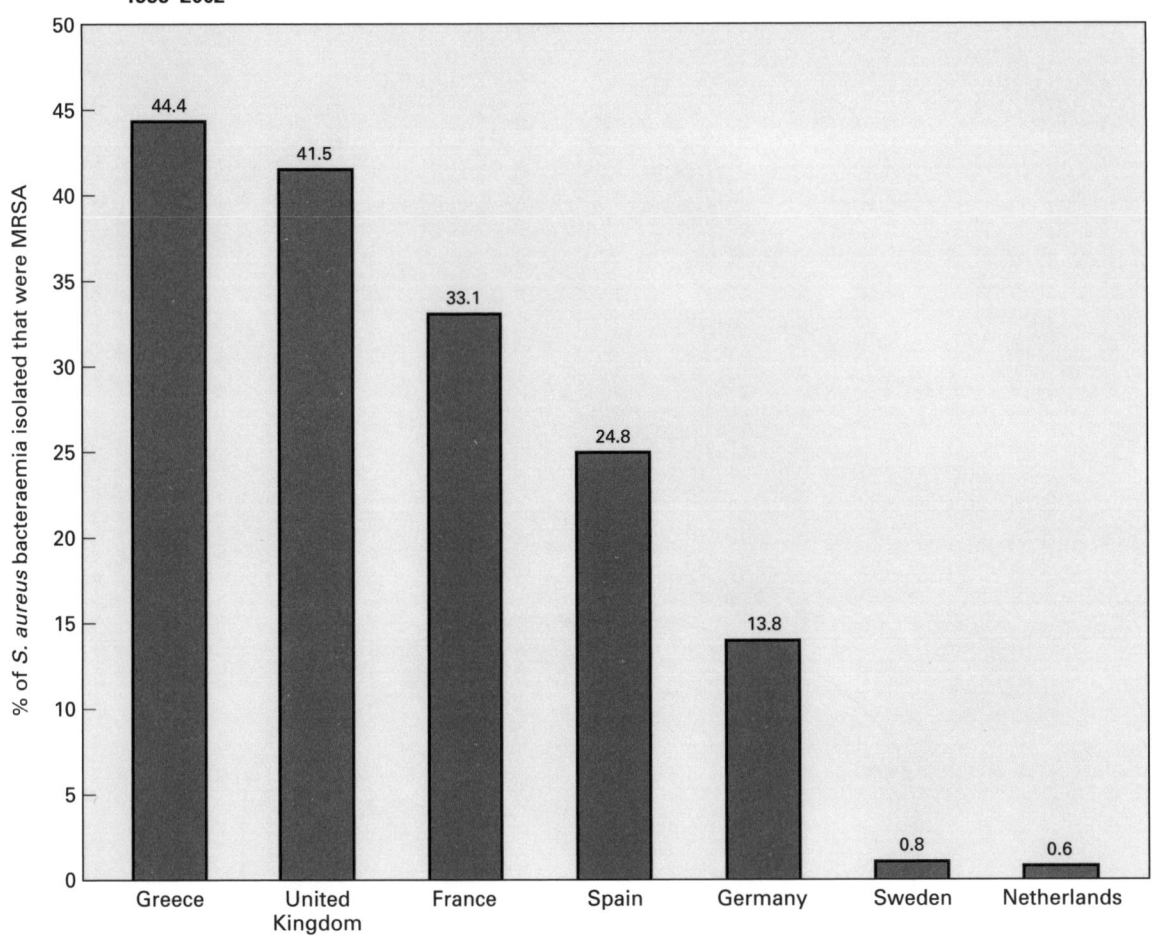

% of *S. aureus* bacteraemia isolated that were MRSA

Greece	44.4
United Kingdom	41.5
France	33.1
Spain	24.8
Germany	13.8
Sweden	0.8
Netherlands	0.6

Chart 4.10 MRSA bacteraemia rates

Methicillin-resistant *Staphylococcus aureus* (MRSA) attracts a high level of public and media concern. It is of such importance that all the countries of the UK operate sophisticated surveillance and reporting schemes to monitor the problem. Bacteraemia (or blood infection) rates are monitored as they reflect true MRSA infections rather than contamination or colonisation. MRSA bacteraemia is difficult to manage because there are so few antibiotics left for effective treatment and because of the potentially serious health consequences of a blood infection with MRSA. The rate of MRSA bacteraemia per 1000 bed days is a robust measure of the amount of MRSA in a hospital population and also serves as a measure of success of infection control policies and hygiene standards. Within the UK, in 2003–04, rates ranged from 0.11 cases per 1000 bed days in Wales to 0.18 cases per 1000 bed days in England.

Sources: Health Protection Agency, NHS Wales, ISD Scotland, NICS.

4.10 MRSA bacteraemias per 1000 bed days, UK countries 2003–04

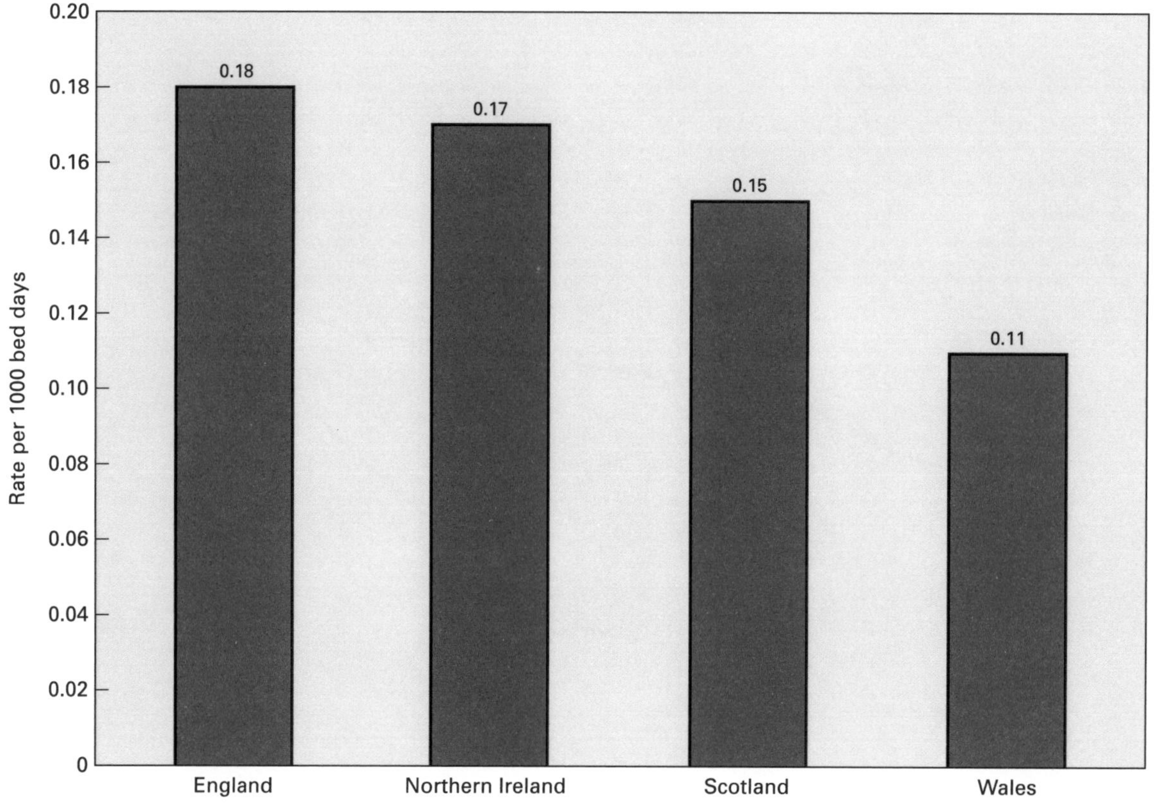

The Quest for Quality in the NHS: a chartbook on quality of care in the UK

103

Chart 4.11 Deaths involving MRSA

The Quest for Quality in the NHS: a chartbook on quality of care in the UK

During the period 1993–2002, MRSA mortality rates in England and Wales increased more than 15-fold (rising from 51 to 800 deaths). MRSA was recorded on death certificates as involved in 0.07% of all deaths and in 0.12% of deaths that occurred in NHS general hospitals (Griffiths *et al.*, 2004). The mortality rates are dwarfed by the rate at which MRSA is isolated from blood cultures. In 2003–04, NHS Trusts in England made 7647 reports of MRSA bacteraemia. This represents a 5% increase over the 2001–02 figure of 7250 (CDR, 2004). These increases may, to some extent, reflect better reporting.

Source: Griffiths *et al.*, 2004.

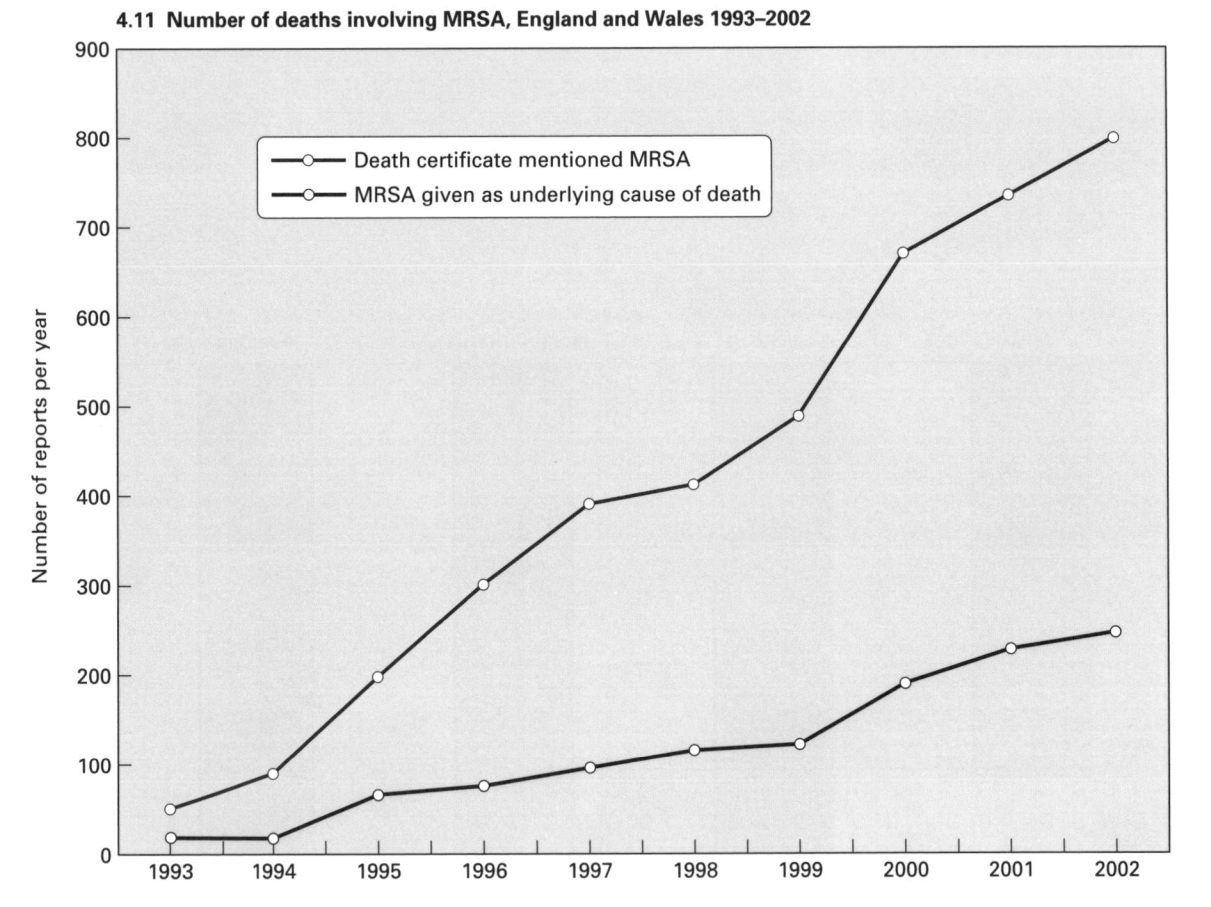

4.11 Number of deaths involving MRSA, England and Wales 1993–2002

Legend:
- Death certificate mentioned MRSA
- MRSA given as underlying cause of death

Y-axis: Number of reports per year

Perceptions about safety issues

Current opinion on safety in healthcare recognises the importance of *system failures* in creating conditions that allow adverse events to occur (Reason, 1997). Experience from other high-risk industries, such as aviation and nuclear power, has shown that highly reliable organisations do not depend on human perfection to achieve high levels of safety. Rather, these industries design 'fault tolerant' systems with attention to the human propensity for error. Such systems can prevent errors from occurring, or mitigate their effects when they do occur. Accordingly the focus for improvement in safety in healthcare has shifted from blaming individuals to designing systems, organisations and operations so that they will better assure patient safety (WHO, 2004).

Within the system view of safety, awareness is growing that organisational culture is a key factor in securing improvements (Walshe and Shortell, 2004). Cultural characteristics such as staff attitudes, beliefs and values have been linked to safety in the aviation industry (Helmreich, 2000) and to improved outcomes in the healthcare sector (Shortell *et al.*, 1994; 1995). For example, taken-for-granted assumptions about appropriate working practices are thought to play a major role in safety issues and willingness (and propensity) to change. The perceptions of healthcare workers are therefore of particular importance in trying to achieve fundamental improvements in safety. The goal is to create an organisational environment in which individuals have the understanding, skills and ability to routinely practise safety-enhancing behaviours, such as observing evidence-based infection control procedures and engaging in effective communication with patients and other members of the care team.

Patients' views are also increasingly recognised as of value in improving safety. Patients can play a vital role in helping to identify and quantify risks and providing options to devise solutions.

The Quest for Quality in the NHS: a chartbook on quality of care in the UK

The Quest for Quality in the NHS: a chartbook on quality of care in the UK

Chart 4.12 Hospital effectiveness at finding and addressing medical error: physicians' views

Physicians play a critically important role in tackling safety issues in healthcare organisations. These charts illustrate physicians' perceptions about the extent to which the systems for identifying and addressing medical error, in the hospitals in which they practise, are effective. Chart 4.12a shows that the UK had the lowest level of 'excellent' ratings across the five countries surveyed. Chart 4.12b amplifies the UK results; the majority of respondents rated their hospitals' ability to deal with medical error as fair or poor.

4.12a Hospital rated excellent at finding and addressing medical error, international comparison, 2000

4.12b Physicians' ratings of hospital effectiveness in finding and addressing medical error, UK 2000

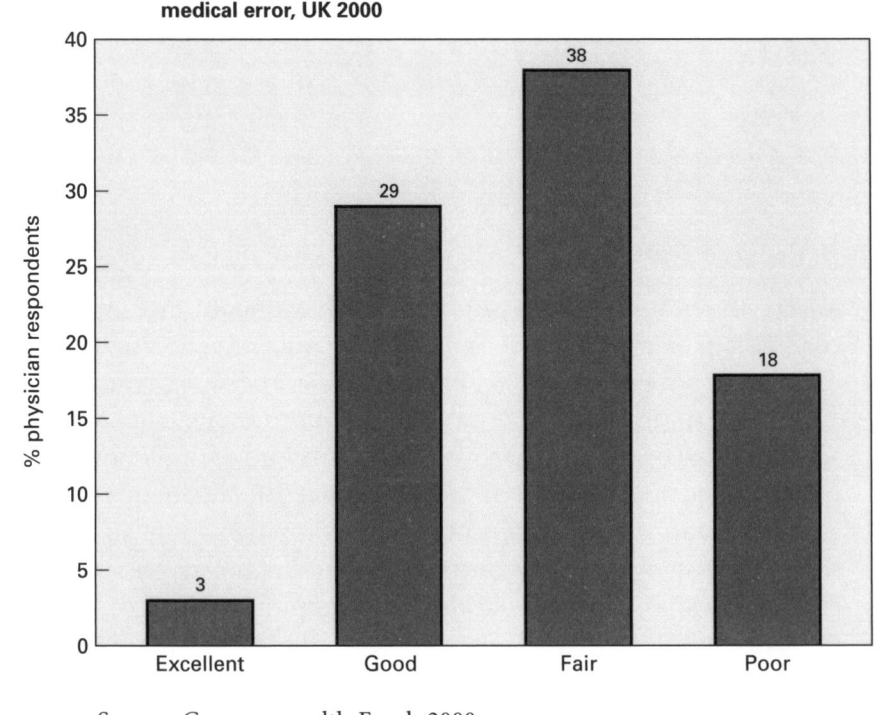

Source: Commonwealth Fund, 2000.

Source: Commonwealth Fund, 2000.

Note: 'Physician' in the Commonwealth Fund surveys is used as a general term to denote doctors.

Chart 4.13 Safety views of hospital executives

These charts provide some insight into the views that hospital executives have of their organisations' capacity and willingness to identify and address safety issues. The relatively high ratings of US and UK executives may reflect the emphasis and policy attention paid to safety issues in both countries in recent years. Chart 4.13a shows that almost one-quarter of hospital executives in the UK, Australia and the US consider their system for identifying and addressing preventable medical errors to be very effective. Chart 4.13b presents the views of hospital executives regarding the engagement of physicians in safety programmes; respondents from the UK and US were most likely to say that physicians in their hospital were very supportive of reporting and addressing medical errors.

4.13a Programme for finding and addressing is very effective, international comparison, 2003

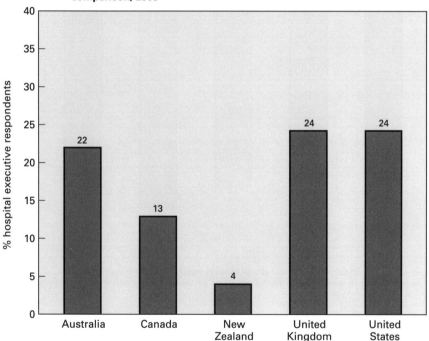

Source: Commonwealth Fund, 2003.

4.13b Physicians very supportive of reporting and addressing errors, international comparison, 2003

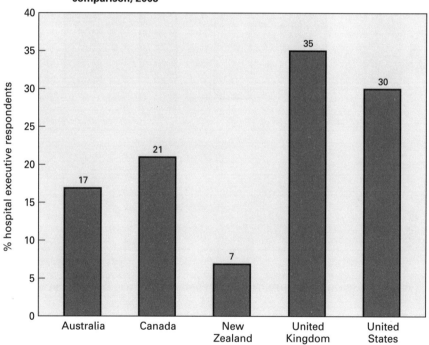

Source: Commonwealth Fund, 2003.

The Quest for Quality in the NHS: a chartbook on quality of care in the UK

Chart 4.14 Medical errors and their consequences: patients' perspective

The Quest for Quality in the NHS: a chartbook on quality of care in the UK

The Commonwealth Fund's 2002 International Health Policy Survey focused on adult patients with health problems. Respondents were asked whether in the past two years they thought that either a medication error or a medical mistake had been made in their treatment or care. The UK sample reported the lowest proportion of incidents: almost one in five respondents indicated that they had experienced a mistake or error. In the UK, half of those respondents who experienced an error or mistake (9% of total sample) reported that the error had serious consequences for their health.

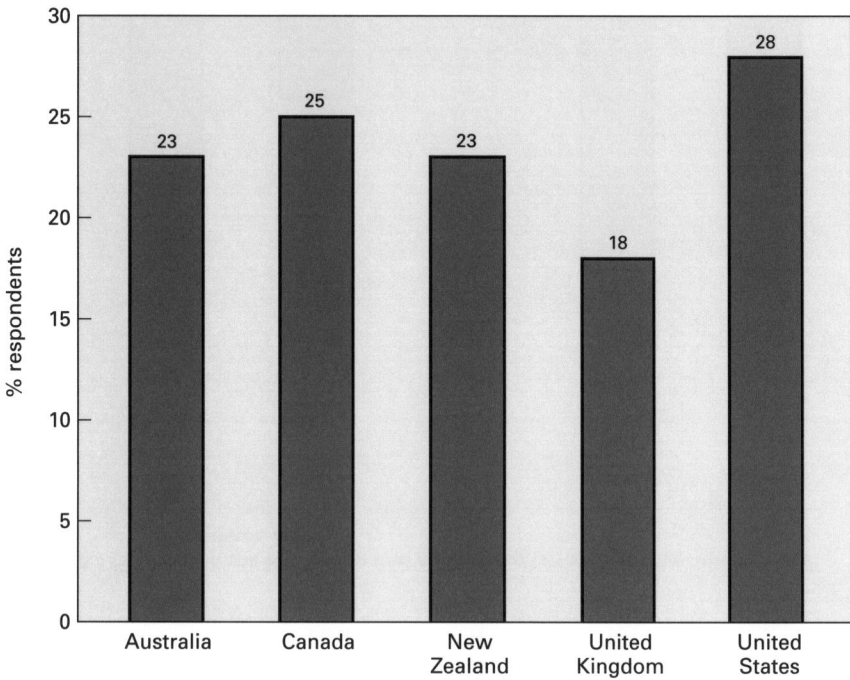

4.14a Either a medication error or medical mistake was made in treatment or care in the past two years, international comparison, 2003

Source: Commonwealth Fund, 2002.

4.14b An error or mistake caused serious problems, international comparison, 2003

Source: Commonwealth Fund, 2002.

Chart 4.15 Medication errors: patients' perspective

This chart provides data from two Commonwealth Fund international surveys, one conducted with adult patients with health problems (in 2002) and one with primary care patients (in 2004). In both surveys, the UK had the lowest rate of reported errors of all the comparison countries. Nonetheless, one in 10 adults with health problems reported that they had experienced a medication error in the two years preceding the survey.

Source: Commonwealth Fund 2002; 2004.

4.15 Respondents given the wrong medication or wrong dose by a doctor, hospital or pharmacist in preceding 2 years, international comparison 2002 and 2004

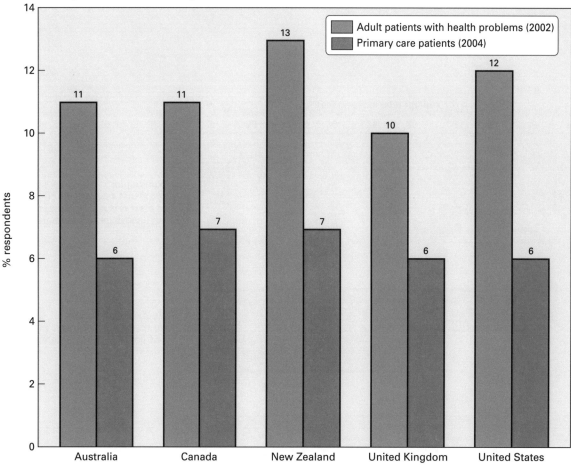

The Quest for Quality in the NHS: a chartbook on quality of care in the UK

Chart 4.16 Safety issues after discharge from hospital

The Quest for Quality in the NHS: a chartbook on quality of care in the UK

The Healthcare Commission undertakes large surveys of NHS patients in England, covering a wide range of issues and aspects of the patient experience. This chart draws on data from two surveys, one of hospital inpatients and one of young patients (in-patients and day cases < 18 yrs) focusing on issues that may arise after discharge. Explanations of the purpose of medications to be taken home were reported to be clear in the vast majority of cases. However, patients were less well informed about potential side effects and health-related 'danger signals' to watch for when they got home.

Source: Healthcare Commission; www.nhssurveys.org.

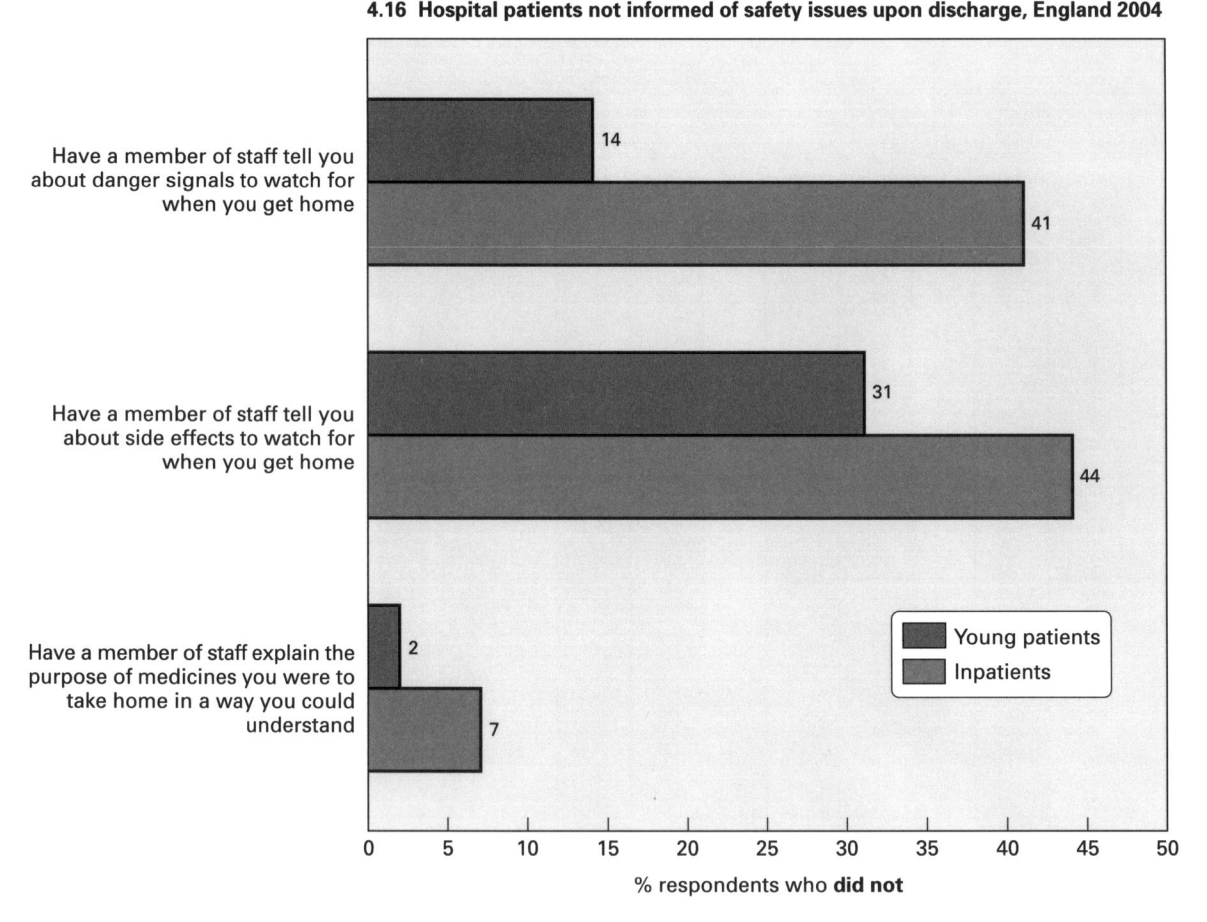

4.16 Hospital patients not informed of safety issues upon discharge, England 2004

Have a member of staff tell you about danger signals to watch for when you get home
- Young patients: 14
- Inpatients: 41

Have a member of staff tell you about side effects to watch for when you get home
- Young patients: 31
- Inpatients: 44

Have a member of staff explain the purpose of medicines you were to take home in a way you could understand
- Young patients: 2
- Inpatients: 7

■ Young patients
■ Inpatients

% respondents who **did not**

Chart 4.17 Managing polypharmacy risks

Polypharmacy refers to the administration of numerous medicines, often for multiple indications, at the same time. It may be *appropriate* when all drugs in the regimen address recognised indications and do not interact. Polypharmacy may be *inappropriate* when more drugs are prescribed than necessary, drugs with unacceptable side effects or toxicity are prescribed (either when used alone or in combination with other medications in the regimen) or redundant drugs are prescribed (American Academy of Family Physicians, 2005). Medications reviews can limit the consequences of inappropriate polypharmacy. This chart shows that more than one-third of all respondents from the UK reported that they had not had a thorough medications review with their GP in the previous two years, the worst performance among the five surveyed countries.

Source: Commonwealth Fund, 2004.

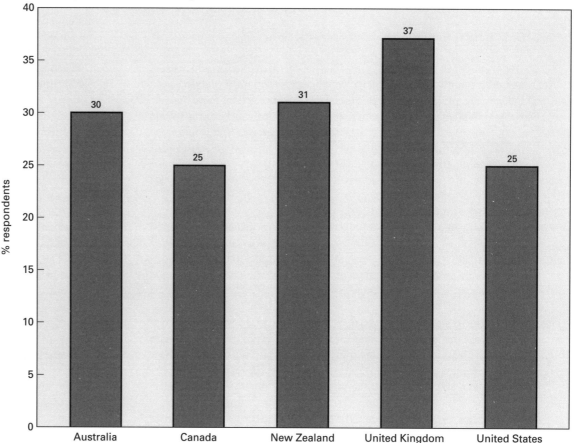

4.17 Regular doctor did NOT review medications (including those prescribed by other doctors) in preceding 2 years, international comparison 2004

The Quest for Quality in the NHS: a chartbook on quality of care in the UK

AHRQ (2001) Reducing and preventing adverse drug events to decrease hospital costs. *Research in Action.* Issue 1. AHRQ Publication Number 01–0020. Agency for Healthcare Research and Quality, Rockville, MD. Available at: www.ahrq.gov/qual/aderia/aderia.htm#14 [last accessed 31 January 2005].

American Academy of Family Physicians (2005) *Polypharmacy: Introduction* [Online]. Available at: www.aafp.org/x28929.xml [last accessed 31 January 2005].

Aylin P, Tanna S, Bottle A *et al.* (2004) Dr Foster's case notes: how often are adverse events reported in English hospital statistics? *BMJ.* **329**: 369.

Baker GR, Norton PG, Flintoft V *et al.* (2004) The Canadian Adverse Events Study: the incidence of adverse events among hospital patients in Canada. *Canadian Medical Association Journal.* **179**(11): 1678–86.

Bates DW, Boyle DL, Vander Vliet MB *et al.* (1995) Relationship between medication errors and adverse drug events. *J Gen Intern Med.* **10**(4): 199–205.

Bates DW, Spell N, Cullen DJ *et al.* (1997) The costs of adverse drug events in hospitalised patients. *JAMA.* **277**(4): 307–11.

Bobb A, Gleason K, Husch M *et al.* (2004) The epidemiology of prescribing errors: the potential impact of computerized prescriber order entry. *Archives of Internal Medicine.* **164**: 785–92.

Brennan TA, Leape LL, Laird NM *et al.* (1991) Incidence of adverse events and negligence in hospitalized patients. Results of the Harvard Medical Practice Study I. *NEJM.* **324**(6): 370–7.

CDR (2004) The third year of regional and national analyses of the Department of Health's mandatory MRSA surveillance scheme in England: April 2001 – March 2004. *CDR Weekly.* **14**(29). Available online at: www.hpa.org.uk/cdr/PDFfiles/2004/cdr2904.pdf [last accessed 31 January 2005].

Chief Medical Officer (2002) *Getting Ahead of the Curve: a strategy for combating infectious diseases.* Department of Health, London.

Chief Medical Officer (2003) *Winning Ways: working together to reduce healthcare associated infection in England.* Department of Health, London.

Chief Pharmaceutical Officer (2004) *Building a Safer NHS for Patients: improving medication safety.* Department of Health, London.

Classen DC, Pestotnik SL, Evans RS *et al.* (1997) Adverse drug events in hospitalized patients. Excess length of stay, extra costs, and attributable mortality. *JAMA.* **277**(4): 301–6.

Commonwealth Fund (2000) *International Health Policy Survey of Physicians.* Commonwealth Fund, New York.

Commonwealth Fund (2002) *International Health Policy Survey of Adults with Health Problems.* Commonwealth Fund, New York.

Commonwealth Fund (2003) *International Health Policy Survey of Hospital Executives.* Commonwealth Fund, New York.

Commonwealth Fund (2004) *International Health Policy Survey of Adults' Experiences with Primary Care.* Commonwealth Fund, New York.

Davis P, Lay-Yee R, Briant R, Ali W, Scott A and Schug S (2002) Adverse events in New Zealand public hospitals I: occurrence and impact. *New Zealand Medical Journal.* **115**(1167): U271.

Department of Health (2000) *An Organisation with a Memory: report of an expert group on learning from adverse events in the NHS.* Department of Health, London.

Department of Health, Social Services & Public Safety (2004) *Statistics on MRSA published by NISRA and CDSC* [Online]. Available at: www.nics.gov.uk/press/hss/041005a-hss.htm [last accessed 31 January 2005].

Edmondson AC (2004) Learning from failure in health care: frequent opportunities, pervasive barriers. *Quality and Safety in Health Care.* **13**: ii3–ii9.

Ferner RE, Langford NJ, Anton C, Hutchings A, Bateman DN and Routledge PA (2001) Random and systematic medication errors in routine clinical practice: a multicentre study of infusions, using acetylcysteine as an example. *Br J Clin Pharmacol.* **52**(5): 573–7.

Griffiths C, Lamagni TL, Crowcroft NS, Duckworth G and Rooney C (2004) Trends in MRSA in England and Wales: analysis of morbidity and mortality data for 1993–2002. *Health Statistics Quarterly.* **Spring**(21): 15–22.

Health Protection Agency (2003) *Surveillance of Surgical Site Infection in English Hospitals 1997–2002: a national surveillance and quality improvement programme.* Available at: www.hpa.org.uk/infections/topics_az/hai/SSIreport.pdf [last accessed 31 January 2005].

Health Protection Agency (2004) *The Third Year of Regional and National Analyses of the Department of Health's Mandatory MRSA Surveillance Scheme in England: April 2001–March 2004.* CDR Weekly [Online]. Available at: www.hpa.org.uk/cdr/PDFfiles/2004/cdr2904.pdf [last accessed 31 January 2005].

Helmreich R (2000) On error management: lessons from aviation. *BMJ.* **320**: 781–5.

Jha AK, Kuperman GJ, Teich JM *et al.* (1998) Identifying adverse drug events: development of a computer-based monitor and comparison with chart review and stimulated voluntary report. *J Am Med Inform Assoc.* **5**(3): 305–14.

Kohn LT, Corrigan JM and Donaldson M (eds) (2000) *To Err Is Human: building a safer health system.* Institute of Medicine, Washington, DC.

Leape LL, Brennan TA, Laird N *et al.* (1991) The nature of adverse events in hospitalised patients: results of the Harvard Medical Practice Study II. *NEJM.* **324**(6): 377–84.

Leape LL, Bates DW, Cullen DJ *et al.* (1995) Systems analysis of adverse drug events. *JAMA.* **274**(1): 35–43.

Lesar TS, Briceland L and Stein DS (1997) Factors relating to errors in medication prescribing. *JAMA.* **277**(4): 312–17.

Millar J, Mattke S and OECD Patient Safety Panel (2004) *Selecting Indicators for Patient Safety at the Health Systems Level in OECD Countries.* OECD, Paris.

National Audit Office (2000) *The Management and Control of Hospital Acquired Infection in Acute Trusts in England* (HC 230 Session 1999–00). TSO, London.

National Audit Office (2004) *Improving Patient Care by Reducing the Risk of Hospital Acquired Infection: a progress report* (HC 876 Session 2003–04). TSO, London.

National Patient Safety Agency (2004) *Standardising and Centralising Infusion Devices: a project to develop safety solutions for NHS Trusts.* Available at: http://81.144.177.110/site/media/documents/527_npsa_eval_summary.pdf [last accessed 31 January 2005].

NHSScotland (2004) *Reports on Methicillin-resistant* Staphylococcus aureus *Bacteraemia in Scotland* [Online]. Available at: www.show.scot.nhs.uk/scieh/infectious/hai/MRSA_Scot.htm [last accessed 31 January 2005].

Plowman R, Graves N, Griffin MA *et al.* (2001) The rate and cost of hospital-acquired infections occurring in patients admitted to selected specialties of a district general hospital in England and the national burden imposed. *J Hosp Infect.* **47**(3): 198–209.

Reason J (1997) *Managing the Risks of Organisational Accidents.* Ashgate Publishing Co., Burlington,Vermont.

Scottish Audit of Surgical Mortality (2002) *Summary Report.* Available at: www.sasm.org.uk/Reports/2002_Report/Scottish_Audit_of_Surgical_Mortality_Summary_2002.pdf [last accessed 31 January 2005].

Scottish Audit of Surgical Mortality (2003) *Summary Report.* Available at: www.sasm.org.uk/Reports/2003Report/Summary_Annual_Report_final_2003_data.pdf [last accessed 31 January 2005].

Shortell SM, Zimmerman JE, Rousseau DM, *et al.* (1994) The performance of intensive care units: does good management make a difference? *Medical Care.* **32**: 508–25.

Shortell SM, O'Brien JL, Carman JM, *et al.* (1995) Assessing the impact of continuous quality improvement/total quality management: concept versus implementation. *Health Services Research.* **30**: 377–401.

Taxis K and Barber N (2003) Ethnographic study of incidence and severity of intravenous drug errors. *BMJ.* **326**(7391): 684.

Thomas EJ, Studdert DM, Newhouse JP *et al.* (1999) Costs of medical injuries in Utah and Colorado. *Inquiry.* **36**(3): 255–64.

Tiemersma EW, Bronzwaer SL, Lyytikainen O *et al.*, European Antimicrobial Resistance Surveillance System Participants (2004) Methicillin-resistant *Staphylococcus aureus* in Europe, 1999–2002. *Emerg Infect Dis.* **10**(9): 1627–34.

US National Coordinating Council for Medication Error Reporting and Prevention [Online]. Available at: www.nccmerp.org [last accessed 31 January 2005].

Vincent C, Neale G and Woloshynowych M (2001) Adverse events in British hospitals: preliminary retrospective record review. *BMJ.* **322**(7285): 517–19.

Walshe K and Shortell SM (2004) When things go wrong: how health care organizations deal with major failures. *Health Affairs.* **23**(3):103–11.

Wilson RM, Runciman WB, Gibberd RW, Harrison BT, Newby L and Hamilton JD (1995) The Quality in Australian Health Care Study. *Medical Journal of Australia.* **163**: 458–71.

World Health Organization (2004) *World Alliance for Patient Safety* [Online]. Available at: www.who.int/patientsafety [last accessed 31 January 2005].

Quality in healthcare requires the use of best available scientific evidence, diagnostic acumen and technical proficiency; all applied in safe and managerially efficient environments. An equally important component in the quest for quality is patient-centredness, that is, a concern for – and responsiveness to – patient preferences, attitudes and experiences.

A responsive health service has been an espoused goal of health policy in the UK for several decades. Progress to date is generally regarded to be modest (Coulter, 2003). This sluggishness is attributed to various factors including resource constraints, rhetorical rather than genuine commitment, and profession-based cultural mores. Recent policy across the countries of the UK has articulated a common goal and set priorities to develop a more patient-centred NHS. Initiatives vary in their emphases: England focuses on patient choice in terms of how, when, and where healthcare is provided; Scotland has established a Scottish Health Council and Patient Information Initiatives; and Wales explicitly encourages each citizen and community to play a role in health policy development and plans to implement patient-centred standards in 2005 (DH, 2003a; NHSScotland, 2001; 2003; NHS Wales, 2001; 2004).

Against this background of a greater focus on the patient's perspective, data that provides insight into patients' views, attitudes and judgements is of great interest. The particular topics selected for inclusion in this chapter are relevant to the characteristics that patient surveys and focus groups consistently identify as necessary for a high-quality service. That is, patients want a National Health Service that:

- is efficient and integrated where access to services is gained quickly
- is reliable and consistent
- has good communication and gives clear information
- treats patients as individuals
- is responsive and flexible
- provides a comfortable and clean environment that puts patients at ease (Wanless, 2002: p90).

This list is noteworthy for the preponderance of concerns with service, convenience and responsiveness rather than issues of clinical effectiveness and safety.

The charts that follow draw on a range of surveys, both national and international in their sampling frames. The charts are grouped according to three themes:

- overall view of the healthcare system
- patient responsiveness
- physical environment.

The Quest for Quality in the NHS: a chartbook on quality of care in the UK

Overall view of system

Healthcare systems are increasingly seen as a network of partnerships connecting a range of disparate stakeholders. At the centre of the network is the patient-citizen – the primary beneficiary, and in the UK, the funder of the healthcare system. It is increasingly recognised that patients' views should be taken into account in decision-making, both at the level of individual care and in issues of management and policy. Moreover, the patient is ultimately best placed to judge many aspects of quality. Patients, and their families, offer an important perspective on health services, one that complements other quality assessment methods such as inspections, clinical audits and routine data collection for management purposes.

This section contains survey data on patients' views about quality and the healthcare system.

Chart 5.1 Extent of change required in healthcare system

The 2004 Commonwealth Fund International Health Policy Survey, which focused on primary care, asked respondents: *Which of these statements comes closest to expressing your overall view of the health care system in this country?* UK respondents were the most satisfied with their healthcare system. As seen in Chart 5.1a, 13% of UK respondents indicated that their healthcare system required a complete rebuild; in contrast, 33% of US respondents indicated this level of dissatisfaction. UK respondents also had the highest proportion of respondents (26%) indicating that only minor change was required. Attitudes across the countries of the UK were fairly similar (Chart 5.1b) although respondents in Northern Ireland were most likely to register complete dissatisfaction with the system.

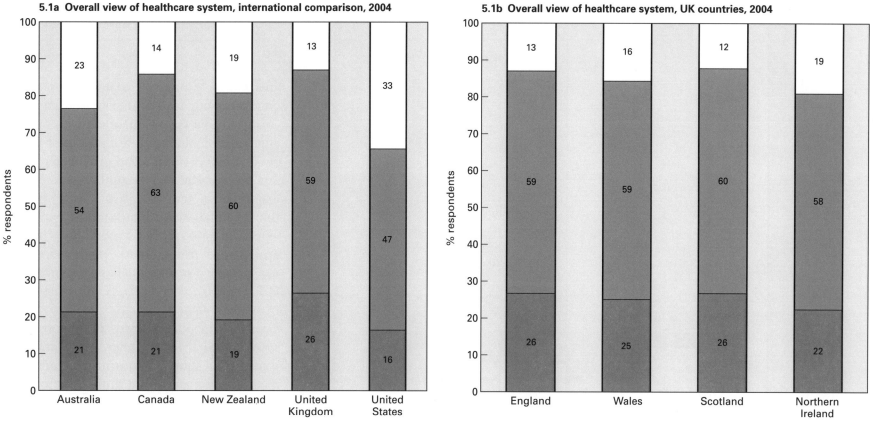

5.1a Overall view of healthcare system, international comparison, 2004

5.1b Overall view of healthcare system, UK countries, 2004

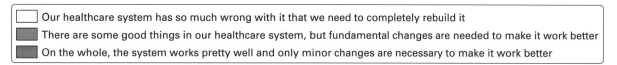

☐ Our healthcare system has so much wrong with it that we need to completely rebuild it

▨ There are some good things in our healthcare system, but fundamental changes are needed to make it work better

■ On the whole, the system works pretty well and only minor changes are necessary to make it work better

Source: Commonwealth Fund, 2004.

Note: In these charts, not all percentage columns tally to 100 due to rounding and missing responses.

The Quest for Quality in the NHS: a chartbook on quality of care in the UK

117

Chart 5.2 Extent of change required in healthcare system, UK time series

The Quest for Quality in the NHS: a chartbook on quality of care in the UK

The Commonwealth Fund International Health Policy Surveys are conducted each year, often focusing on a particular set of stakeholders within healthcare systems, such as hospital executives or adults with health problems. This chart reports results over time concerning UK respondents' answers to the question: *Which of these statements comes closest to expressing your overall view of the healthcare system in this country?* No particular trend is obvious: consistently around one-quarter of respondents indicated that minor change was required, and around 15% answered that a complete rebuild was required. The absence of any marked change in perceptions over a 16-year period is interesting given the considerable changes in investment, access and performance that have occurred over the same time frame (*see* Chapters 1, 2 and 3, in particular).

Source: Commonwealth Fund 2001; 2004.

Note: In this chart, not all percentage columns tally to 100 due to rounding and missing responses.

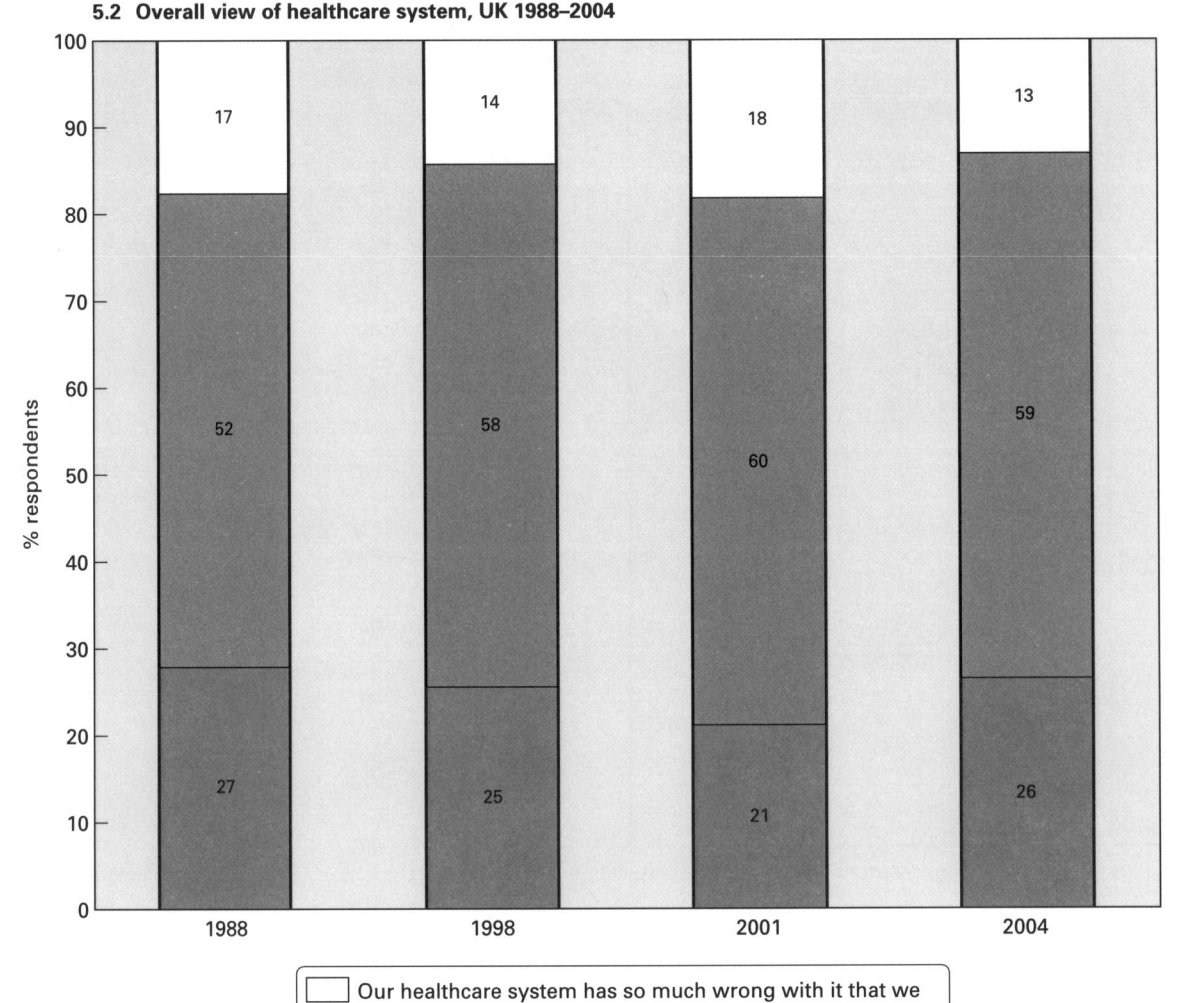

5.2 Overall view of healthcare system, UK 1988–2004

% respondents

	1988	1998	2001	2004
	17	14	18	13
	52	58	60	59
	27	25	21	26

Our healthcare system has so much wrong with it that we need to completely rebuild it

There are some good things in our healthcare system, but fundamental changes are needed to make it work better

On the whole, the system works pretty well and only minor changes are necessary to make it work better

Chart 5.3 Getting better or worse? Public perceptions of the NHS in Scotland

The Public Attitudes to the NHS in Scotland Survey was conducted in 2000 and 2004. Chart 5.3a illustrates responses to the question: *Overall when you think about the NHS over the last few years, would you say it has been getting better, worse or staying the same?* The view of NHS performance was more positive in 2004 than in 2000. Chart 5.3b illustrates responses to the question: *Thinking about the NHS over the next few years, do you expect it to get better, worse or stay the same?* Of the respondents in 2004, 39% were optimistic about the future of the NHS in Scotland and 23% were pessimistic.

5.3a Public ratings of the NHS over preceding few years, Scotland 2000 and 2004

Source: Public Attitudes to the NHS in Scotland Surveys (Scottish Executive Central Research Unit, 2001; Rose *et al.*, 2004).

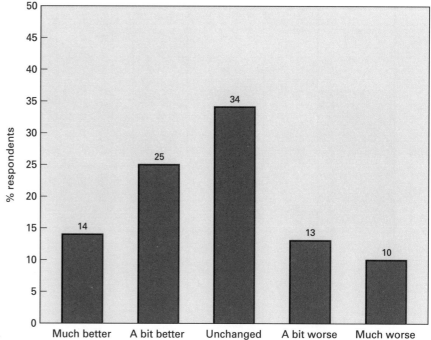

5.3b Public expectations for the NHS in future years, Scotland 2004

Source: Public Attitudes to the NHS in Scotland Surveys (Rose *et al.*, 2004)

The Quest for Quality in the NHS: a chartbook on quality of care in the UK

5 Patient-centredness

Chart 5.4 Patient ratings of hospital and mental healthcare in England

The Quest for Quality in the NHS: a chartbook on quality of care in the UK

The Healthcare Commission conducts large-scale patient surveys in England across different patient groups in the NHS. This chart illustrates the responses to the question: *Overall, how would you rate the care you received?* It was asked in four separate surveys: adult inpatients in 2002 and 2004 (allowing for comparison over time), young patients (aged 0–17; inpatients and day cases) in 2004, and adult mental health patients in 2004. For the three surveys that focused on hospital care, the overall rating was high, with between 74% and 79% of respondents indicating that care was excellent or good. Mental health patients were less satisfied with the care they received, with 54% rating it excellent or good.

Source: Healthcare Commission.

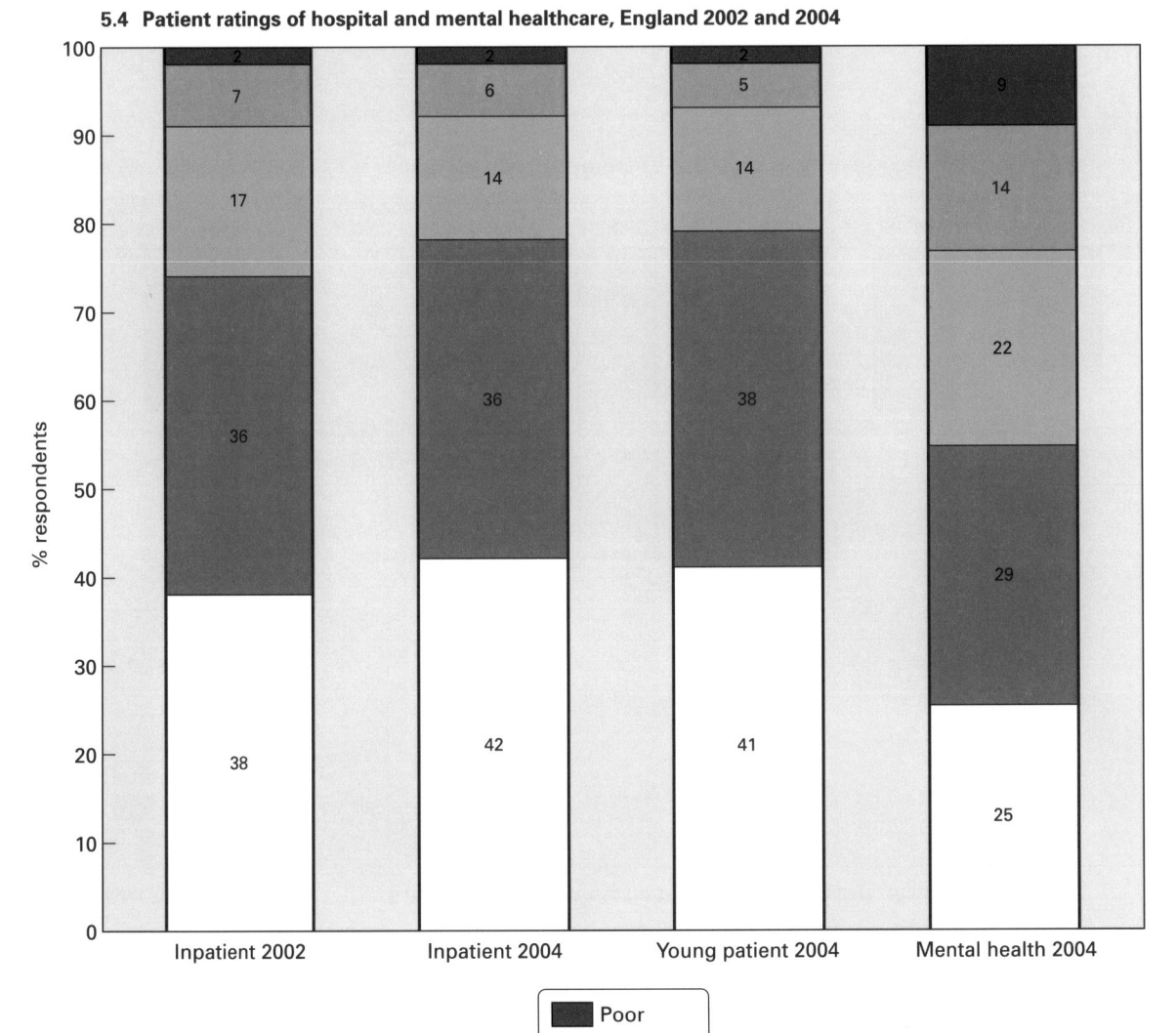

5.4 Patient ratings of hospital and mental healthcare, England 2002 and 2004

Legend:
- Poor
- Fair
- Good
- Very good
- Excellent

Chart 5.5 Public ratings of healthcare services in Northern Ireland

This chart is based on the Public Attitudes to Health and Personal Social Services in Northern Ireland Survey, 2004. The vast majority of respondents were satisfied with the care they received on an individual level: ratings of very satisfied or satisfied were 95% for GP services, 90% for outpatient services and 89% for inpatient services (percentages refer to the proportion of respondents that had used the particular service). Fewer respondents (78%), however, indicated that they were either very satisfied or satisfied with health and social services overall.

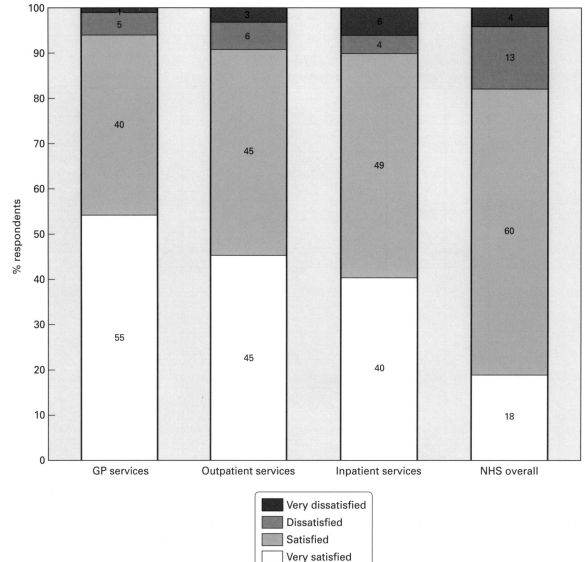

5.5 Public ratings of healthcare services, Northern Ireland 2004

Source: DHSSPS.

Note: In this chart, not all percentage columns tally to 100 due to rounding and missing responses.

The Quest for Quality in the NHS: a chartbook on quality of care in the UK

Chart 5.6 Public ratings of healthcare services in Scotland

The Quest for Quality in the NHS: a chartbook on quality of care in the UK

The Public Attitudes to the NHS in Scotland Survey in 2004 found high levels of satisfaction with the NHS in Scotland. The percentages of respondents indicating that they were very or fairly satisfied with the NHS services they had used in the previous 12 months were as follows: 93% for GP services; 90% for inpatient services; 88% for out-of-hours services; 86% for outpatient services; and 85% for the NHS overall. However, the percentage of respondents who were *very* satisfied with the NHS overall was much lower (37%) than that for specific services (53% to 62%).

Source: Rose *et al.*, 2004.

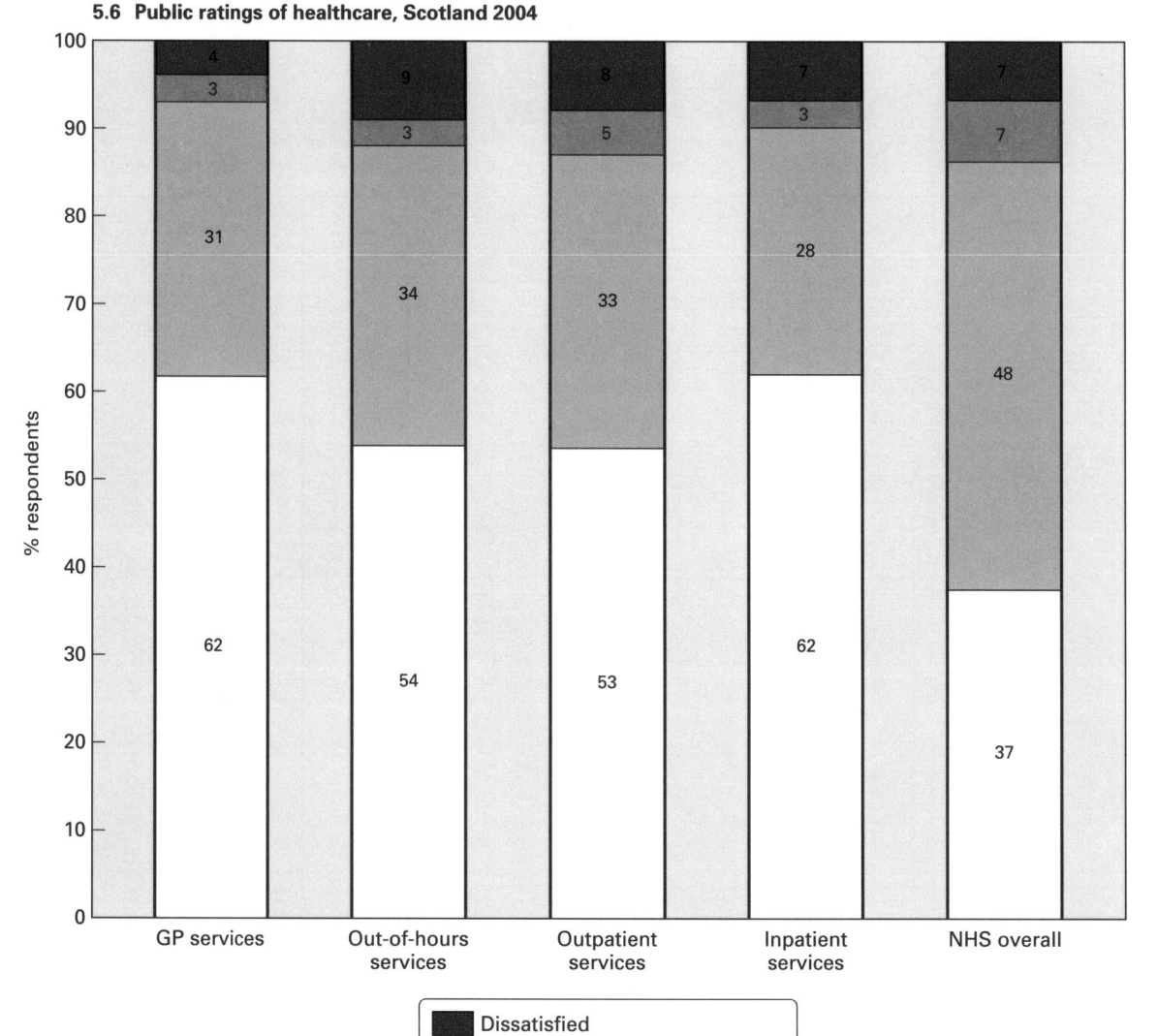

5.6 Public ratings of healthcare, Scotland 2004

% respondents

Legend:
- Dissatisfied
- Neither satisfied nor dissatisfied
- Fairly satisfied
- Very satisfied

Responsiveness to patient needs and expectations

Patient responsiveness encompasses several different factors:

- choice in time, place and provider of healthcare services
- involvement in decision-making: at the level of individual treatment plans and at a system level with citizen involvement in shaping policy and service delivery
- communication and information flow between patients and professionals
- attitudes and behaviour of NHS staff, including issues of respect and dignity.

Making meaningful choices and being involved in shared decision-making depend heavily upon the quality of information available. Evidence-based information is needed both before health problems arise, allowing individuals to take action to protect and improve their own health proactively; and after diagnosis of a particular condition. Providing such information, together with access to the patient's own medical records, is seen as central to achieving high quality care. The Bristol Inquiry (2001) recommended that patients should be involved as much as possible in decisions about their treatment and care, and that health professionals should receive training in the principles of good communication and shared decision-making. However, in 2003 a DH consultation exercise, *Choice, Responsiveness and Equity in the NHS and Social Care* (DH, 2003b), found that health information was widely regarded by patients to be problematic, patchy and of variable quality; these results corroborated patient survey findings that highlighted patients' dissatisfaction with the amount of information they receive about their illness and its treatment (Coulter, 2003).

Clearly, information underpins choice and is key to building patient trust and confidence in healthcare services. However, the potential value of information flow is not unidirectional. The perspectives and experiences of service users provide valuable insights into quality of healthcare and may reveal potential means of improvement (Farrell, 2004). Further, in publicly funded health systems such as the NHS, there is a growing acknowledgement that those who fund the service, that is the citizens, should inform, shape and participate in its development.

In terms of interpersonal interactions, the landmark report *Crossing the Quality Chasm* (Institute of Medicine, 2001: p63) identified several key features that patients should expect from their healthcare. It highlighted the importance of:

- **individualisation:** patients should be known and respected as individuals; choices and preferences should be sought and respected; in the case of special needs, care should be adapted accordingly
- **anticipation:** care should anticipate patients' needs, help should be proactive rather than reactive
- **cooperation:** healthcare professionals and their organisations should cooperate and coordinate their work with each other and with the patient: patient experiences should be seamless and patients should never feel lost.

This section presents data pertaining to the key aspects of responsiveness: choice, decision-making, communication, and staff interactions.

The Quest for Quality in the NHS: a chartbook on quality of care in the UK

Chart 5.7 Importance of more choice over hospital

The Quest for Quality in the NHS: a chartbook on quality of care in the UK

The Government has in recent times become increasingly focused on choice as a central policy theme. In England the most tangible commitments to patient choice to date have focused on issues of access and convenience. In 2003 the Government pledged that, by Summer 2004, patients waiting longer than six months will be offered the choice of an alternative hospital for faster treatment and that, by December 2005, all patients in England will be offered four or five places for elective care (DH, 2003a). Chart 5.7 draws on data from a YouGov survey and displays responses to the question: *How important is it to you to have more choice over which hospital treated you and your family?* More than one-quarter of respondents indicated that more choice in hospitals was very important to them; almost two-thirds said more choice was very or fairly important.

Source: Economist/YouGov Poll, 2004.

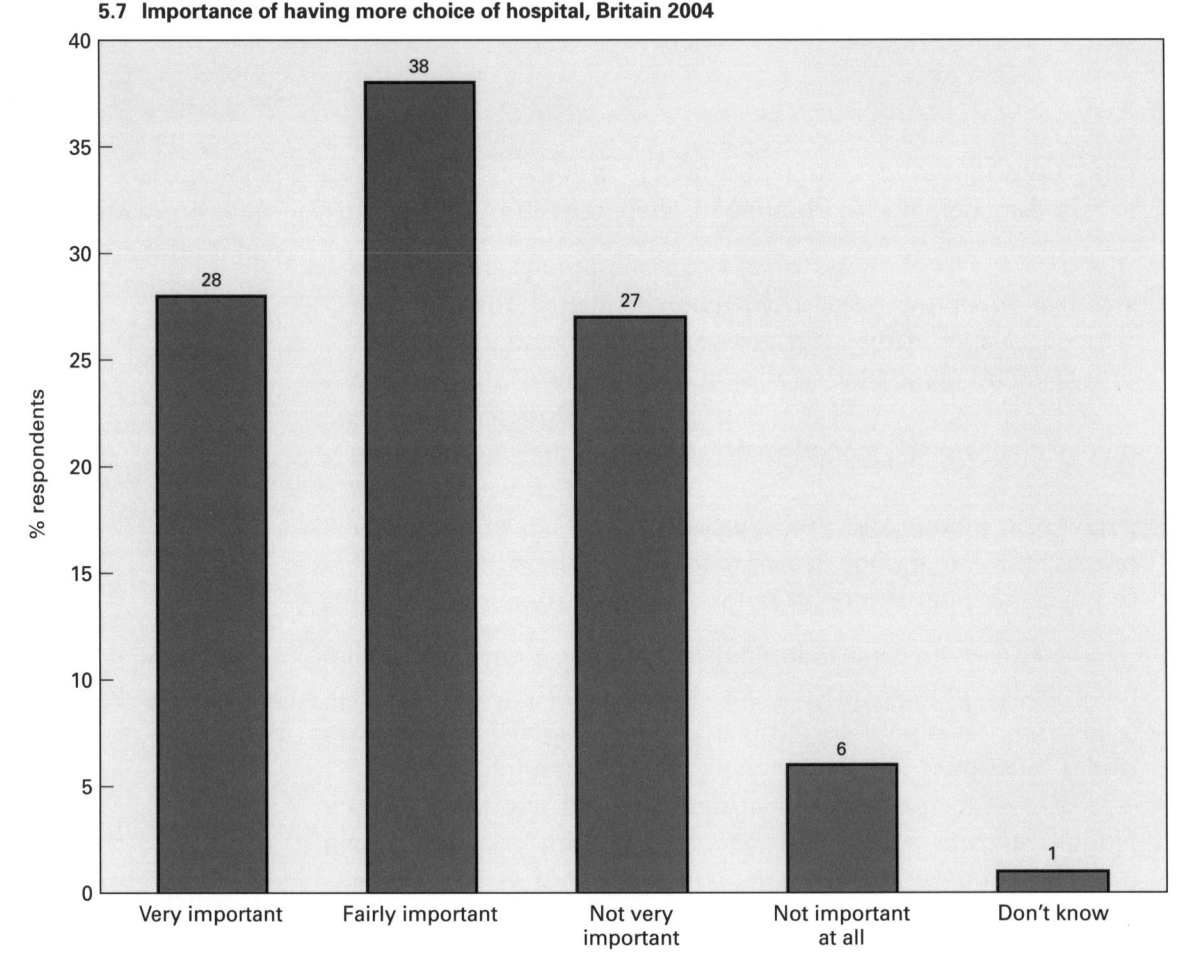

5.7 Importance of having more choice of hospital, Britain 2004

Chart 5.8 Choice of doctor

From the 2004 Commonwealth Fund International Health Policy Survey, which focused on primary care, we report on responses to the question: *How satisfied are you with the amount of choice you have in the doctors you see?* Of the UK respondents, 80% indicated that they were satisfied with that aspect of care. This was broadly in line with the responses from the comparator countries.

Source: Commonwealth Fund, 2004.

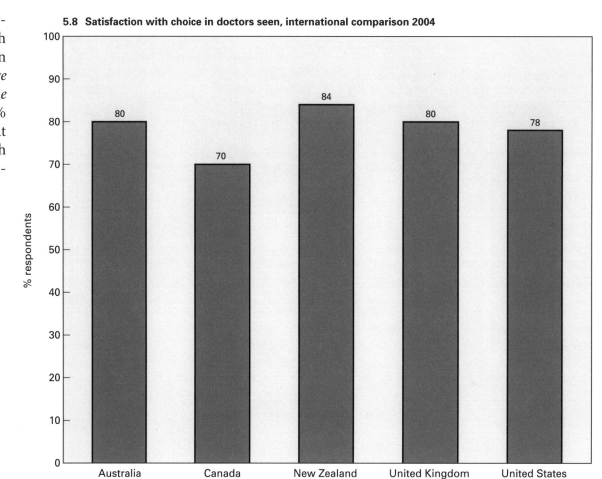

5.8 Satisfaction with choice in doctors seen, international comparison 2004

% respondents

Australia	Canada	New Zealand	United Kingdom	United States
80	70	84	80	78

Chart 5.9 Choice in referrals

Charts 5.9a and b illustrate responses from two different sets of patients surveyed in 2004. Data in Chart 5.9a reflects responses to questions asked of hospital patients admitted as elective cases: *Were you given a choice of admission dates?* (asked of English and Scottish respondents) and *Were you given a choice about which hospital you were referred to?* (English respondents only). Almost one-quarter of English respondents indicated that they had been given a choice of admission date, as did about one-third of Scottish respondents. Few

(9%) of the English patients were offered a choice of hospital. Chart 5.9b focuses on a question asked of English primary care patients that were referred to secondary care: *Were you given a choice about where you were referred to?* Of these respondents, 74% indicated that they had not been offered such a choice. However, just 16% of all respondents would have welcomed such a choice but did not receive one.

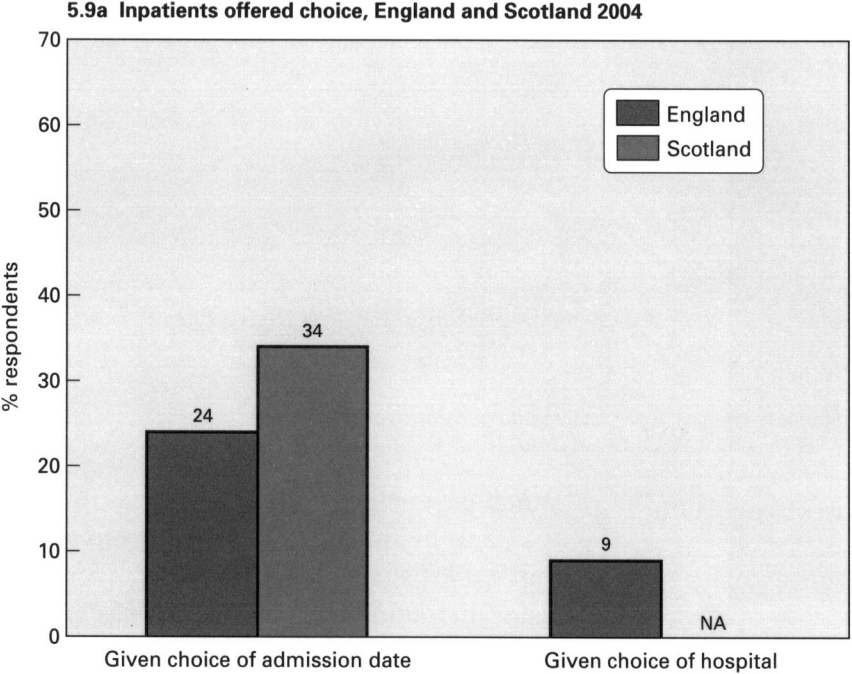

5.9a Inpatients offered choice, England and Scotland 2004

Source: Healthcare Commission, Rose *et al.*, 2004.

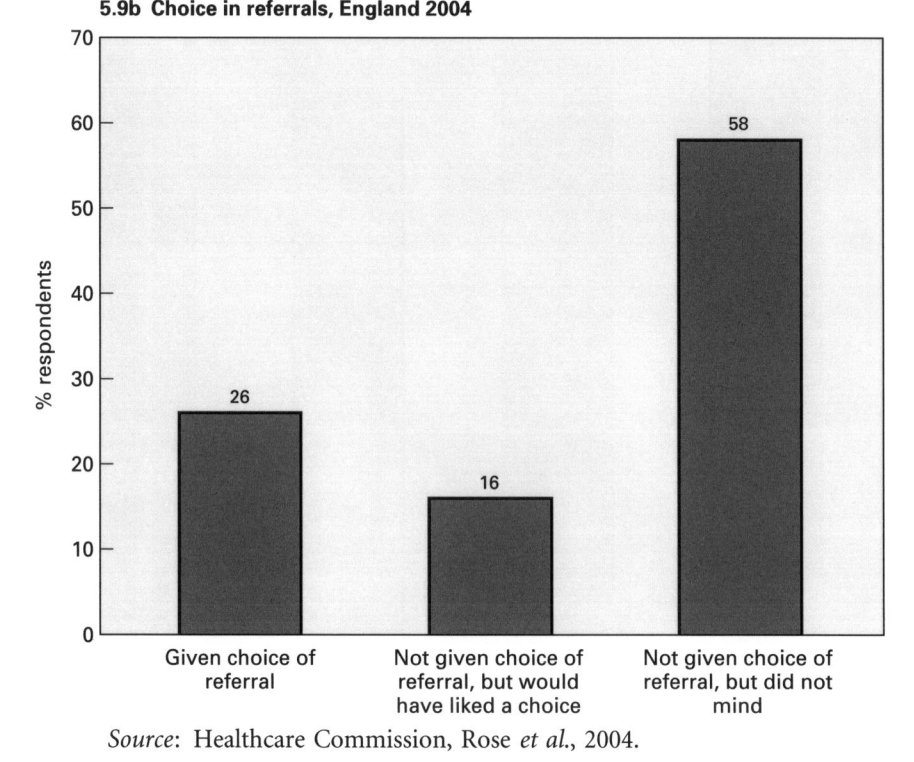

5.9b Choice in referrals, England 2004

Source: Healthcare Commission, Rose *et al.*, 2004.

The Quest for Quality in the NHS: a chartbook on quality of care in the UK

Chart 5.10 Involvement in decision-making

The Healthcare Commission conducts large-scale patient surveys in England across different patient groups in the NHS. The surveys regularly ask: *Were you involved as much as you wanted to be in decisions about your care and treatment?* Data in this chart is drawn from four separate surveys: primary care 2004; young patients 2004 (both inpatients and day cases; directly surveyed for ages 12–17 and completed by parent or guardian for ages 0–11); inpatients 2004; and mental health patients 2004. Only just over half of adult inpatient and young patient respondents indicated that they were definitely involved as much as they wanted to be in decisions about their care and even fewer, 41%, of mental health patients indicated that they were.

Source: Healthcare Commission.

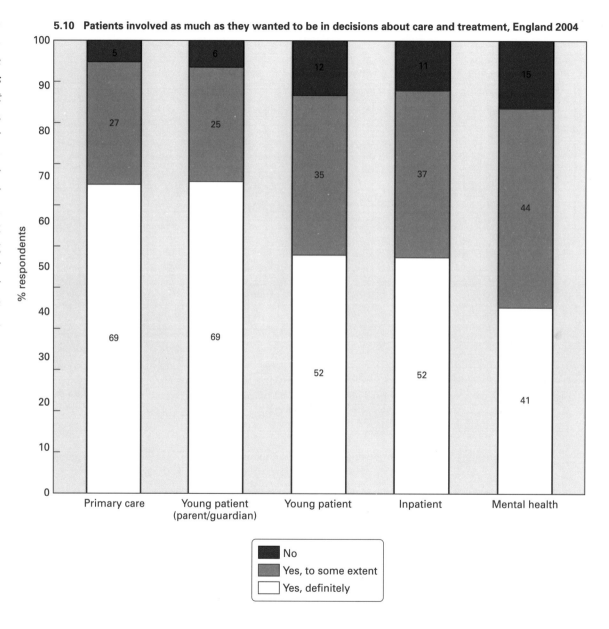

5.10   Patients involved as much as they wanted to be in decisions about care and treatment, England 2004

	No	Yes, to some extent	Yes, definitely
Primary care	5	27	69
Young patient (parent/guardian)	6	25	69
Young patient	12	35	52
Inpatient	11	37	52
Mental health	15	44	41

The Quest for Quality in the NHS: a chartbook on quality of care in the UK

The Quest for Quality in the NHS: a chartbook on quality of care in the UK

Chart 5.11 Interactions with general practitioners

In the 2004 Commonwealth Fund International Health Policy Survey, three questions focused on the quality of interactions between patients and general practitioners (GPs): *When you visit your doctor, does he or she always: 1. listen carefully to you; 2. explain things in a way you can understand; and 3. spend enough time with you?* Ratings were generally high, although time pressures may be affecting patients' perceptions of quality. Only 66% of respondents from New Zealand, 63% from Australia, 58% from the UK, 55% from Canada and 44% from the US indicated that their doctors always spend enough time with them. Within the UK, results were fairly uniform, except for London where all scores were considerably lower than in the rest of the country.

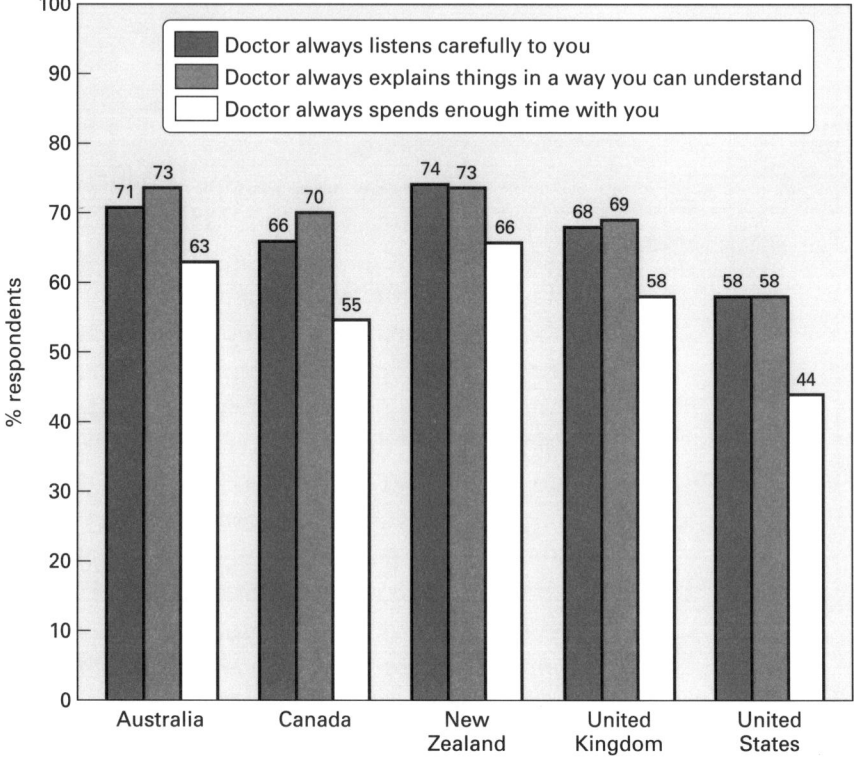

5.11a Patient perceptions of interactions with GPs, international comparison 2004

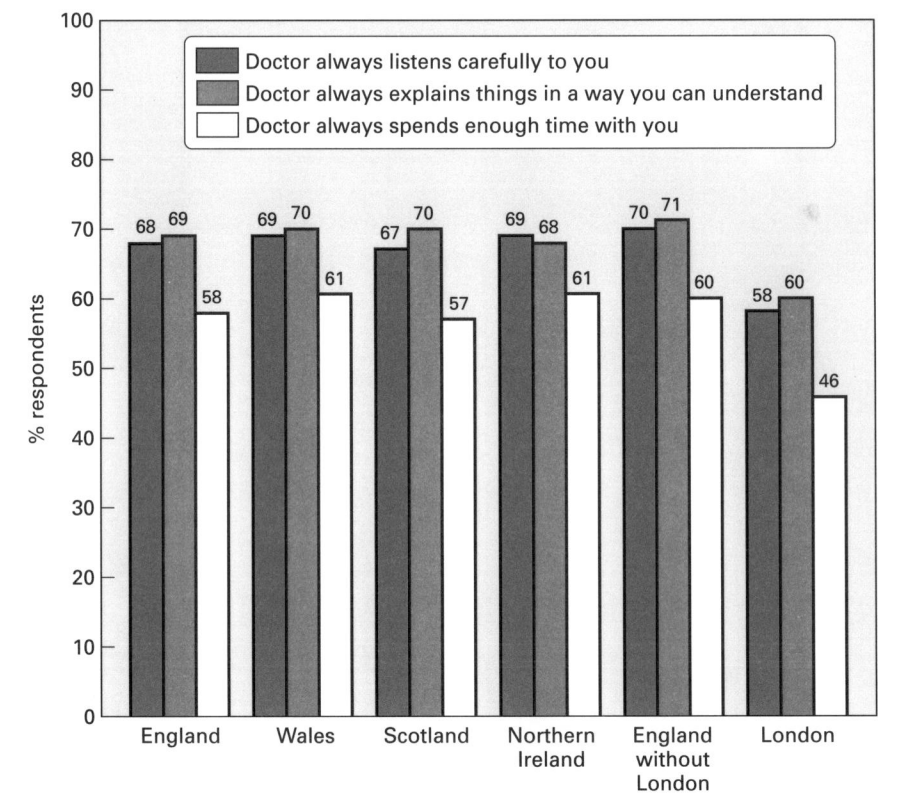

5.11b Patient perceptions of interactions with GPs, UK countries 2004

Source: Commonwealth Fund, 2004.

Source: Commonwealth Fund, 2004.

Chart 5.12 Communicating about treatment options in primary care

The 2004 Commonwealth Fund International Health Policy Survey asked about three primary care communication issues: *When you visit your doctor, does he or she* **always:** *1. tell you about treatment choices and ask for your ideas and opinions; 2. make clear the specific goals and plan for your treatment; 3. give clear instructions so that you know what to do or what symptoms to look for?* About two-thirds of respondents in each country indicated that instructions were always given clearly; about one-half were told of specific goals and plans. In contrast, only about one-quarter (except in Australia) indicated that an active dialogue was always taking place (i.e. asking for patients' ideas and opinions).

Source: Commonwealth Fund, 2004.

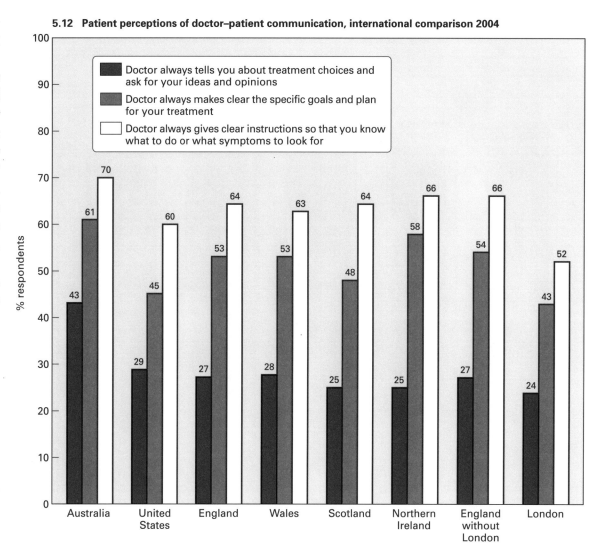

5.12 Patient perceptions of doctor–patient communication, international comparison 2004

Legend:
- Doctor always tells you about treatment choices and ask for your ideas and opinions
- Doctor always makes clear the specific goals and plan for your treatment
- Doctor always gives clear instructions so that you know what to do or what symptoms to look for

Country	Treatment choices	Goals and plan	Clear instructions
Australia	43	61	70
United States	29	45	60
England	27	53	64
Wales	28	53	63
Scotland	25	48	64
Northern Ireland	25	58	66
England without London	27	54	66
London	24	43	52

y-axis: % respondents

The Quest for Quality in the NHS: a chartbook on quality of care in the UK

Chart 5.13 Patient access to medical record: achieved and desired

The Quest for Quality in the NHS: a chartbook on quality of care in the UK

The 2004 Commonwealth Fund International Health Policy Survey asked respondents: *Do you have access to your own medical record?* Of the five countries surveyed, UK respondents reported the lowest rates of access (28%). However, UK respondents were also the least likely to express a desire to see their own medical record.

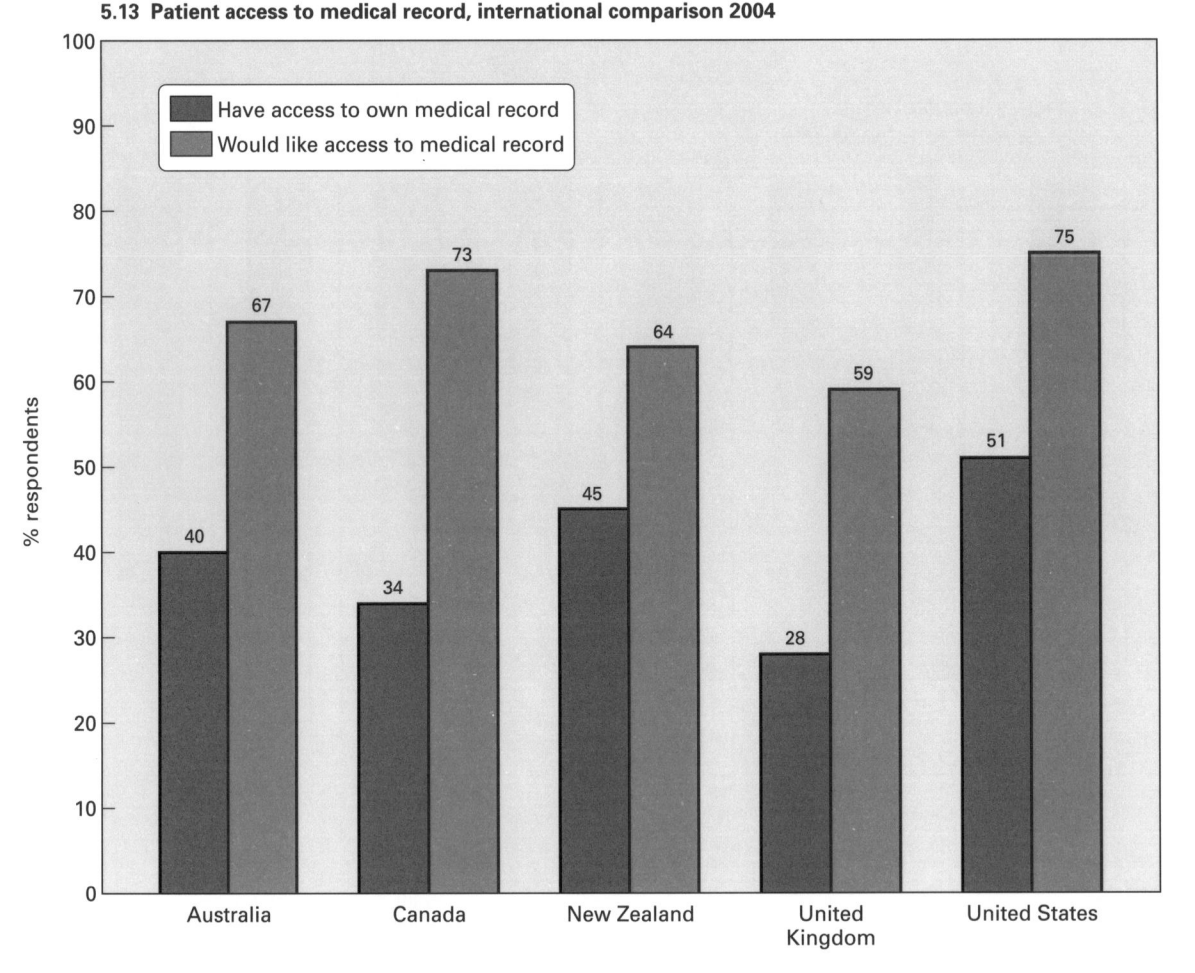

5.13 Patient access to medical record, international comparison 2004

Legend:
- Have access to own medical record
- Would like access to medical record

Source: Commonwealth Fund, 2004.

Chart 5.14 Extent of public influence on NHS in Scotland

Recent health policy documents have emphasised the importance of public involvement in shaping services at a local level (NHS Wales, 2001; NHSScotland 2001; DH, 2003b). The Public Attitudes to the NHS in Scotland Surveys found big discrepancies, in 2000 and 2004, between percentages of respondents who want such involvement and percentages who perceive they have it. Between 2000 and 2004, the extent of influence that respondents felt they had on the NHS decreased considerably. This finding is of interest given that political devolution became established in the same time frame.

Source: Scottish Executive Central Research Unit, 2001; Rose *et al.*, 2004.

Note: Response options differed slightly between 2000 and 2004; *see* Technical Appendix for details.

Note: In this chart, not all percentage columns tally to 100 due to rounding and missing responses.

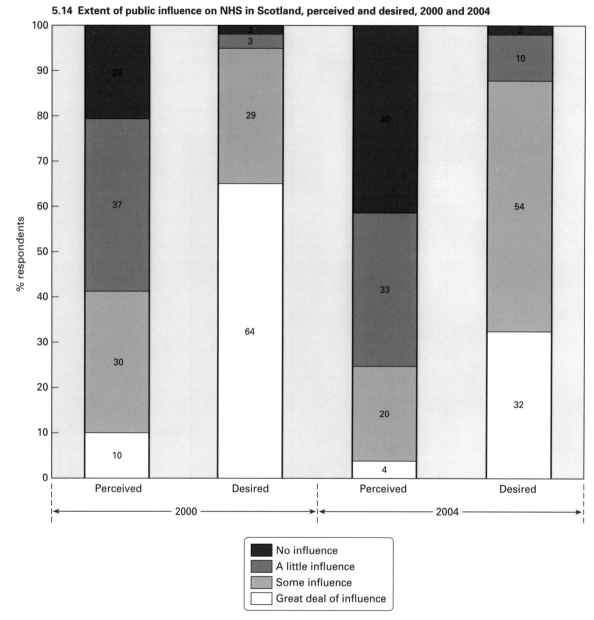

5.14 Extent of public influence on NHS in Scotland, perceived and desired, 2000 and 2004

Legend:
- No influence
- A little influence
- Some influence
- Great deal of influence

The Quest for Quality in the NHS: a chartbook on quality of care in the UK

5 Patient-centredness

Chart 5.15 Patient perceptions: treated with respect and dignity

The Quest for Quality in the NHS: a chartbook on quality of care in the UK

The Healthcare Commission surveys in England gauge opinion among different patient groups in the NHS. The question: *Overall, did you feel you were treated with respect and dignity?* was asked of primary care patients, inpatients, young patients (both inpatients and day cases, aged 0–17 years),* and mental health patients in 2004. A large majority of respondents indicated that they were treated with respect and dignity at all times. While these results are commendable, the finding that over one-fifth of inpatient, young patient and mental health patients (referring to psychiatrists) felt that they were not treated with dignity and respect at all times is of concern.

Source: Healthcare Commission.

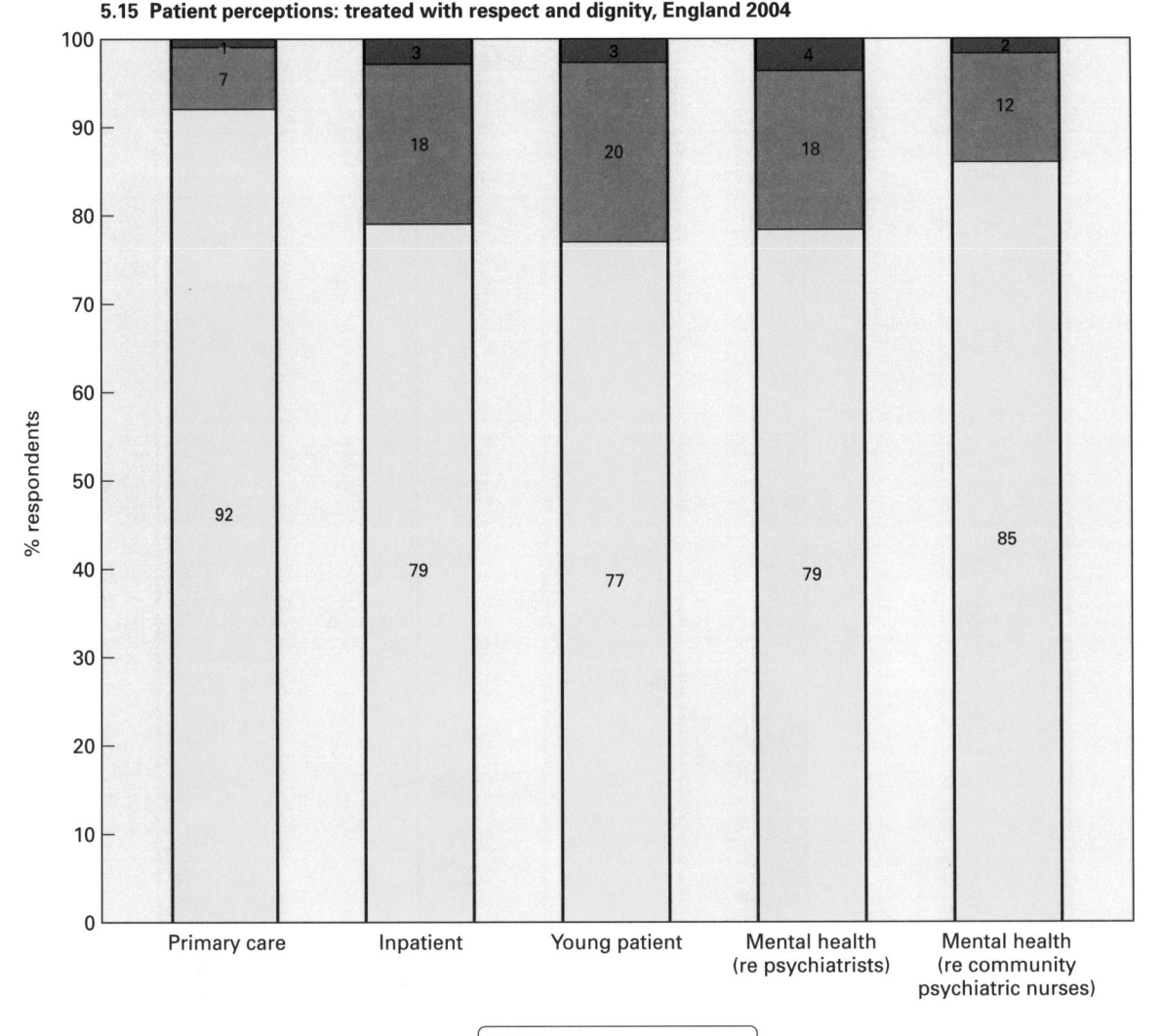

5.15 Patient perceptions: treated with respect and dignity, England 2004

* In cases where young patients were under 12 years of age, their parents or guardians were surveyed.

Chart 5.16 Patient perceptions: confidence and trust

Many Healthcare Commission surveys include the question: *Did you have confidence and trust in the doctors treating you?* Three-quarters or more of respondents in the surveys of inpatients, primary care patients and young patients indicated that they had complete confidence and trust in their doctors. In contrast, among those responding to the mental health survey, only 59% indicated that they had complete trust and confidence in the doctors treating them.

Source: Healthcare Commission.

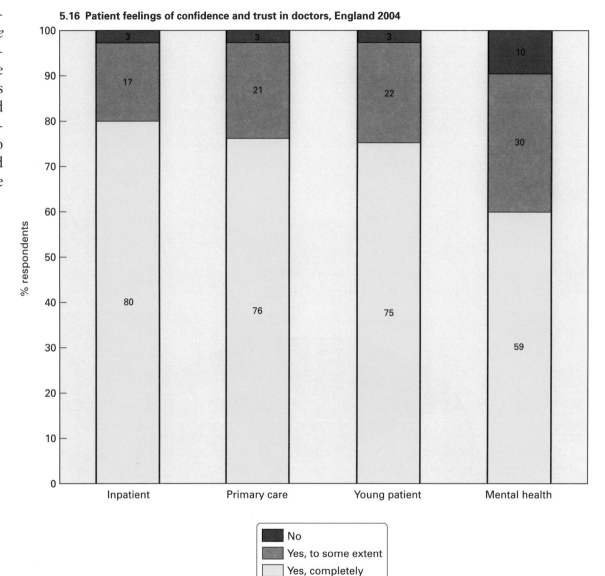

5.16 Patient feelings of confidence and trust in doctors, England 2004

% respondents

	No	Yes, to some extent	Yes, completely

Inpatient · Primary care · Young patient · Mental health

The Quest for Quality in the NHS: a chartbook on quality of care in the UK

Chart 5.17 Fair treatment

The Public Attitudes to Health and Personal Social Services in Northern Ireland Survey, 2004, surveyed the public on a wide range of issues. This chart shows the responses to the question: *Do you feel that health and social services treat all groups fairly?* Only 71% of respondents answered yes with 14% saying they did not know. Supplemental questions ascertained that, of the 15% who said no, 63% (i.e. 9% of total sample) indicated that the elderly were treated less fairly than other groups.

Source: DHSSPS, 2004.

5.17 Patient perceptions of fairness, Northern Ireland 2004

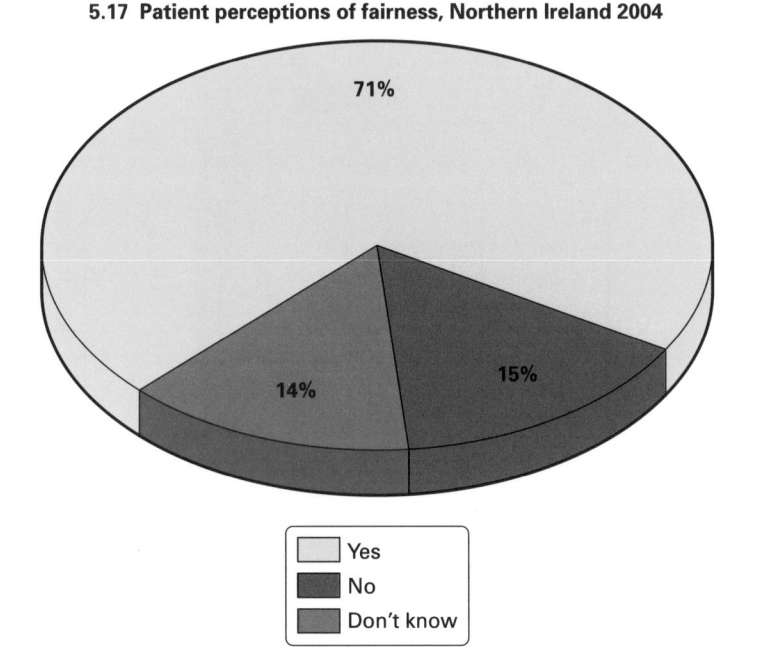

71%

15%

14%

Yes
No
Don't know

Physical environment

The wellbeing of patients can be markedly influenced by the environment in which they are cared for. Factors such as cleanliness, the quality of food and other physical characteristics such as excessive noise are an important part of the patient experience and can impact upon recuperation and recovery processes (www.chi.nhs.uk/ratings/).

One of the greatest concerns of patients is that when they are admitted to hospital, they wish to be cared for in single-sex rooms. In response, the Government manifesto made a commitment to eliminate mixed-sex wards in 95% of NHS Trusts by 2002 (www.chi.nhs.uk/Ratings/Trust/Indicator/IndicatorDescriptionShort.asp?IndicatorId=1046).

Chart 5.18 Cleanliness of healthcare facilities

The Quest for Quality in the NHS: a chartbook on quality of care in the UK

Research carried out among various interest groups in advance of the launch of *The NHS Plan* identified that cleanliness had become a major issue of concern among the public.* This concern has recently been heightened by the association between shortcomings in standards of cleanliness and increases in the incidence of healthcare-acquired infections (*see* Charts 4.7–4.11, pages 100–4). *The NHS Plan* (2000) pledged extra funds for cleaning and established specialist inspection teams, known as Patient Environment Action Teams (PEAT), to conduct unannounced visits to gauge cleanliness of NHS Trusts. This chart draws on Healthcare Commission patient surveys and illustrates the responses to the question: *In your opinion how clean was the room/ward/toilet/bathroom?* General practice surgeries scored the highest percentage of very clean ratings (73%). In the surveys of hospital patients, only about one-half of the respondents indicated that the facilities were very clean. In general, toilets and bathrooms were judged to be less clean than wards.

Source: Healthcare Commission.

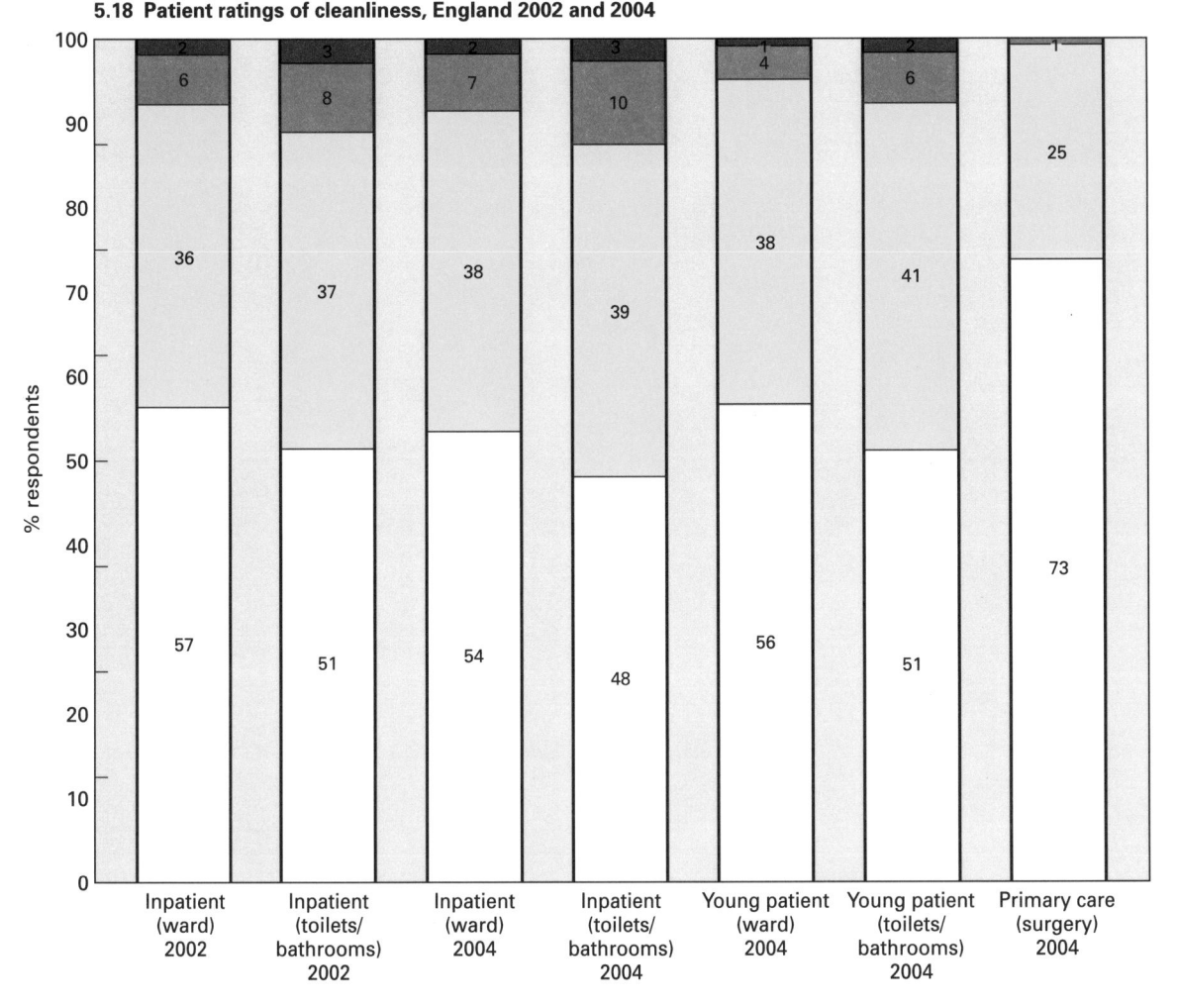

5.18 Patient ratings of cleanliness, England 2002 and 2004

Legend:
- Not at all clean
- Not very clean
- Fairly clean
- Very clean

* www.chi.nhs.uk/Ratings/Trust/Indicator/IndicatorDescriptionShort.asp?IndicatorId=1006

Chart 5.19 Mixed-sex wards

This chart is based on a Healthcare Commission survey of inpatients in England in 2004. It illustrates the responses to the question: *During your [current] hospital stay did you ever share a room or bay with a patient of the opposite sex?* Of all respondents, 22% indicated that they were in mixed accommodation during their stay. These results should be interpreted in the light of commitments made by the Government to eliminate mixed-sex accommodation in 95% of NHS Trusts by 2002.

Source: Healthcare Commission.

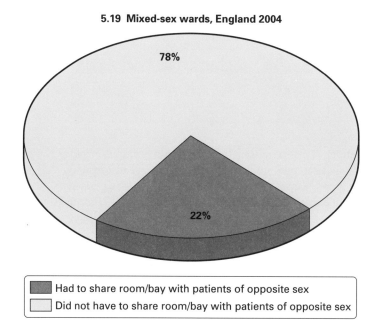

5.19 Mixed-sex wards, England 2004

78%

22%

| | Had to share room/bay with patients of opposite sex |
| | Did not have to share room/bay with patients of opposite sex |

References

Bristol Royal Infirmary Inquiry (2001) *Learning from Bristol: The report of the public inquiry into children's heart surgery at the Bristol Royal Infirmary 1984–1995*. The Stationery Office, London.

Commonwealth Fund (2001) *International Health Policy Survey*. Commonwealth Fund, New York.

Commonwealth Fund (2004) *International Health Policy Survey of Adults' Experiences with Primary Care*. Commonwealth Fund, New York.

Coulter A (2003) Engaging patients and citizens. In: S Leatherman and KI Sutherland. *The Quest for Quality in the NHS: a mid-term evaluation of the ten-year quality agenda*. TSO, London.

Department of Health (2003a) *Building on the Best: choice, responsiveness and equity in the NHS*. Department of Health, London. Available online at: www.dh.gov.uk/assetRoot/04/06/84/00/04068400.pdf [last accessed 31 January 2005].

Department of Health (2003b) *Choice, Responsiveness and Equity in the NHS and Social Care: a national consultation*. Department of Health, London. Available online at: www.dh.gov.uk/assetRoot/04/07/53/08/04075308.pdf [last accessed 31 January 2005].

Department of Health, Social Services and Public Safety (2004) *Public Attitudes to Health and Personal Social Services in Northern Ireland Survey*. Department of Health, Social Services and Public Safety, Belfast. Available online at: www.dhsspsni.gov.uk/publications/2004/pas/pas-report.asp [last accessed 31 January 2005].

Economist/YouGov Poll (2004) Choosing to choose. *The Economist*. 7 **April**.

Farrell C (2004) *Patient and Public Involvement in Health: the evidence for policy implementation*. Department of Health, London. Available online at: www.dh.gov.uk/assetRoot/04/08/23/34/04082334.pdf [last accessed 31 January 2005].

Institute of Medicine, Committee on Quality Healthcare in America (2001) *Crossing the Quality Chasm: a new health system for the 21st century*. National Academies Press, Washington, DC.

NHSScotland (2001) *Patient Focus and Public Involvement*. Scottish Executive, Edinburgh. Available online at: www.scotland.gov.uk/library3/health/pfpi.pdf [last accessed 31 January 2005].

NHSScotland (2003) *Partnership for Care: Scotland's health white paper*. Scottish Executive, Edinburgh. Available online at: www.scotland.gov.uk/library5/health/pfcs-00.asp [last accessed 31 January 2005].

NHS Wales (2001) *Improving Health in Wales: a plan for the NHS and its partners*. The National Assembly for Wales, Cardiff. Available online at: www.wales.gov.uk/healthplanonline/health_plan/content/nhsplan-e.pdf [last accessed 31 January 2005].

NHS Wales (2004) *A Statement of Healthcare Standards: standards for NHS care and treatment in Wales. Consultation document*. The National Assembly for Wales, Cardiff. Available online at: www.wales.nhs.uk/sites/documents/465/English.pdf [last accessed 31 January 2005].

Rose N, Glendinning R and Carr-Hill R (2004) *Public Attitudes to the NHS in Scotland Survey*. Scottish Executive, Edinburgh. Available online at: www.scotland.gov.uk/library5/government/panhss-00.asp [last accessed 31 January 2005].

Scottish Executive Central Research Unit (2001) *Public Attitudes to the NHS in Scotland Survey*. Scottish Executive, Edinburgh. Available online at: www.scotland.gov.uk/cru/kd01/purple/panhs-00.asp [last accessed 31 January 2005].

Wanless D (2002) *Securing our Future Health: taking a long-term view. Interim report*. The Public Inquiry Unit, HM-Treasury, London. Available online at: www.hm-treasury.gov.uk./consultations_and_legislation/wanless/consult_wanless_interimrep.cfm [last accessed 31 January 2005].

Disparities refer to differences in health status and differences in access to healthcare services across subgroups within a population. Disparities in healthcare systems have long been a central concern of policymakers around the world (Kunst and Mackenbach, 1999; WHO, 2000; Morrisson, 2002; Smedley, *et al.*, 2003).

This chapter presents charts on two types of disparities: disparities in health status and disparities in healthcare services.

- **Disparities in health status** are variations in measures of 'healthiness' or health outcomes across different groups or sub-populations. These variations are often attributed to socio-economic status and are influenced by a wide range of contributory factors such as educational attainment, employment and housing. Such social and economic differences are often compounded by differences in health-maintenance and health-care-seeking behaviours. Widely referred to in the UK as *health inequalities*, disparities in health status are measured with indicators such as gaps in life expectancy between different socio-economic groups or incidence of coronary heart disease, stratified by deprivation.

- **Disparities in healthcare services** are variations in the provision of healthcare services and are of two principal types. The first type is a function of resource availability and distribution and encompasses issues such as geographical remoteness. The second type is a result of inconsistent and inequitable clinical decision-making

based on discrimination, both conscious and unconscious, on the grounds of age, gender, social class, or race. Disparities in healthcare services may be manifested in variability in the type and volume of healthcare provided or in the convenience, timeliness, and cultural appropriateness of services. Examples include denying revascularisation procedures to elderly patients on the basis of their age; or failing to provide translators for patients who do not speak English.

Disparities have proven to be a widespread and enduring problem in healthcare systems around the world. They are a result of a complex mix of patient behaviour (compliance, lifestyle, etc.), environmental context (socio-economic deprivation, geographic remoteness, social and cultural influences, etc.) and clinician behaviour and decision-making (variable thresholds for referral or treatment, etc.). While there is a wealth of data and research on the extent of disparities that exist, and a growing list of their underlying causes, there is far less information available to help policymakers tackle the factors that create specific disparities.

Many of the charts contained in this section refer to deprivation quintiles which separate a population into five bands according to the level of deprivation ranging from least deprived ('richest') to most deprived ('poorest'). The stratification into quintiles is often done on a geographical rather than an individual basis. For a fuller explanation, *see* the Statistical Glossary on page 172.

The Quest for Quality in the NHS: a chartbook on quality of care in the UK

Disparities in health status

Inequalities in health have long been a problem in the UK (Alison, 1840; Chadwick, 1882). The health status of the entire population has improved greatly over time as a result of advances in health technologies and public health interventions, but this improvement has not always been achieved at the same rate across all social groups or in all parts of the UK. In 1998, the Acheson Report asserted that:

the weight of scientific evidence supports a socio-economic explanation of health inequalities. This traces the roots of ill health to such determinants as income, education and employment as well as to the material environment and lifestyle.

A significant health gap exists between 'rich' and 'poor' and for many parameters, the gap is widening.

In the early 1970s death rates among men of working age were almost twice as high for unskilled groups as they were for professional groups. By the early 1990s, death rates were almost three times higher among unskilled groups. There are regional differences too. In 1999/2001, the difference between areas with the highest (North Dorset) and lowest (Manchester) life expectancy at birth was 9.5 years for boys and 6.9 years for girls. The highest life expectancy for girls was in West Somerset and the lowest was in Manchester. In smaller communities within these areas, the differences can be even greater.   DH, 2003

In recent years, health policy throughout the UK has reiterated its commitment to reducing health inequalities.* In England, DH and the Treasury agreed a Public Service Agreement (HM Treasury, 2002) target for reducing health inequalities. It stated the intention, by 2010, to reduce inequalities in health outcomes by 10% as measured by life expectancy at birth and infant mortality.

The charts in this section illustrate the impact that deprivation has on a range of health outcomes, both in terms of mortality, and in terms of the impact and severity of diseases such as cancer, asthma and diabetes. Outcome measures such as those displayed in the charts reflect the influence of many more factors than the quality of medical care provided. However, they contextualise the performance of the healthcare system and inform the development of strategies for improving health in particular populations, health conditions and geographic areas.

---

* Including *Independent Inquiry into Inequalities in Health* [Acheson Report] (Acheson, 1998); *Saving Lives: our healthier nation* (Department of Health, 1999); *The NHS Plan* (Department of Health, 2000); *Tackling Health Inequalities: a programme for action* (Department of Health, 2003); *Choosing Health* (Department of Health, 2004); *Towards a Healthier Scotland* (Scottish Office, 1999); *Health Inequalities in the New Scotland* (Blamey *et al.*, 2002); *Better Health, Better Wales* (Welsh Office, 1998); *New Targeting Social Need: action plan* (DHSSPS, 2001); *Investing for Health* (DHSSPS, 2002).

Chart 6.1 Life expectancy

The charts below display two perspectives on life expectancy in the UK. Chart 6.1a shows that, in the past 10 years, life expectancy has generally increased although there are considerable differences between males and females and between the countries of the UK. Chart 6.1b provides a more detailed picture and illustrates the disparities that underlie any one country's results. Arraying English data on life expectancy at a local authority level according to level of socio-economic deprivation, the pattern clearly demonstrates that the higher the level of deprivation, the lower the population's life expectancy for both sexes.

6.1a Life expectancy, UK countries 1991–93 and 2001–03

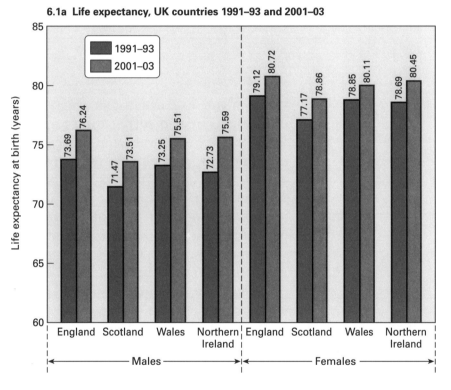

Source: ONS.

6.1b Pooled life expectancy, by local authority, vs deprivation, England 2001–03

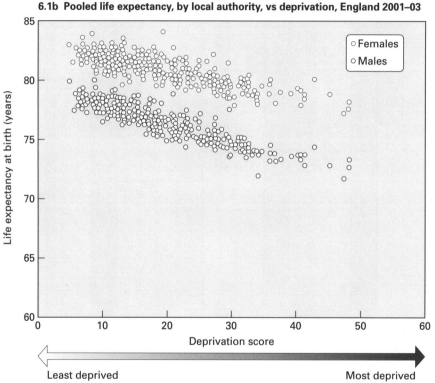

Source: ONS, Healthcare Commission (analysis by Raleigh, Sims, Irons).

The Quest for Quality in the NHS: a chartbook on quality of care in the UK

Chart 6.2 Infant mortality by socio-economic classification

The Quest for Quality in the NHS: a chartbook on quality of care in the UK

Deprivation levels are known to affect infant mortality rates. In its drive to tackle health inequalities, the Government has pledged 'by 2010 [to] reduce by at least 10% the gap in infant mortality between routine and manual groups and the population as a whole' (HM Treasury, 2002), using 1997–99 as the baseline (i.e. a difference of 0.4 deaths per 1000 live births). The data displayed opposite shows a generalised improvement, that is, a decrease in infant mortality rates in England and Wales. However, infant mortality rates in routine and manual groups have not shown consistent improvement and the gap between rates for routine and manual groups and for the population as a whole is widening (in 2001–03 the difference was 0.8 deaths per 1000 live births). This pattern indicates an exacerbation rather than a decline in disparities.*

Source: ONS.

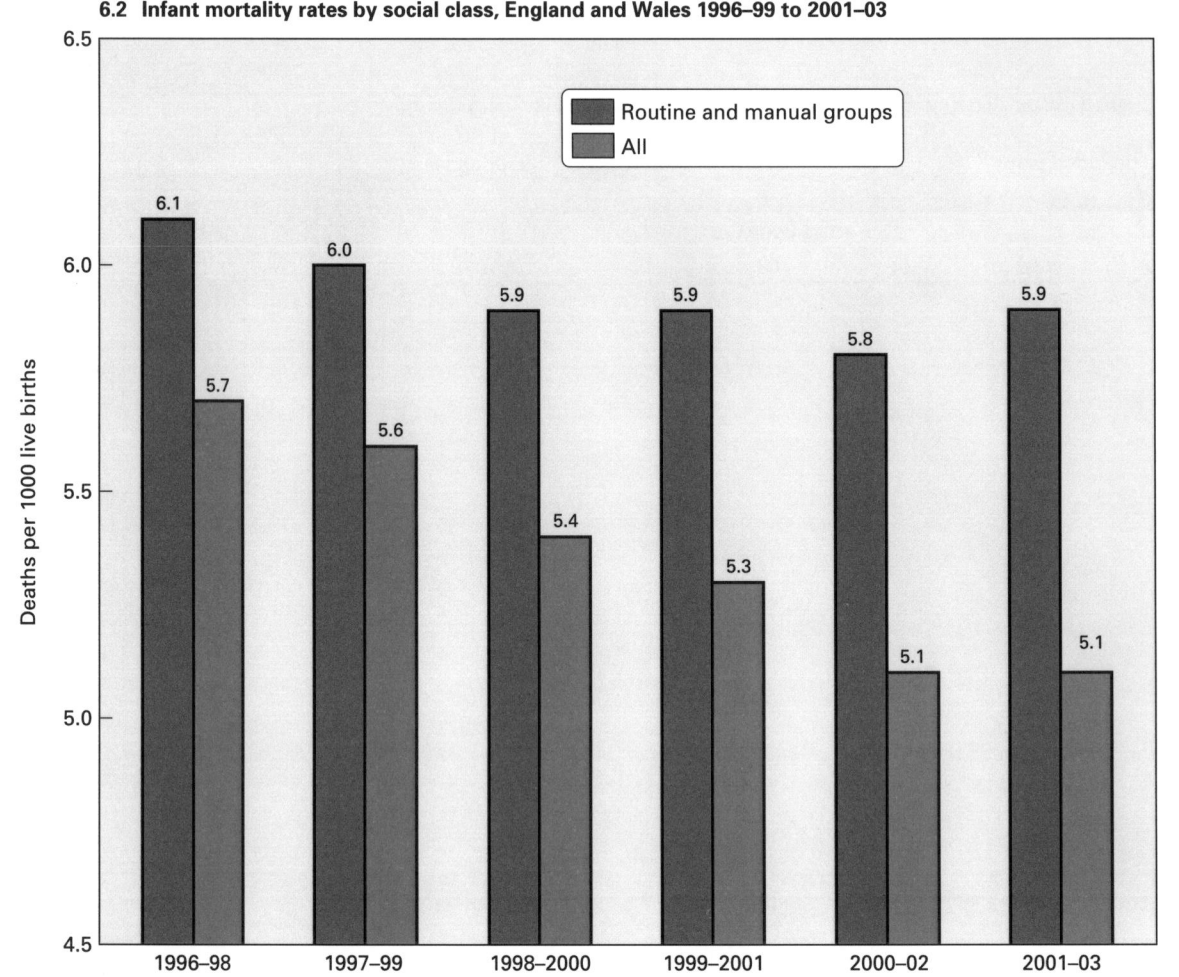

6.2 Infant mortality rates by social class, England and Wales 1996–99 to 2001–03

* Figures exclude sole registrations, i.e. births registered by mother only. Note: 2001–03 figures for England only; social class classification scheme change to NS-SEC in 2000–02, *see* Technical Appendix and Statistical Glossary.

Chart 6.3 Low birth weight by deprivation

Low birth weight (< 2500 grams) is associated with an increased risk of infant mortality and can lead to varied and enduring health problems (Stevens-Simon and Orleans, 1999). Chart 6.3 illustrates the impact that deprivation can have on birth weight. Evidence suggests that interventions such as smoking cessation programmes can help prevent low birth weight; however, there is little evidence-based information about how to design and implement effective interventions for use in the most affected, deprived subpopulations (Bull *et al.*, 2003).

Source: ONS; Healthcare Commission (analysis by Raleigh, Irons, Sims).

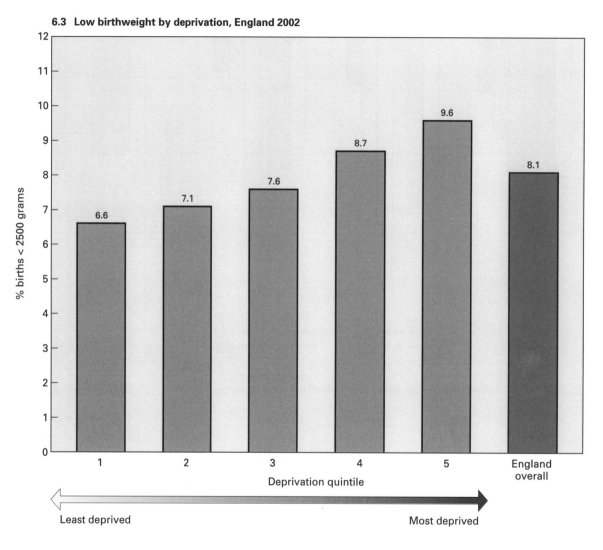

6.3 Low birthweight by deprivation, England 2002

% births < 2500 grams

Bar values: 1: 6.6, 2: 7.1, 3: 7.6, 4: 8.7, 5: 9.6, England overall: 8.1

Deprivation quintile

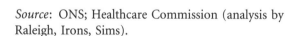

Least deprived — Most deprived

The Quest for Quality in the NHS: a chartbook on quality of care in the UK

143

Chart 6.4 Smoking in pregnancy

The Quest for Quality in the NHS: a chartbook on quality of care in the UK

Smoking in pregnancy can lead to obstetric complications and serious health problems in newborns. *Smoking Kills: a white paper on tobacco* (DH, 1998) announced a UK-wide target to reduce the percentage of women who smoke during pregnancy from 23% to 15% by 2010, with an intermediate target of 18% by 2005. Across the entire population, the association between smoking and socio-economic classification is strong (Hamlyn *et al.*, 2002). This association is echoed in the data for pregnant women, Chart 6.4a is based on data from a survey of mothers of babies born in the UK in 2000 and shows that, for the UK as a whole, women who have never worked are most likely to smoke in pregnancy (36%); among women in 'lower occupations' such as routine sales, production and agricultural work, 29% smoked, while within the 'higher occupations' such as traditional professions, only 8% smoked during pregnancy. Across the countries of the UK (Chart 6.4b), rates of smoking in pregnancy are highest in Northern Ireland (23%). The differences in rates of smoking between socio-economic groups are greater in Scotland and Northern Ireland than in England and Wales.

6.4a Smoking rates in pregnancy by mother's socio-economic group (NS-SEC), UK 2000

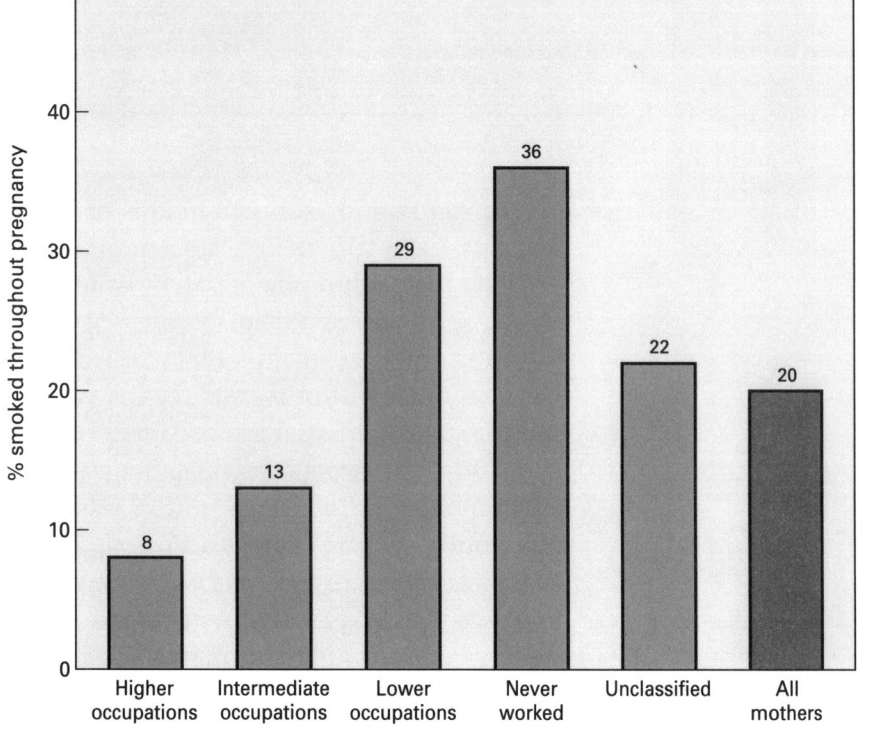

Source: Hamlyn *et al.*, 2002.

6.4b Smoking rates in pregnancy by mother's socio-economic group (NS-SEC), UK countries 2000

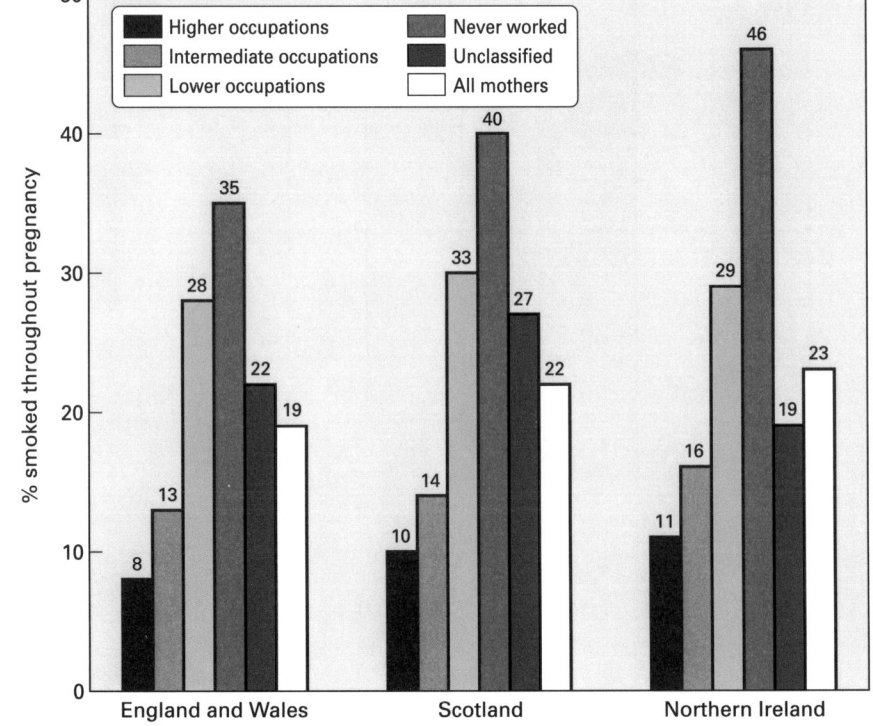

Source: Hamlyn *et al.*, 2002.

This chart depicts differences in five-year cancer survival rates in England and Wales by socio-economic status. Patients were classified into one of five categories of socio-economic deprivation, based on their electoral ward at the time of diagnosis (1996–99). The chart illustrates the 'deprivation gap' i.e. the difference, in terms of the percentages of patients surviving five years post diagnosis, between patients from least socio-economically deprived areas (the richest 20% of the population) and most deprived areas (the poorest 20% of the population). For example, the five-year survival rate for males with colon cancer from the least deprived socio-economic areas was 5.7% higher than for those from the most deprived areas. The study focused on 20 types of cancer (only common cancers are shown here). Overall, the association between higher deprivation and lower survival rates was strong, although in a few cases, less deprived groups had lower five-year survival rates than more deprived (e.g. women with pancreatic cancer, men with brain cancer).

Source: Coleman *et al.*, 2004.

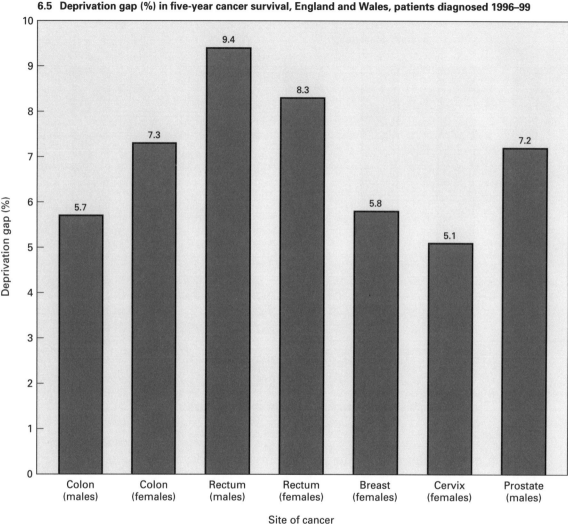

6.5 Deprivation gap (%) in five-year cancer survival, England and Wales, patients diagnosed 1996–99

The Quest for Quality in the NHS: a chartbook on quality of care in the UK

Chart 6.6 Avoidable admissions by deprivation

The Quest for Quality in the NHS: a chartbook on quality of care in the UK

These charts show the relationship between levels of deprivation and rates of admission for two potentially avoidable adverse health events in England in 2002–03. High quality primary care should reduce admissions for chronic conditions such as asthma and diabetes (Giuffrida *et al.* 1999). Asthma admissions and diabetic amputations may reflect suboptimal outpatient care or poor patient compliance or both. The charts show an association between poor outcomes and deprivation; rates of asthma-related hospital admis-sions and diabetes-related amputations in the two most deprived quintiles are above the standardised rate for England as a whole. The extent to which the variation in admissions between deprivation quintiles is affected by differences in prevalence is not known. To set the data in context, in England in 2002–03 there were a total of 345 932 admissions with at least one diagnosis of asthma; and 4313 lower leg amputations in patients with a diagnosis of diabetes.

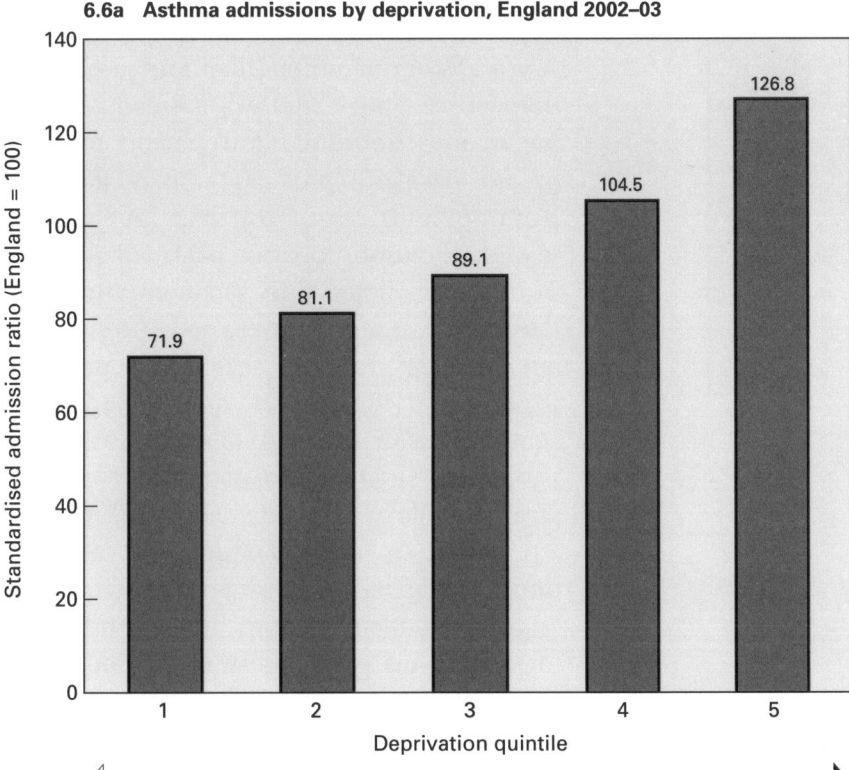

6.6a Asthma admissions by deprivation, England 2002–03

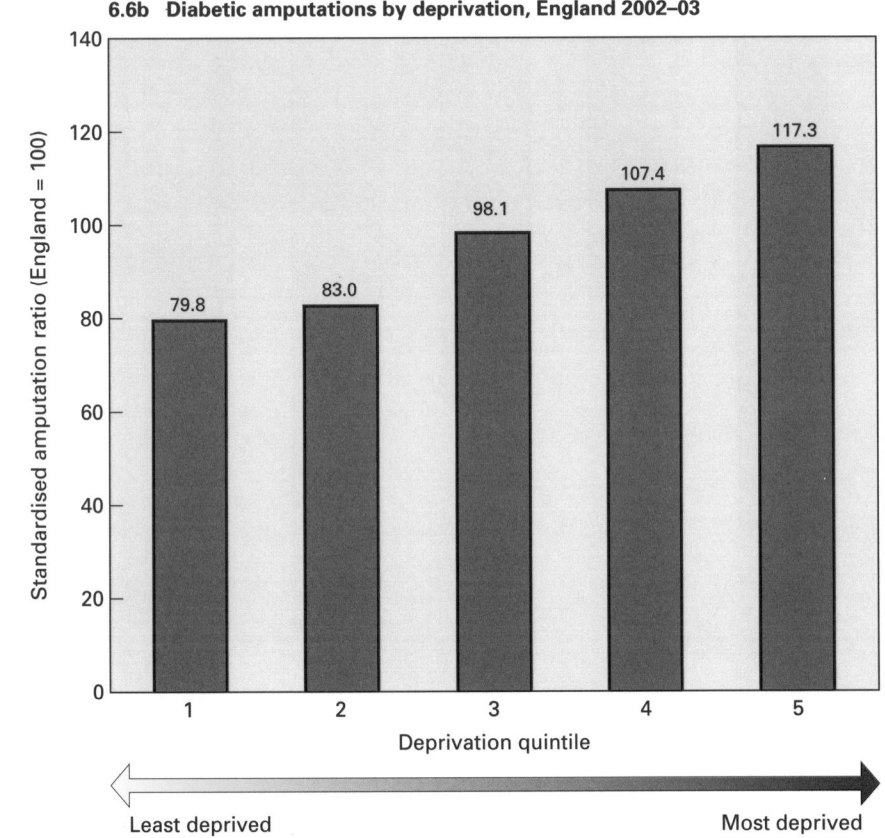

6.6b Diabetic amputations by deprivation, England 2002–03

Source: DH, Healthcare Commission (analysis by Raleigh, Sims, Irons).

Source: DH, Healthcare Commission (analysis by Raleigh, Sims, Irons).

Chart 6.7 Diabetic control in children by deprivation

See Diabetes pp35–8

Glycated haemoglobin (HbA1c) provides a measure of average blood sugar over the 60 to 90 days preceding the test. NICE clinical guidelines for type 1 (insulin dependent) diabetes recommend that the HbA1c level should be less than 7.5%.* This chart draws on 2002 audit data for 11 696 children under 16 years of age with type 1 diabetes in England, Wales, Northern Ireland and Jersey. Diabetic control, in general, did not comply with the NICE guidelines. Patients from more deprived areas had slightly poorer control than other groups, although the mean HbA1c for the most deprived group was only 0.3% higher than the mean for the least deprived. In all groups, even the most advantaged, there is a substantial gap between the target and actual HbA1c levels.

Source: National Paediatric Diabetes Audit, 2004.

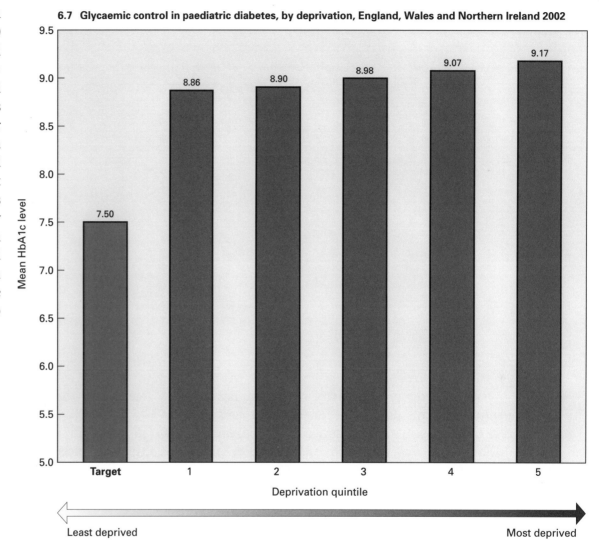

6.7 Glycaemic control in paediatric diabetes, by deprivation, England, Wales and Northern Ireland 2002

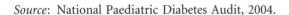

Least deprived   Most deprived

The Quest for Quality in the NHS: a chartbook on quality of care in the UK

* However, NICE notes that targets should be individualised to the lowest achievable HbA1c without causing severe hypoglycaemia.

147

The Quest for Quality in the NHS: a chartbook on quality of care in the UK

Disparities in healthcare services

Equity, one of the founding principles of the NHS, remains an explicit priority today. An equitable system provides health services to a consistent standard, on the basis of individual patients' particular medical and psychosocial needs rather than personal or demographic characteristics unrelated to their health status. The availability and quality of care should not differ because of characteristics such as gender, race, age, ethnicity, income, education, disability, sexual orientation or place of residence.

Differences in the extent to which patients receive appropriate healthcare services may be explained by a number of factors, including

- inconsistent provision of care on the basis of criteria other than clinical need
- unequal geographic distribution of resources and/or other barriers to convenience of access
- reluctance on the part of patients to seek care, as a result of individual preferences, social and cultural influences, or a perceived inability to cover any anticipated costs.

Chart 6.8 Anticipated costs as a barrier to care

The 2004 Commonwealth Fund International Health Policy Survey, which focused on primary care, asked: *During the past 12 months, was there a time when you had a medical problem but did not visit a doctor because of the medical care costs of the doctor's visit?* Data for the entire sample from each country is shown, alongside data from a subset of respondents, those with below-average income. The results are striking in their variation across countries. In the UK, despite the aforementioned problems with health inequalities, patients encounter few cost barriers in visiting a doctor. Further, the UK has the smallest difference between overall responses and those from respondents with below-average income, indicating that income disparity has little impact on primary care visits.

Source: Commonwealth Fund, 2004.

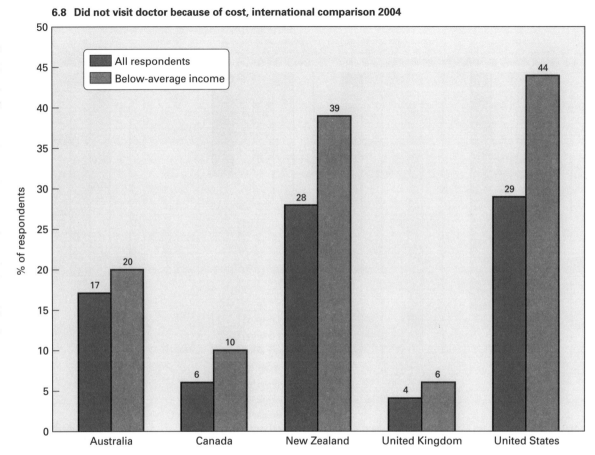

6.8 Did not visit doctor because of cost, international comparison 2004

Chart 6.9 Cost-related barriers to medical, pharmaceutical or dental care

The Quest for Quality in the NHS: a chartbook on quality of care in the UK

Internationally, cost is a frequent factor in inhibiting equitable access to medical care when needed. These charts array data from the patients' perspective regarding cost-related barriers to care. Chart 6.9a shows that UK patients perceived fewer cost barriers to accessing tests or treatments compared to patients in other countries (particularly the US). However, more than two in five UK patients indicated that they had not filled a prescription or had skipped doses because of cost concerns, and about one in five indicated that cost was an issue for dental care. Chart 6.9b shows data from respondents with below-average income only. Comparing across the two charts, the UK has the smallest difference between all respondents and those with below-average income (i.e. the UK had the smallest cost-related barriers) in accessing recommended medical tests and dental treatment.

6.9a Cost-related barriers to healthcare, all respondents, international comparison 2004

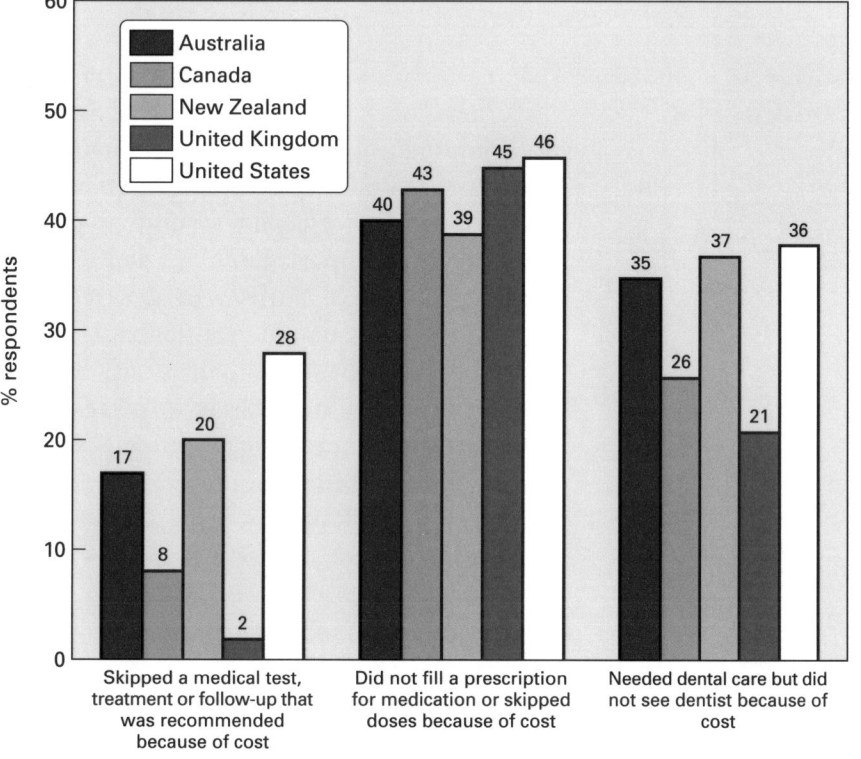

Source: Commonwealth Fund, 2004.

6.9b Cost-related barriers to healthcare, below-average income, international comparison 2004

Source: Commonwealth Fund, 2004.

Chart 6.10 Influenza vaccination rates by deprivation

See Infectious diseases pp39–40

This data, drawn from NHS Trusts in England in 2003, shows that 71% of people over 65 years of age were vaccinated against influenza. When coverage rates are arrayed by levels of deprivation, a slight discrepancy emerges; more deprived areas achieve a lower vaccination rate. However, a difference of just 4% between the lowest and highest quintiles of deprivation could be interpreted as a relatively positive finding and an indication of the equity of service provision in the NHS.

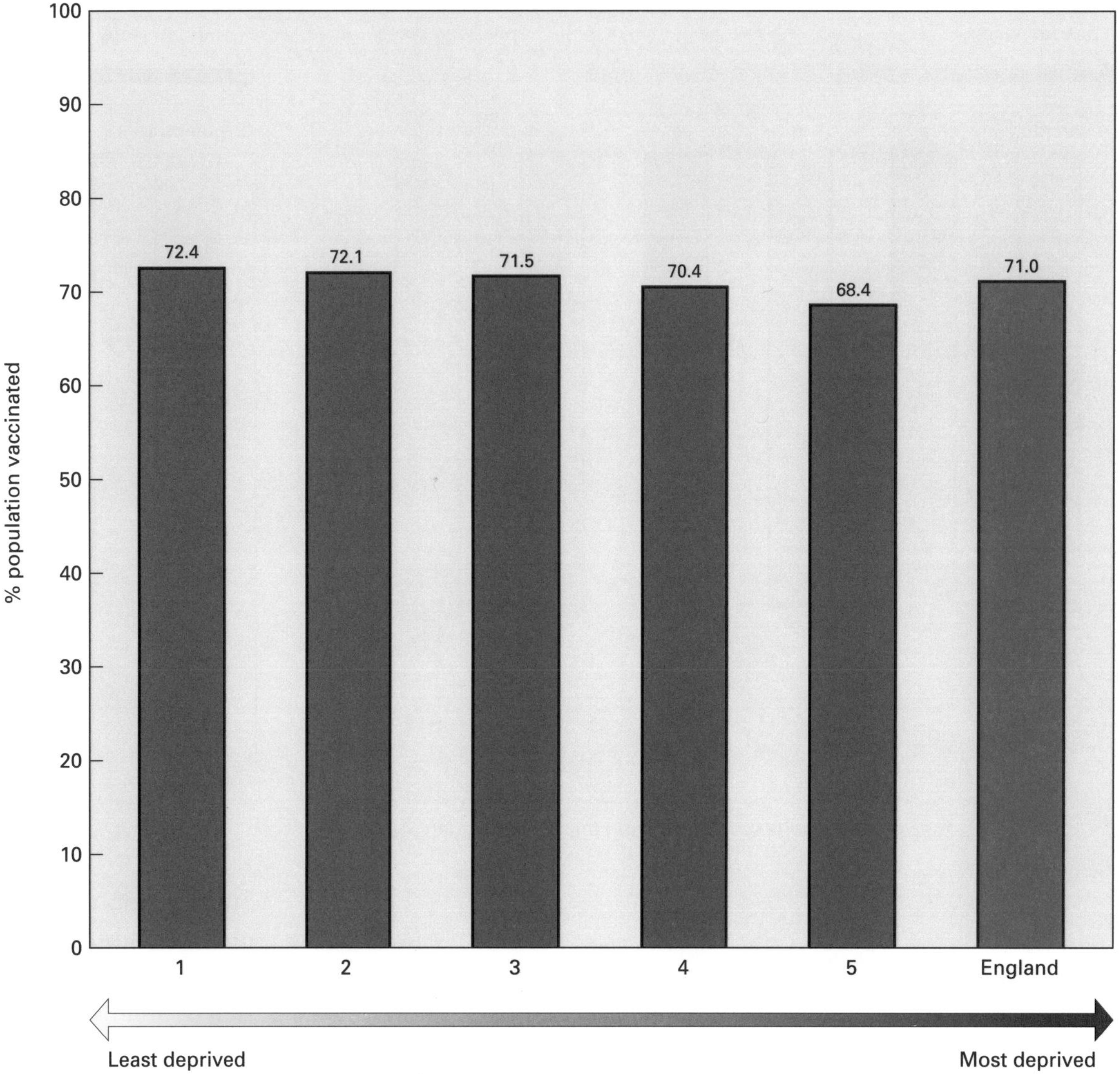

Source: DH, Healthcare Commission (analysis by Raleigh, Irons, Sims).

6.10 Influenza vaccination rate (people > 65 years) by deprivation, England 2003

Quintile	% population vaccinated
1	72.4
2	72.1
3	71.5
4	70.4
5	68.4
England	71.0

% population vaccinated

Least deprived → Most deprived

Chart 6.11 Cancer screening rates by deprivation

The Quest for Quality in the NHS: a chartbook on quality of care in the UK

These charts indicate that women from more deprived areas are less likely to receive recommended screening for cancer than those of more affluent areas. In the case of breast cancer screening (Chart 6.11a), the difference in uptake between the least and most deprived is 7.2%; for cervical cancer screening (Chart 6.11b) the difference in uptake is 4.1%. Small differentials between deprivation quintiles are an indicator of equitable provision of care. Nevertheless, lower rates of uptake in preventive health interventions such as cancer screening have important, but as yet unquantified, implications for the health of people living in the most challenging socio-economic conditions in England.

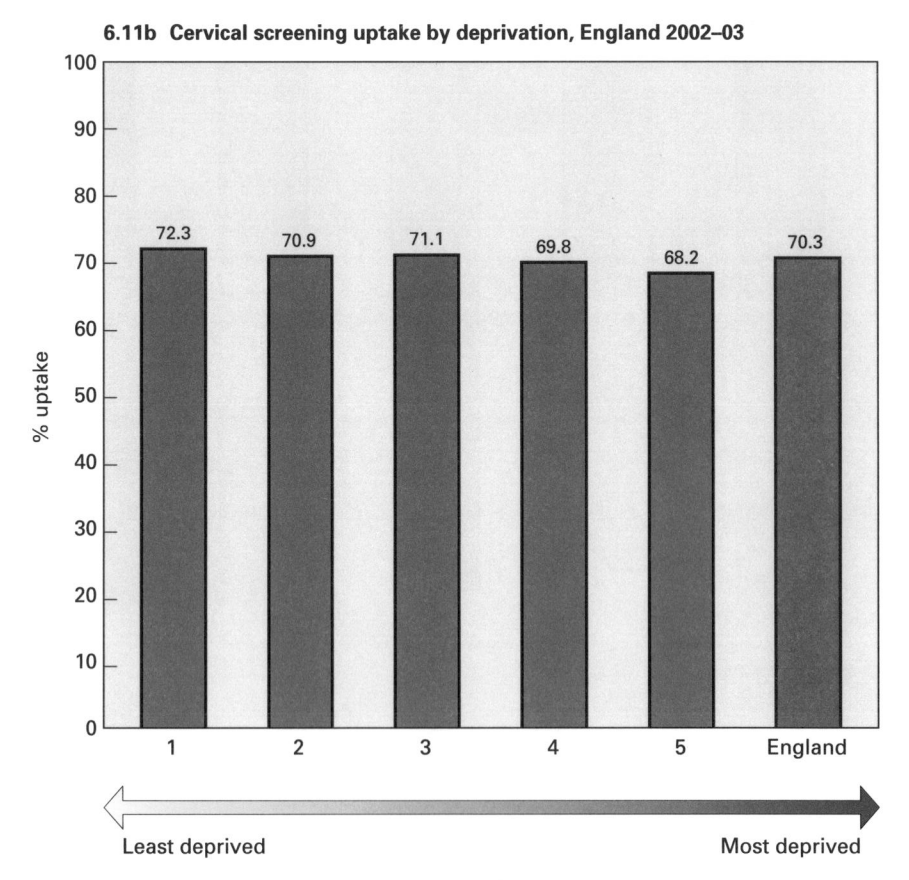

6.11a Breast cancer screening uptake by deprivation, England 2002–03

6.11b Cervical screening uptake by deprivation, England 2002–03

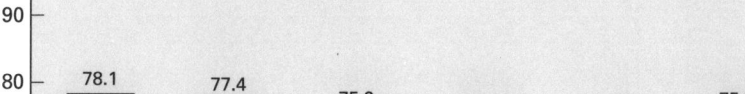

Source: DH, Healthcare Commission (analysis by Raleigh, Irons and Sims).

Source: DH, Healthcare Commission (analysis by Raleigh, Irons and Sims).

Chart 6.12 Socio-economic deprivation and heart failure: incidence, consultations and survival

See Coronary heart disease (CHD) p19

In a study of 2186 adults with heart failure in 53 general practices in Scotland, age- and sex-standardised incidence of heart failure increased with deprivation. Further, more deprived patients saw their GPs less frequently and had lower estimated survival times than less deprived patients. Prescribing data was available for 1007 patients with heart failure (439 men and 568 women). Prescribing rates (for diuretics, beta-blockers, angiotensin-converting enzyme (ACE) inhibitors, digoxin and spironolactone) did not differ across socio-economic gradients. No data was available on the proportion of prescriptions that were actually filled but, as Chart 6.9 shows, many patients do not fill prescriptions or skip doses because of cost concerns.

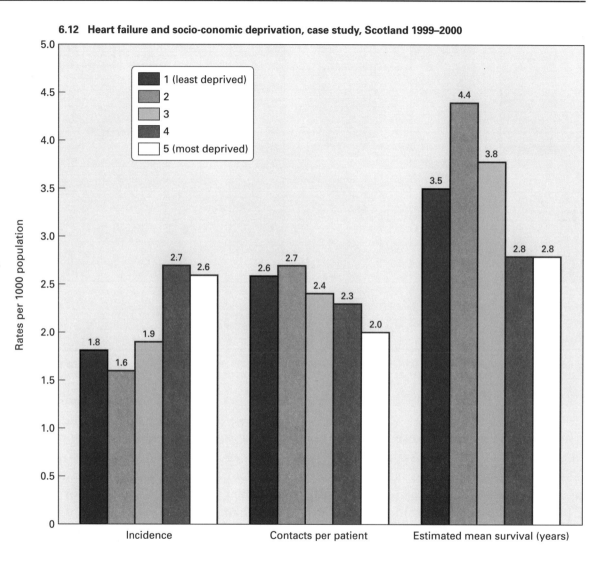

6.12   Heart failure and socio-conomic deprivation, case study, Scotland 1999–2000

Legend:
- 1 (least deprived)
- 2
- 3
- 4
- 5 (most deprived)

Rates per 1000 population

Incidence: 1.8, 1.6, 1.9, 2.7, 2.6
Contacts per patient: 2.6, 2.7, 2.4, 2.3, 2.0
Estimated mean survival (years): 3.5, 4.4, 3.8, 2.8, 2.8

Source: McAlister *et al.* (2004).

The Quest for Quality in the NHS: a chartbook on quality of care in the UK

Chart 6.13 Gender-based disparities in revascularisation rates in patients ≥ 65 years

See Coronary heart disease (CHD) p19
Revascularisation pp27–9

These charts draw on a recently published study into gender disparity in the treatment of coronary heart disease. Based on retrospective analysis of Government health databases for 1997–99, the study found that, in both England and the US, women were consistently less likely than men to undergo revascularisation procedures. Rates of coronary artery bypass graft (CABG) surgery per acute myocardial infarction (AMI or heart attack), a measure that controls for differences in incidence of heart disease, were around twice as high for men as for women in both countries. Rates of coronary angioplasty (PTCA) procedures per AMI were one and a half times higher in English men and two and a half times higher in American men than in women in the two countries, respectively. The data also highlights the differences between revascularisation rates in England and the US, a finding corroborated by data shown in Chart 1.19.

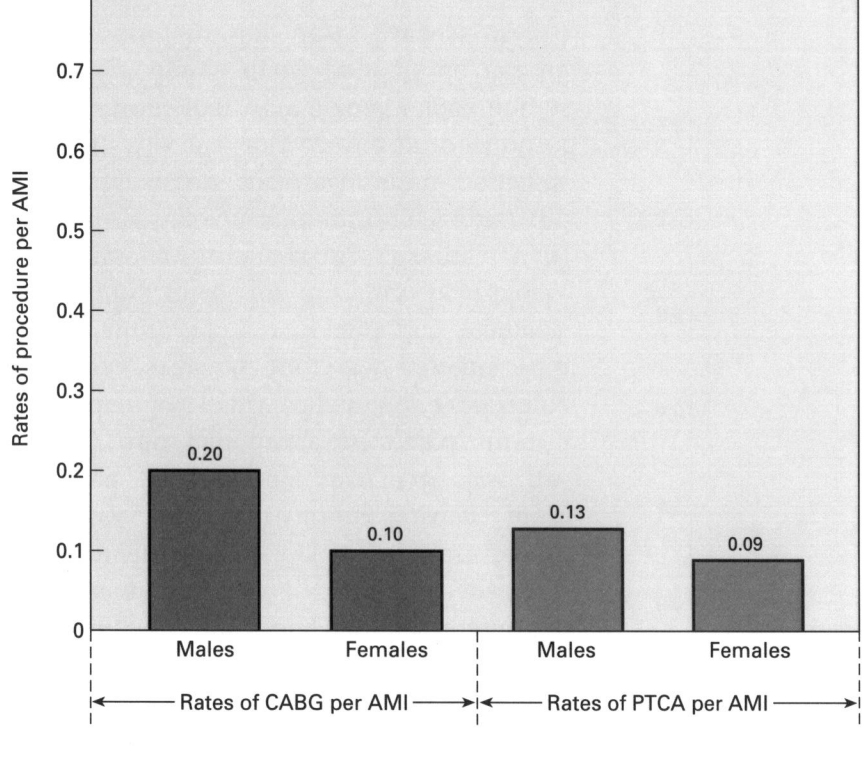

6.13a Rates of revascularisation in men and women, England 1997–99

Source: Weisz *et al.*, 2004.

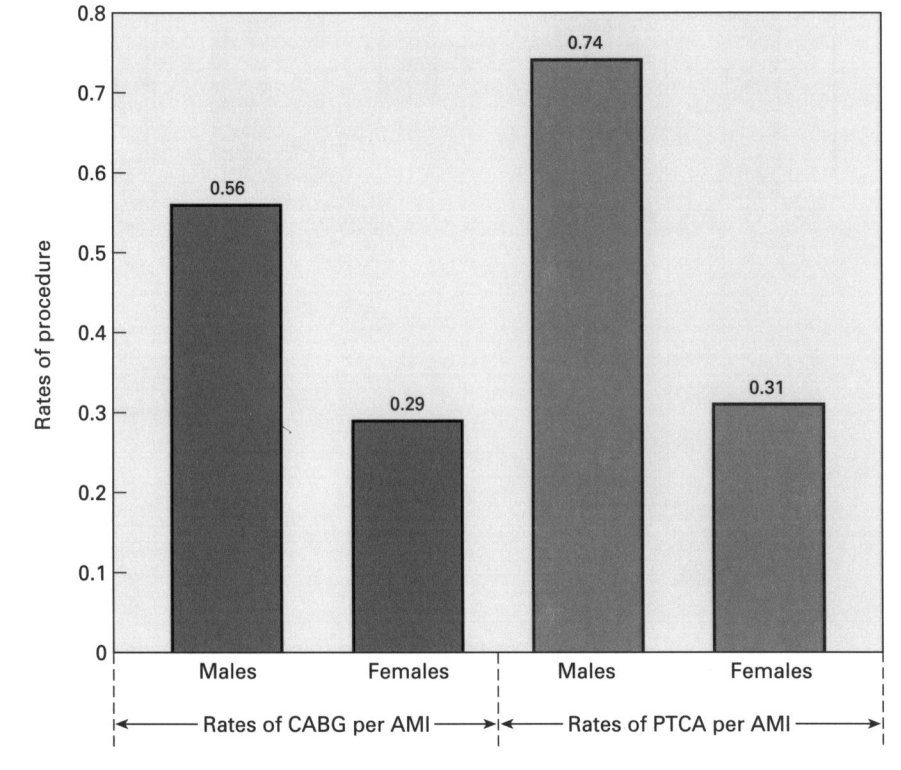

6.13b Rates of revascularisation in men and women, United States 1997–99

Source: Weisz *et al.*, 2004.

The Quest for Quality in the NHS: a chartbook on quality of care in the UK

Chart 6.14 Prescribing for older people

Some studies suggests that older patients receive suboptimal care both in terms of underuse of beneficial treatments (Dudley *et al.*, 2002; Fahey *et al.*, 2003; Reid *et al.*, 2002; Hippisley-Cox *et al.*, 2001) and of overuse of treatments, particularly excessive prescribing (RCP, 1997). However, the studies we found that measured the differences in care given to different age groups in the UK used data that was about five years old on publication.* This chart does not catalogue differences in care between different age groups, but instead provides a picture of the standard of care provided to older patients. The chart is based on clinical audits of 100 consecutive medical inpatients aged ≥ 65 years admitted to 62 hospitals in England in 1999 and in 2000. One in 10 patients were put at risk of paracetamol overdose (> 4000 mg/day); fewer than half of the patients receiving benzodiazepines (a class of sedatives) were being prescribed them appropriately. More than one-third of prescriptions written on an 'as required' [PRN] basis did not have a maximum frequency recorded, contravening British National Formulary guidance and creating the potential for overdose. More positively, more than 90% of patients with angina were receiving aspirin appropriately.

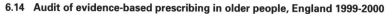
6.14 **Audit of evidence-based prescribing in older people, England 1999-2000**

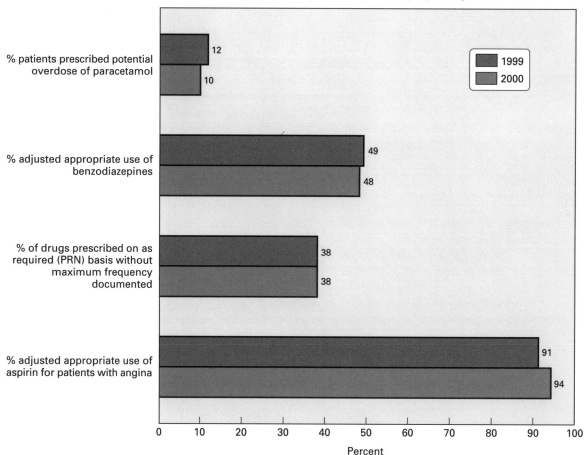

Source: *National Sentinel Clinical Audit for Evidence-based Prescribing for Older People* (Batty, 2003, 2004); Royal College of Physicians.

The Quest for Quality in the NHS: a chartbook on quality of care in the UK

---

* For example, the clinical literature contains numerous studies focused on age discrimination in the treatment of CHD, in particular the use of statins (e.g. Majeed *et al.*, 2000; Reid, *et al.* 2002; DeWilde *et al.*, 2003). However, the available studies draw on data from 1998 or before and, as Chart 1.22 shows, statin usage has increased significantly since that time. Lacking data on any changes in prescribing patterns across age groups over the same time period, we have not charted the findings emanating from those studies.

References

Acheson D (1998) *Independent Inquiry into Inequalities in Health.* The Stationery Office, London. Available online at: www.archive.official-documents.co.uk/document/doh/ih/ih.htm [last accessed 2 February 2005].

Alison WP (1840) *Observations on the Management of the Poor in Scotland and its Effect on the Health in the Great Towns.* Bell, Edinburgh.

Batty GM, Grant RL, Aggarwal R, Lowe D, Potter JM, Pearson MG and Jackson SH (2003) Using prescribing indicators to measure the quality of prescribing to elderly medical in-patients. *Age Ageing.* 32(3): 292–8.

Batty GM, Grant RL, Aggarwal R *et al.* (2004) National Clinical Sentinel Audit of Evidence-based Prescribing for Older People. *Journal of Evaluation in Clinical Practice.* 10(2): 273–9.

Blamey A, Hanlon P, Judge K and Muirie J (eds) (2002) *Health Inequalities in the New Scotland.* Public Health Institute of Scotland, Glasgow. Available online at: www.dph.gla.ac.uk/hppu/publns/HealthInequalitiesReport.pdf [last accessed 2 February 2005].

Bull J, Mulvihill C and Quigley R (2003) *Prevention of Low Birth Weight: assessing the effectiveness of smoking cessation and nutritional interventions.* HDA Evidence briefing. Health Development Agency, London. Available online at: www.hda-online.org.uk/documents/low_birth_weight_summary.pdf [last accessed 2 February 2005].

CEEU (2001) *National Sentinel Clinical Audit for Evidence-based Prescribing for Older People.* Clinical Effectiveness and Evaluation Unit, Royal College of Physicians, London. Available online at: www.rcplondon.ac.uk/college/ceeu/ceeu_ebpop_report.pdf [last accessed 2 February 2005].

Chadwick E (1882) *A Report on the Sanitary Conditions of the Labouring Population in Scotland.* The Poor Law Commission, London.

Coleman MP, Rachet B, Woods LM, Mitry E, Riga M, Cooper N, Quinn MJ, Brenner H and Esteve J (2004) Trends and socioeconomic inequalities in cancer survival in England and Wales up to 2001. *Br J Cancer.* 90(7): 1367–73.

Commonwealth Fund (2004) *International Health Policy Survey of Adults' Experiences with Primary Care.* Commonwealth Fund, New York.

Department of Health (1998) *Smoking Kills: a white paper on tobacco.* The Stationery Office, London. Available online at: www.archive.official-documents.co.uk/document/cm41/4177/4177.htm [last accessed 2 February 2005].

Department of Health (1999) *Saving Lives: our healthier nation.* The Stationery Office, London. Available online at: www.archive.official-documents.co.uk/document/cm43/4386/4386.htm [last accessed 2 February 2005].

Department of Health (2000) *The NHS Plan: a plan for investment, a plan for reform.* The Stationery Office, London. Available online at: www.dh.gov.uk/assetRoot/04/05/57/83/04055783.pdf [last accessed 2 February 2005].

Department of Health (2003) *Tackling Health Inequalities: a programme for action.* The Stationery Office, London. Available online at: www.dh.gov.uk/assetRoot/04/01/93/62/04019362.pdf [last accessed 2 February 2005].

Department of Health (2004) *Choosing Health: making healthier choices easier.* The Stationery Office, London. Available online at: www.dh.gov.uk/PublicationsAndStatistics/Publications/PublicationsPolicyAndGuidance/PublicationsPolicyAndGuidanceArticle/fs/en?CONTENT_ID=4094550&chk=aN5Cor [last accessed 2 February 2005].

Department of Health, Social Services and Public Safety (2001) *New Targeting Social Need: action plan.* DHSSPS, Belfast. Available online at: www.dhsspsni.gov.uk/publications/archived/2001/tsneeds.pdf [last accessed 2 February 2004].

Department of Health, Social Services and Public Safety (2002) *Investing for Health.* DHSSPS, Belfast. Available online at: www.dhsspsni.gov.uk/publications/2002/invest1.pdf [last accessed 2 February 2005].

DeWilde S, Carey IM, Bremner SA *et al.* (2003) Evolution of statin prescribing 1994–2001: a case of ageism but not of sexism? *Heart.* 89: 417–21.

Dudley NJ, Bowling A, Bond M *et al.* (2002) Age- and sex-related bias in the management of heart disease in a district general hospital. *Age and Ageing.* 31: 37–42.

Fahey T, Montgomery AA, Barnes J *et al.* (2003) Quality of care for elderly residents in nursing homes and elderly people living at home: controlled observational study. *BMJ.* 326: 580–84.

Giuffrida A, Gravelle H and Roland M (1999) Measuring quality of care with routine data: avoiding confusion between performance indicators and health outcomes. *BMJ.* 319(7202): 94–8.

Hamlyn B, Brooker S, Oleinikova *et al.* (2002) *Infant Feeding 2000.* The Stationery Office, London. Available online at: www.dh.gov.uk/assetRoot/04/05/97/63/04059763.pdf [last accessed 2 February 2005].

Hippisley-Cox J, Pringle M, Crown N *et al.* (2001) Sex inequalities in ischaemic heart disease in general practice: cross sectional survey. *BMJ.* 322: 832–7.

HM Treasury (2002) *Public Service Agreement.* HM Treasury, London. Available online at: www.hm-treasury.gov.uk/Spending_Review/spend_sr02/psa/spend_sr02_psaindex.cfm [last accessed 2 February 2005].

Kunst A and Mackenbach J (1999) *Measuring Socioeconomic Inequalities in Health*. WHO Europe, Copenhagen. Available online at: www.euro.who.int/Document/PAE/Measrpd416.pdf [last accessed 2 February 2005].

Majeed A, Moser K and Maxwell R (2000) Age, sex and practice variations in the use of statins in general practice in England and Wales. *Journal of Public Health Medicine*. 22(3): 275–9.

McAlister FA, Murphy NF, Simpson CR *et al.* (2004) Influence of socioeconomic deprivation on the primary care burden and treatment of patients with a diagnosis of heart failure in general practice in Scotland: a population based study. *BMJ*. 328: 1110 (originally published online 23 April 2004 doi.1136/bmj.38043.414074.EE).

Morrisson C (2002) *Health, Education and Poverty Reduction*. OECD, Policy Brief 19. Available online at: www.oecd.org/dataoecd/59/57/1851366.pdf [last accessed 2 February 2005].

National Paediatric Diabetes Audit (2004) *Results from the Audit Year 2002*. Diabetes UK. Available online at: www.diabetes.org.uk/audit/downloads/PaediatricAuditReport.pdf [last accessed 2 February 2005].

Reid FD, Cook DG and Whincup PH (2002) Use of statins in the secondary prevention of coronary heart disease: is treatment equitable? *Heart*. 88(1):15.

Royal College of Physicians (1997) *Medication for Older People* (2e). Royal College of Physicians, London.

The Scottish Office (1999) *Towards a Healthier Scotland – A White Paper on Health*. The Stationery Office, Edinburgh. Available online at: www.scotland.gov.uk/library/documents-w7/tahs-00.htm [last accessed 2 February 2005].

Smedley BD, Stith AY and Nelson AR (eds) (2003) *Unequal Treatment: confronting racial and ethnic disparities*. National Academies Press, Washington, DC.

Stevens-Simon C and Orleans M (1999) Low birthweight prevention programs: the enigma of failure. *Birth*. 26: 184–91.

Weisz D, Gusmano MK and Rodwin VG (2004) Gender and the treatment of heart disease in older persons in the United States, France and England: a comparative, population-based view of a clinical phenomenon. *Gender Medicine*. 1 (1): 29–40.

Welsh Office (1998) *Better Health, Better Wales*. The Stationery Office, London. Available online at: www.archive.official-documents.co.uk/document/cm39/3922/3922.htm [last accessed 2 February 2005].

World Health Organization (2000) Inequalities in health. *WHO Bulletin*. (Special Issue) 78: 1–152.

6 Disparities

Chart 1.1 Mortality from causes considered amenable to healthcare

Age-standardised rates per 100 000 population, age 0–74.

Chart 1.1a Source data from national statistics. European data published in Nolte and McKee, 2004; Australian data in Korda and Butler, 2004. For list of ISD codes included in causes of death considered amenable to health, refer to Nolte and McKee (2004: p66). Data including and excluding ischaemic heart disease (IHD) is shown because IHD is considered amenable to healthcare. However, because of the high incidence of IHD, its inclusion can obscure the effects of other diseases.

Chart 1.1b Source data from ONS, analysis from NCHOD.
www.nuffieldtrust.org.uk/policy_themes/docs/avoidablemortality.pdf
http://nceph.anu.edu.au/Publications/Working_Papers/WP49.pdf

Chart 1.2 Cancer mortality rates: international comparison

Includes all ages. The number of deaths according to sex and selected causes are extracted from the World Health Organization Mortality Database. Age-standardised death rates per 100 000 population for selected causes are calculated by the OECD Secretariat, using the total OECD population for 1980 as the reference population. Malignant neoplasms are coded C00-C97 in *OECD Health Data 2004* and Tenth revision of the International Classification of Diseases.

Chart 1.3 Mortality rates from common cancers, UK

Data from ONS, age-standardised to European Standard Population.
www.statistics.gov.uk/StatBase/Expodata/Spreadsheets/D7461.xls

Chart 1.4 Premature deaths from cancer: progress against a target, England

Age-standardised using European standard population; three-year rolling averages (to smooth any anomalous years); people under 75. ICD-9 data for 1995 to 1998 and 2000 have been adjusted to be comparable with ICD-10 data for 1999 and 2001 onwards.
www.dh.gov.uk/assetRoot/04/08/35/76/04083576.pdf

Chart 1.5 Five-year relative survival rates for common cancers

England and Wales data (*see* for confidence intervals): www.statistics.gov.uk/statbase/ssdataset.asp?vlnk=7091
Scotland data: www.isdscotland.org/isd/files/Survival_summary_7701.pdf

Chart 1.6 Breast cancer mortality rates

Age-standardised to an OECD standard 1980 population using the direct method.
www.cmwf.org/publications/publications_show.htm?doc_id=227628

Chart 1.7 Breast cancer survival and screening rates

Data on breast cancer screening differed as shown in table below.

	Age of screened population	Screened within	Year of data
Australia	50–69	Past 2 years	2001 (survey)
Canada	50–69	Past 2 years	2000–01 (survey)
England	50–64	Past 3 years	1999–2001 (programme)
New Zealand	50–64	Past 3 years	2001 (programme)
United States	40+	Past 2 years	1999 (survey)

Survival rate data was for slightly different time frames: Australia (1992–97); Canada (1992–97); England (1993/95–1998/2000); New Zealand (1992–97); United States (1992–97).
www.cmwf.org/publications/publications_show.htm?doc_id=227628
Intra-UK data from ONS. Data for NI 2000 differs from that shown in Regional Trends tables as the data for that year referred to uptake rather than coverage. 'Uptake' refers to the percentage of women invited for screening who attend. This figure differs from 'coverage' which is the percentage of eligible women who have been screened.
www.statistics.gov.uk/downloads/theme_compendia/regional_trends_2001/rt36.pdf
www.statistics.gov.uk/StatBase/Product.asp?vlnk=836&Pos=&ColRank=1&Rank=422

Chart 1.8 Colorectal cancer mortality rates

1.8a Data for Canada and New Zealand are from 1998, not 1999. There may be some differences between countries in attribution of mortality to colorectal cancer versus other causes.
www.cmwf.org/publications/publications_show.htm?doc_id=227628
1.8b Data from ONS, published by Cancer Research UK.
www.cancerresearchuk.org/aboutcancer/statistics/statsmisc/pdfs/factsheet_bowel_apr2004.pdf

Chart 1.9 Colorectal cancer survival rates: Scotland

ICD-9 153-154; ICD-10 C18-C21. Rates are directly standardised to the World Standard Cancer Patient Population. Cases diagnosed 1999–2001 do not have five years' follow-up and cases diagnosed in 1994–2001 do not have 10 years' follow-up. Data extracted August 2004.

www.isdscotland.org/isd/files/cancer_colorectal_surv7701.xls

Chart 1.10 Childhood leukaemia survival rates

Observed rates. Data for Australia from 1992–97; Canada 1992–97; England and Wales 1991–95 to 1996–2000; New Zealand 1994–99; US 1992–98.

www.cmwf.org/publications/publications_show.htm?doc_id=227628

Chart 1.11 Circulatory disease mortality rates

1.11a OECD data from Health Data 2004. The number of deaths according to sex and selected causes are extracted from the World Health Organization Mortality Database.

Age-standardised death rates per 100 000 population for selected causes are calculated by the OECD Secretariat, using the total OECD population for 1980 as the reference population.

1.11b ONS data is for all ages and has been age-standardised using the European standard population. Standardised rates, and International Classification of Diseases. Data for 2000 are for England and Wales only.

www.statistics.gov.uk/StatBase/ssdataset.asp?vlnk=7433&Pos=3&ColRank=2&-Rank=272

Chart 1.12 Premature deaths from circulatory disease: progress against a target, England

Age-standardised using European standard population; three-year rolling averages (to smooth any anomalous years); people under 75.

www.dh.gov.uk/assetRoot/04/08/35/76/04083576.pdf

Chart 1.13 Mortality from coronary heart disease

Age-standardised using the European standard population; persons aged 35–74 years. Data from WHO Mortality Database. Data for France, Germany, Australia, Sweden and US from 1999; UK data from 2000.

www.heartstats.org/temp/Mortalityspchapter.pdf

Chart 1.14 Coronary heart disease mortality rates: UK time series

Data from ONS, published by heartstats.org.uk. Age-standardised using the European standard population.

www.heartstats.org/temp/Mortalityspchapter.pdf

Chart 1.15 Explaining the decline in CHD mortality

Used IMPACT mortality model to combine and analyse data on uptake and effectiveness of cardiological treatments and risk factor trends.

From Unal *et al.*, 2004.

Chart 1.16 Mortality from acute myocardial infarction

Age-standardised to the OECD population in 1980. Canada and New Zealand data are for 1998 not 1999.

www.cmwf.org/publications/publications_show.htm?doc_id=227628

Chart 1.17 Managing acute AMI
Chart 1.18 Thrombolysis rates after AMI

MINAP is coordinated by the Clinical Effectiveness and Evaluation Unit of the Royal College of Physicians. Based on data from: 214 hospitals in England in 2002; 210 hospitals in England in 2003; 210 hospitals in England and 17 hospitals in Wales in 2004.

www.rcplondon.ac.uk/pubs/books/minap04/HowHospitalsManageHeartAttacks June2004.pdf

Chart 1.19 Revascularisation rates and mortality from heart disease: international comparison

Age-standardised death rates per 100 000 population are calculated using the total OECD population for 1980 as the reference population. CABG data from the US is from 1999.

Chart 1.20 Appropriateness of revascularisations

Prospective study of consecutive patients undergoing coronary angiography at three London hospitals. Data was collected on patients undergoing elective or emergency coronary angiography between April 1996 and April 1997. A total of 2552 patients were followed for a median of 30 months after angiography. Before patients were recruited, a 9-member panel rated the appropriateness of PTCA and CABG on a 9-point scale (1 = highly inappropriate; 9 = highly appropriate) for specific clinical indicators. These ratings were then applied to a population of patients with coronary artery disease. The patients were treated without regard to the ratings.

Chart 1.21 Deaths following CABG, England

Indirectly age, sex and method of admission standardised rates of deaths within 30 days of a coronary artery bypass graft (CABG), per 100 000 patients of all ages (includes deaths in hospital and after discharge). For first CABG (OPCS4 K40-K46), except after PTCA (K49-K50 other than K50.2, K50.3) and/or alongside heart valve procedure (K25-K38)

Chart 1.22 Statin use in Europe

Rate use in defined daily doses/1000 population per day. Data sources were governmental or major insurance or sickness funds.

www.dhsspsni.gov.uk/publications/2004/COMPARATIVE_DATA_12MAY04.pdf

Chart 1.23 Stroke mortality rates

1.23a All rates were age-standardised to the OECD population in 1980. Australia data is for 2001; England 2001; New Zealand 1999; US 1999. Diagnosis codes: Australia used ICD-10-AM163 and i64. UK, New Zealand and the US used ICD-9 433, 434 and 436.

www.cmwf.org/publications/publications_show.htm?doc_id=227628

1.23b Trends in mortality from stroke (underlying cause ICD-9 430-438 adjusted, ICD-10 I60-I69). Directly standardised rates (and 95% confidence intervals), 1993 to 2003 annually, ages under 75 years (rates are presented per 100 000 European Standard Population).

www.isdscotland.org/isd/files/m2.xls

Chart 1.24 Mortality from diabetes

DH Mortality Extracts 1993–2003, ONS; Mid-Year Population Estimates 1993–2003, ONS. Rates produced by NCHOD.

Chart 1.25 Diabetic control in children

1.25a The number of children aged (0–16 yrs) with diabetes in 2002 was estimated at: England 1.62 per 1000; Wales 1.80 per 1000; Northern Ireland 2.08 per 1000 (Paediatric Diabetes Audit). Chart draws on audit data from 11 696 children under 16 years of age with type 1 (insulin dependent) diabetes in England, Wales, Northern Ireland and Jersey. If a target figure of ≤ 9.0 is used instead of 7.5, the achievement rate increases to 60%.

1.25b Emergency admissions were identified from Scottish Morbidity Records (SMR01). Emergency admissions occurring between 1 April 1993 and 31 March 2003 were included.

www.diabetes.org.uk/audit/downloads/PaediatricAuditReport.pdf
www.show.scot.nhs.uk/indicators/Outcomes/2004_Health_Indicators_Report.pdf

Chart 1.26 Measures indicating poor diabetic control

Source of data: Hospital Episodes Statistics. Indirectly age and sex standardised rates of admissions to hospital per 100 000 persons of all ages. Rates are standardised to the Person – England rate for 2000–01. 1.26a Any diagnosis – ICD-10 codes: E10-E14 with 4th digit codes .0 and .1 only. 1.26b Any diagnosis – ICD-10 codes: E10-E14, Any Procedure – OPCS4 codes: X09, X10, X11.

Chart 1.27 Influenza vaccinations (for people > 65 yrs)

The Commonwealth Fund 2004 survey focused on primary care experiences among adults and consisted of telephone interviews with random, representative samples of people aged 18 and older: AUS 1400; CAN 1410; NZ 1400; UK 3061; US 1401. The margin of sampling error is approximately plus or minus three percentage points for differences between countries and plus or minus two percentage points for country averages at the 95% confidence level. Poststratification weights were applied in each country to adjust for variations between the sample demographics and known population parameters. Analysis compared responses between or within countries using t-tests and chi-square tests.

www.cmwf.org/surveys/surveys_list.htm?attrib_id=9121&attrib_filter=1

Communicable Disease Surveillance Centre reports that in 2003–04, 71% of people aged 65 or over England & Wales received influenza vaccination.

www.publications.doh.gov.uk/public/sb0416tables.xls

Chart 1.28 Childhood vaccinations by age two

Chart 1.28a shows average vaccination rates across the different diseases. Data drawn from Health Protection Agency.

www.hpa.org.uk/infections/topics_az/vaccination/vac_coverage.htm
Based on UK country datasets:
www.dh.gov.uk/assetRoot/04/09/95/78/04099578.xls
www.show.scot.nhs.uk/scieh/infectious/vaccine/table4.html
www.wales.gov.uk/keypubstatisticsforwalesheadline/content/health/2003/hdw200311272-e.htm
www.cdscni.org.uk/surveillance/Coveragestats/24months.htm

Chart 1.29 Antibiotic prescribing patterns

1.29a Data taken from Clinical Outcomes Indicators, 2004.
www.show.scot.nhs.uk/indicators/Outcomes/2004_Health_Indicators_Report.pdf

1.29b Data drawn from the General Practice Research Database (GPRD) for 1994–98. Prescribing information for 1.4 million patients, registered with 210 general practices in England and Wales, was included.

www.statistics.gov.uk/downloads/theme_health/HSQ14_v4.pdf

Chart 1.30 Suicide rates

England and Wales use a broader definition of suicide for national statistics, one that includes 'open' verdicts; the rate for all ages using that definition was 8.5. The age band in England and Wales is for 14–19 years not 15–19 years. The age band in the US is for 20–24 years not 20–29 years. Diagnosis codes ICD-9 E950-E959, except ICD-10: X60-X84 in Australia. Data is for Australia 2000; Canada 1998; England and Wales 2000; New Zealand 2000–01; US 1998.

www.cmwf.org/publications/publications_show.htm?doc_id=227628

Chart 1.31 Suicide rates: countries within the UK

The definition used for counting suicides in the UK includes those recorded as 'open verdict' deaths. This definition may include some deaths that are not suicides. However, the more inclusive definition is considered to be a more accurate reflection of the likely incidence of suicide. Codes ICD-10 E950-E959 plus E980-E989 excluding E988.8.

www.samaritans.org

Chart 1.32 Emergency psychiatric readmissions

The indicator supports the Public Service Agreement and National Priorities Guidance target to reduce nationally the psychiatric readmission rate by 2% from the 1997–98 baseline, by 2001–02.

www.publications.doh.gov.uk/paf/

Chart 1.33 Surgical outcomes, Scotland

1.33a The range of procedures included accounts for around half of all 'non-minor' elective procedures carried out in Scottish hospitals. Surgery types included are: aortic aneurysm repair, cataract extraction, cholecystectomy, colectomy, herniorrhaphy, hysterectomy, knee replacement, mastectomy, oesophagectomy, prostatectomy, total hip replacement, gastrectomy. Data was standardised for the age and sex composition of the patients operated on, and also for the Carstairs deprivation quintile of patients' postcode sector of residence. Additionally for this indicator the results are standardised for type of surgery, to take account of the fact that Trusts and hospitals perform varying proportions of higher and lower risk procedures.

1.33b The procedures included in abdominal and pelvic surgery data are: colectomy, cholecystectomy, hysterectomy, herniorrhaphy and prostatectomy. Those included in the lower limb arthroplasty set are total hip replacement, knee replacement, other hip arthroplasty, other joint replacements and arthroplasties indicating procedure on lower limb.

www.show.scot.nhs.uk/indicators/July_trends/Winter2/Main.htm

www.show.scot.nhs.uk/indicators/Outcomes/Clinical_Outcome_Indicators_Report_2003.pdf

Chart 1.34 Caesarean section rates

1.34a Data collection: 213 NHS consultant-led units, 20 NHS midwifery-led units and three private maternity hospitals. Sample size: 152 413 births May–July 2000 were audited. For information, the audit showed that in England and Wales 37% of caesarean sections are elective.

1.34b Number of caesareans defined as count of episodes where at least one procedure field = R17 or R18. Results exclude any providers with less than 10 deliveries per week. Analysis was carried out using HES2002/03.

Chart 2.1 Waiting for elective surgery: international comparison

The 1998 Commonwealth Fund International Health Policy Survey consisted of telephone interviews with adults > 18 years of age between April and June 1998. Sample sizes were Australia 1001; Canada 1006; New Zealand 999; United Kingdom 1043; and the United States 1010. The survey randomly selected an adult in each household and asked him or her a series of questions about recent personal healthcare experiences, recent use of services, health status, socio-economic status, and views or concerns about the national healthcare system.

The 2001 Commonwealth Fund International Health Policy Survey consisted of telephone interviews with adults > 18 years of age in April and May 2001. Sample sizes were AUS 1412; CAN 1400; NZ 1400; UK 1400; and the US 1401.

OECD data was taken from a report investigating waiting times in OECD countries. Data was also presented on mean waiting times. These figures were generally higher, e.g. in England, hip replacement mean waits were 244 days; cataract 281 days; CABG 213 days.

www.oecd.org/dataoecd/24/32/5162353.pdf

www.oecd.org/dataoecd/31/10/17256025.pdf

Chart 2.2 Proportion of population waiting: UK countries 2004
Chart 2.3 Excessive inpatient waits: intra-UK comparison

Data for England is commissioner-based. Commissioner-based data excludes all patients living outside England and all privately funded patients waiting for treatment in NHS hospitals. However, it does include NHS funded patients living in England who are waiting for treatment in Scotland, Wales and Northern Ireland, abroad and at private hospitals. Data for Scotland excludes those patients waiting with an Availability Status Code (ASC). An ASC refers to certain specified circumstances in which it may not be possible to meet a waiting time standard, e.g. where the patient refuses a reasonable offer of admission.

www.performance.doh.gov.uk/waitingtimes/index.htm

www.wales.gov.uk/keypubstatisticsforwales/content/publication/health/2003/hsw2004/hsw2004-ch6/hsw2004-ch6.htm

www.isdscotland.org/isd/info3.jsp?pContentID=1196&p_applic=CCC&p_service=Content.show&

www.dhsspsni.gov.uk/stats&research/order.asp

Chart 2.4 Numbers of patients waiting for hospital admission and median length of waits: England

Chart 2.4a uses commissioner-based data (*see* Chart 2.2).

Chart 2.4b Median waits are for end March each year. Department of Health official waiting list returns and records the length of time a patient has been *waiting* at a particular return date. This differs from the median total time *waited* by patients admitted over a period of time calculated from Hospital Episode Statistics (HES). Differences in trends mainly reflect the reductions in the proportions of long waiters on hospital lists. A detailed technical paper 'Trends in waiting time to date and total time waited: are the sources compatible?' is available in *Health Statistics Quarterly* (November 2004) at www.statistics.gov.uk/statbase/Product.asp?vlnk=6725&More=N.

For information, median wait data is also available for Scotland. In 1997 median wait was 31 days and in 2044 was 41 days; *see* www.isdscotland.org/isd/files/Annual_trends_in_activity_March_2004_NovRelease.xls.

Chart 2.5 Cancelled operations and rescheduling: England

Data taken from:
www.performance.doh.gov.uk/hospitalactivity/data_requests/cancelled_operations.htm

Chart 2.6 Delayed discharges: England and Scotland

2.6a Since January 2004, local authorities in England have been required to reimburse the NHS for delays in hospital discharge which result from failure to provide necessary assessments or services for a patient. The Cash for Change programme, which started in October 2001, provided £300m to local councils over two years to ensure that they had the capacity to care for people being discharged from hospital who need extra support. Councils also receive an additional £100m per year under the Delayed Discharges Grant.

2.6b To calculate the percentage of acute beds occupied by a delayed discharge, published figures for average available acute beds (annual) were used as the denominator and data from delayed discharge project as numerator. It is interesting to note that there was a target set in March 2002 to increase by 1000 the number of patients transferred to more appropriate care by April 2003, and the corresponding dip in the data at that time.
www.isdscotland.org/isd/info3.jsp?pContentID=1208&p_applic=CCC&p_service=Content.show&
Data for England taken from Chief Executive's Report to the NHS December 2004: www.dh.gov.uk/assetRoot/04/09/75/40/04097540.pdf

Chart 2.7 Outpatient waits: intra-UK comparison

2.7a 2004–05 data is for three-quarters only. NI data is for calendar year, England and Scotland is for financial year.

2.7b Wales reports on waits over three months (rather than 13 weeks). NI data from CH3.
www.performance.doh.gov.uk/waitingtimes/index.htm
www.statswales.wales.gov.uk/TableViewer/tableView.aspx

www.isdscotland.org/isd/info3.jsp?pContentID=1196&p_applic=CCC&p_service=Content.show&
www.dhsspsni.gov.uk/stats&research/order.asp

Chart 2.8 Waiting in A&E: international comparison
Chart 2.9 Waits for primary care
Chart 2.11 Using A&E for primary care

The Commonwealth Fund 2004 survey focused on primary care experiences among adults and consisted of telephone interviews with random, representative samples of people aged 18 and older: AUS 1400; CAN 1410; NZ 1400; UK 3061; US 1401. The Health Foundation partnered with the Commonwealth Fund to expand the UK and enable analysis by UK country. The margin of sampling error is approximately plus or minus three percentage points for differences between countries and plus or minus two percentage points for country averages at the 95% confidence level. Poststratification weights were applied in each country to adjust for variations between the sample demographics and known population parameters. Analysis compared responses between or within countries using t-tests and chi-square tests. The Healthcare Commission is currently undertaking a patient survey of A&E patients which will provide data from a much larger sample of patients.

Chart 2.9 Waits for primary care: international survey data

See entry for Chart 2.8.

Chart 2.10 Waits for primary care appointments: England

Over 123 000 patients in 304 primary care trusts (PCTs) in England were involved in the local health services survey in 2003 (for the question shown, n = 102 152). Over 122 000 registered patients were involved in the 2004 primary care trust (PCT) survey. The survey asked patients from 303 primary care trusts in England about their recent experience of local health services (for the question shown, n = 100 316).
www.healthcarecommission.org.uk/NationalFindings/Surveys/PatientSurveys/fs/en?CONTENT_ID=4000117&chk=XPJRIh

Chart 2.11 Using A&E for primary care

See entry for Chart 2.8.

Chart 2.12 Coronary heart disease waits: Scotland

Data released by ISD Scotland is numbers waiting longer than standards (8 weeks and 12 weeks), compared to total on waiting list. Data is presented in the chart as % patients seen within standard.
www.isdscotland.org/isd/info3.jsp?pContentID=2371&p_applic=CCC&p_service=Content.show&

Chart 2.13 Cancer waits: England

Data from the Department of Health (provider based). Additional context is provided by the number of urgent cancer referrals which increased by 5.4% in the year to September 2004 from 117 118 to 123 391.

www.dh.gov.uk/PolicyAndGuidance/HealthAndSocialCareTopics/Cancer/CancerArticle/fs/en?CONTENT_ID=4001800&chk=dpRNWQ

Chart 3.1 Spending on health: international comparison

OECD data. Total expenditure on health is defined as the sum of expenditure on activities that – through application of medical, paramedical, and nursing knowledge and technology – has the goals of:

- promoting health and preventing disease
- curing illness and reducing premature mortality
- caring for persons affected by chronic illness who require nursing care
- caring for persons with health-related impairments, disability, and handicaps who require nursing care
- assisting patients to die with dignity
- providing and administering public health
- providing and administering health programmes, health insurance and other funding arrangements.

Chart 3.2 Practising physicians per 1000 population

The OECD defines practising physicians as 'The number of physicians, general practitioners and specialists (including self-employed) who are actively practising medicine in public and private institutions. The data should exclude dentists, stomatologists, qualified physicians who are working abroad, working in administration, research and industry positions. Data should include foreign physicians licensed to practice and actively practising medicine in the country.' Data is based on head counts; data shown as 2002 for Australia and the US are 2001 figures; US and French data includes non-practising physicians.

There is no accepted figure for the necessary density of physician numbers required to ensure adequate access to care. High physician density may lead to unnecessary increases in service provision, or 'supplier-induced demand', particularly where payments are on a fee-for service basis. On the other hand, OECD analyses have identified an inverse relationship between physician density and waiting times for elective surgery, indicating the consequences of low density rates for access to care (OECD, Towards high performing health systems, 2004).

Chart 3.3 Staffing: number of consultants

3.3a Numbers of consultants were retrieved from each country's database and the total numbers were divided by the population estimates provided by ONS.

3.3b England data includes Directors of Public Health within consultant numbers. England data generally refers to counts at September each year but for 2004 only, it is the June figure. The corresponding differences in head counts in England is 24 401 consultants in 2000, and 30 171 in 2004 (an increase of 5770 or 24%).

www.dh.gov.uk/PublicationsAndStatistics/Statistics/StatisticalWorkAreas/StatisticalWorkforce/fs/en
www.isdscotland.org/isd/files/WFB08_040825_SH.xls;
www.dhsspsni.gov.uk/stats&research/workforcecen2003.asp
www.wales.gov.uk/keypubstatisticsforwales/content/publication/health/2003/hsw2004/hsw2004-ch14/hsw2004-t14-1.xls;

Chart 3.4 Staffing: number of GPs

3.4a Numbers of GPs were retrieved from each country's database and the total numbers were divided by the population estimates provided by ONS. All figures refer to unrestricted principals or equivalents (UPEs) – a practitioner who is in contract with a PCT or StHA to provide the full range of medical services and whose list is not restricted to any particular group of people. Most people have an Unrestricted Principal as their GP. UPEs also include GMS Unrestricted Principals, PMS Contracted or PMS Salaried Doctors.

3.4b England figures refer to Unrestricted Principals or Equivalents (UPEs). Data in text refers to Practitioners (excluding retainers), these include GP registrars, Restricted Principals, Assistants, Salaried Doctors, Flexible Career Scheme Doctors and GP Returners. NHS Plan group refers to All Practitioners but excludes retainers and registrars.

www.dh.gov.uk/assetRoot/04/10/21/80/04102180.xls
www.wales.gov.uk/keypubstatisticsforwales/content/publication/health/2004/sb58-2004/sb58-2004.htm#uk
www.isdscotland.org/isd/info3.jsp?pContentID=1348&p_applic=CCC&p_service=Content.show&#HCHS

Chart 3.5 Staffing: number of nurses

3.5a Numbers of nurses were retrieved from each country's database and the total numbers were divided by the population estimates provided by ONS. Wales and Northern Ireland data is from 2002.

3.5b Figures include practice nurses. In England, around 6% of wte are midwives; 4% district nurses; 3% health visitors; and 3% registered sick children's nurses.

Chart 3.6 Staffing number of dentists

The OECD data used for international comparators is from 2001. The intra-UK data is based on ONS data and ONS population estimates for 2001. Figures for dentists include principals, assistants and vocational dental practitioners. Salaried dentists, Hospital Dental Services and Community Dental Services are excluded. Further to the data shown, the distribution of dentists is not uniform, ranging from 0.88 per 1000 people in Westminster to 0.16 per 1000 in Ellesmere Port & Neston, although the proportion of time each dentist devotes to NHS patients is unknown (Boulos and Picton-Phillips, 2004).

www.statistics.gov.uk/StatBase/Expodata/Spreadsheets/D5945.xls

www.statistics.gov.uk/downloads/theme_compendia/Regional_Trends_38/rt38.pdf

Chart 3.7 Beds per 1000 population

UK country data is based on reported bed numbers divided by mid-2003 population estimates provided by ONS. International comparators are published by Eurostat and OECD.

www.performance.doh.gov.uk/hospitalactivity/data_requests/download/beds_open_overnight/bed_04_summary.xls

www.dhsspsni.gov.uk/publications/2004/poc-contents.pdf

www.wales.gov.uk/keypubstatisticsforwalesheadline/content/health/2004/hdw20040908-e.htm

www.isdscotland.org/isd/files/Annual_trends_in_available_beds_March_2004_NovRelease.xls

http://epp.eurostat.cec.eu.int/cache/ITY_PUBLIC/3-08032004-AP/EN/3-08032004-AP-EN.HTML

Chart 3.8 Critical care beds

3.8a Data taken from:

www.performance.doh.gov.uk/hospitalactivity/data_requests/critical_care_beds.htm

www.wales.gov.uk/keypubstatisticsforwales/content/publication/health/2003/sb92-2003/sb92-2003-tables.xls

www.dhsspsni.gov.uk/publications/archived/2000/cmointcare.pdf (note NI data is from 2000)

Direct communication from ISD Scotland.

Rates per 100 000 population were calculated using published intensive care bed numbers and mid 2003 population estimates from ONS.

3.8b England data refers to number of beds, and use, on census day.

Chart 3.9 Imaging equipment

Computed tomography (CT or CAT) scanners image anatomical information from a cross-sectional plane of the body. Each image is generated by a computer synthesis of X-ray transmission data obtained in many different directions in a given plane. UK data is for England and Scotland NHS.

Magnetic resonance imaging (MRI) units are a diagnostic modality in which the magnetic nuclei (especially protons) of a patient are aligned in a strong, uniform magnetic field, absorb energy from tuned radio frequency pulses, and emit radio frequency signals as their excitation decays. These signals, which vary in intensity according to nuclear abundance and molecular chemical environment, are converted into sets of tomographic images by using field gradients in the magnetic field, which permit 3-D localisation of the point sources of the signals. Unlike conventional radiography or CT, MRI does not expose patients to ionising radiation. UK data is for 2002 and is from England and Scotland only.

Chart 3.10 Percutaneous coronary interventions: intra-UK comparison

Based on data from 141 Interventional and Diagnostic Centres across the UK.

www.bcis.org.uk/cgi-bin/item.cgi?id=218&d=1&h=28&f=29&dateformat=%o%20%B%20%Y

Chart 3.11 Stroke units

This chart is based on the Royal College of Physicians' National Sentinel Stroke Audit (Clinical Effectiveness and Evaluation Unit) which has taken place on a two-year cycle since 1998. Data was collected within Trusts using a standardised method. Data collection was overseen at a Trust level by a lead clinician for stroke who was responsible for the quality of data supplied. In 2004, the audit achieved 100% participation in England, Wales and Northern Ireland. A stroke unit is defined as a multidisciplinary team including specialist nursing staff based in a discrete ward which has been designated for stroke patients. A Cochrane Review of the evidence base, conducted in 2001 (Stroke Unit Trialists Collaboration), concluded that stroke patients who receive organised inpatient care on a stroke unit are more likely to be alive, independent and living at home one year after the stroke. The benefits were most apparent in units based in a discrete ward.

www.rcplondon.ac.uk/pubs/books/strokeaudit/strokeaudit2004.pdf

Chart 3.12 Acute stroke units: facilities audit

See entry for Chart 3.11 for audit details. Stroke units include the following sub-divisions:

a *Acute stroke units*, which accept patients acutely but discharge early (usually within seven days). This could include an 'intensive' model of care with continuous monitoring and high nurse staffing levels.

b *Rehabilitation stroke units*, which accept patients after a delay of usually seven days or more and focus on rehabilitation.

c *Combined* (i.e. no separation between acute and rehabilitation beds) stroke units that accept patients acutely but also provide rehabilitation for at least several weeks if necessary.

Chart 3.13 Mental health services teams

Data was provided to the Department of Health from the Annual Service Mapping Exercise, University of Durham. 2004 entry is for Spring, all other years refer to Autumn data.

www.dur.ac.uk/service.mapping/amh/

www.dh.gov.uk/assetRoot/04/09/75/40/04097540.pdf

Chart 4.1 Adverse events: routine data source

Researchers examined four years of routinely collected HES data for 1999–00 to 2002–03 (comprising 50 215 687 episodes of care) for any of the 41 three-digit ICD-10 diagnosis codes with an indication of an adverse event. It is noted that hospital-acquired infections are poorly represented within ICD-10 and obstetric complications were excluded from this study. In England and Wales, the National Patient Safety Agency (NPSA) launched the National Reporting and Learning System (NRLS) in 2004. This will be an alternative source of adverse event data. NRLS aims to identify system failures and guide efforts both to understand the problems that underlie those failures and to develop practical solutions. There are plans for the NPSA to publish statistics on trends and issues identified through the NRLS.

http://bmj.bmjjournals.com/cgi/content/full/329/7462/369

Chart 4.2 Adverse events: case notes review

The study was conducted at two acute London hospitals. 500 randomly selected medical records from site 1 were reviewed between July and September 1999; and 514 records from site 2 between December 1999 and February 2000. In both sites the index admissions occurred in two months in 1998. Screening of records was performed by research nurses using predefined screening criteria. Records that screened positive (n = 405) were then reviewed by medically qualified assessors who identified any adverse events and completed a detailed questionnaire.

Chart 4.3 Adverse events under surgical care, Scotland

Based on Scottish Audit of Surgical Mortality (SASM) data. In 2003, there were 4478 deaths identified, of which 4084 were audited. 1.5% of patients admitted to a surgical service died (0.27% of elective admissions and 2.19% of emergency admissions). 344 (8.4%) of the audited deaths had developed a hospital-acquired infection. Delays in obtaining imaging information were noted in 70 patients who died. A fuller analysis of the data is at www.sasm.org.uk.

Chart 4.4 Errors in the preparation of intravenous infusions: observational study

Study design was prospective observation; subjects were 113 nurses and 1 doctor over 76 days; 2 sites, one teaching hospital and one non-teaching. 'Intravenous drug error' was defined as a deviation in preparation or administration of a drug from a doctor's prescription, the hospital's intravenous drug policy, or the manufacturer's instructions. The study used a validated scale to assess clinical importance of errors. Briefly, four healthcare professionals scored the potential clinical importance of each error on a scale between 0 (no harm) and 10 (death). The mean score was calculated, scores < 3 were labelled minor; 3–7 moderate; and > 7 severe.

Chart 4.5 Errors in the preparation of intravenous infusions: acetylcysteine

Prospective collection of pre- and post-infusion samples from acetylcysteine infusion bags and subsequent assay. The median difference between pre- and post-infusion samples was 0% but 9% showed a disparity of greater than ± 50%, suggesting poor mixing of the infusion bag. Systematic calculation errors occurred in 5% of cases (95% confidence interval 2–8%); major errors in drawing up in 3% (1–7%); and inadequate mixing in 9% (4–14%).

Chart 4.6 Infusion error incident study: NPSA

The NPSA set up a project to find out the root causes of incidents involving infusion devices, when no fault with the equipment was identified. The data is drawn from a pilot study in six acute trusts and identified a lack of competency-based staff training and unsystematic purchasing and management of infusion devices as key factors contributing to infusion device incidents. The chart shows the nature of infusion device incidents that occurred in the pilot sites over the period of a year. The two largest participant Trusts identified 82% of all incidents which may indicate poor reporting culture in the smaller sites.

http://81.144.177.110/site/media/documents/541_npsa_full_eval.pdf

Chart 4.7 Surgical healthcare-associated infections: England

Chart is based on data collected between October 1997 and September 2002 from 168 hospitals that participated in the surgical site infection (SSI) module of the Nosocomial Infection National Surveillance Service (NINSS).

www.hpa.org.uk/infections/topics_az/hai/SSIreport.pdf

Chart 4.8 HAIs as a factor in surgical mortality: Scotland

Chart is based on Scottish Audit of Surgical Mortality (SASM) data. In 2003, there were 4478 deaths identified of which 4084 were audited. 1.5% of patients admitted to a surgical service died (0.27% of elective admissions and 2.19% of emergency admissions). www.sasm.org.uk

Chart 4.9 MRSA as a proportion of all *Staphylococcus aureus* bacteraemias: a European comparison

Data provided by European Antimicrobial Resistance Surveillance System (EARSS). Data was collected between January 1999 and December 2000. Reports from 50 759 blood isolates from 27 countries were received. Overall 20% of isolates were reported as methicillin-resistant.
www.earss.rivm.nl/

Chart 4.10 MRSA bacteraemia rates within the countries of the UK

Data was provided separately by each country. The data is based on the number of cases of MRSA bacteraemia in the period, divided by the number of 'acute occupied bed days' (AOBD) for the period. One patient in one bed for one night is one AOBD. The rate is the number of MRSA bacteraemias per 1000 bed days. This rate gives an indication of the number of cases relative to the size of the population at risk (www.show.scot.nhs.uk). The denominator data for Wales was obtained from the Health Solutions Wales database, Quest 1.
www.show.scot.nhs.uk/scieh/infectious/hai/MRSA_Scot.htm
www.wales.nhs.uk/sites/documents/379/S.aureus%20bacteraemia%20Report%20up%20to%20310304%20anon.pdf
www.hpa.org.uk/cdr/PDFfiles/2004/cdr2904.pdf
www.nics.gov.uk/press/hss/041005a-hss.htm

Chart 4.11 Deaths involving MRSA

Since 1993 ONS has stored the text of death certificates on its database, along with the ICD coding relating to causes identified on the death certificate. The authors undertook a 3 stage process to extract deaths mentioning *S. aureus* and then MRSA. 1. All deaths with a code that related to *S. aureus* on the death certificate were extracted and manually searched for any mention of MRSA. 2. All deaths with a non-specific code relating to infection were manually searched for both *S. aureus* and MRSA. 3. Neonatal deaths were searched for separately. For fuller details of ICD codes see:
www.statistics.gov.uk/downloads/theme_health/HSQ21.pdf

Chart 4.12 Hospitals' effectiveness at finding and addressing medical error: physicians' views

The 2000 Commonwealth Fund International Health Policy Survey focused on ascertaining physicians' views about their healthcare organisations and systems. Approximately 400 randomly selected generalist physicians and 100 specialist physicians (cardiologists, gastroenterologists, and oncologists) were interviewed in each country. Sample sizes were AUS 517; CAN 533; NZ 493; UK 500; US 528. The surveys were conducted by a combination of mail, telephone, and Internet during the period 27 April–27 July 2000. Samples of 500 respondents are associated with sampling errors of approximately ± 4%. Sources of non-sampling error include potential non-response bias, question wording and ordering effects, and cross-cultural differences in question interpretation.
www.cmwf.org/publications/publications_show.htm?doc_id=221237

Chart 4.13 Safety views of hospital executives

The 2003 Commonwealth Fund International Health Policy Survey consisted of interviews with hospital executives of larger hospitals in Australia, Canada, New Zealand, the United Kingdom and the United States. The survey drew random samples from lists of the largest general or paediatric hospital in each country, excluding specialty hospitals. The largest hospitals in Australia and Canada had 100 or more beds; and in the UK and US had 200 or more beds. In New Zealand the study included hospitals in the country's 34 District Health Boards, regardless of size. Final survey size was AUS 100; CAN 102; NZ 28; UK 103; US 205.
www.cmwf.org/surveys/surveys_list.htm?attrib_id=9121&attrib_filter=1

Chart 4.14 Medical errors and their consequences: patients' perspective
Chart 4.15 Medication errors: patients' perspective

The Commonwealth Fund 2002 International Health Policy Survey consisted of telephone interviews with adults with health problems. The survey screened initial random samples of adults 18 or older to identify those who met at least one of four criteria: reported their health as fair or poor; or in the past two years had serious illness that required intensive medical care, major surgery or hospitalisation for something other than a normal birth. These questions resulted in final survey samples of: AUS 844; CAN 750; NZ 750; UK 750; and US 755. These samples represent one-quarter to one-third of the adults initially contacted.
www.cmwf.org/surveys/surveys_list.htm?attrib_id=9121&attrib_filter=1

Chart 4.15 Medication errors: patients' perspective
Chart 4.17 Managing polypharmacy risks

The Commonwealth Fund 2004 survey focused on primary care experiences among adults and consisted of telephone interviews with random, representative samples of people aged 18 and older: AUS 1400; CAN 1410; NZ 1400; UK 3061; US 1401. The margin of sampling error is approximately plus or minus three percentage points for differences between countries and plus or minus two percentage points for country averages at the 95% confidence level. Poststratification weights were applied in each country to adjust for variations between the sample demographics and known population parameters. Analysis compared responses between or within countries using t-tests and chi-square tests.
www.cmwf.org/surveys/surveys_list.htm?attrib_id=9121&attrib_filter=1

Chart 4.16 Safety issues after discharge from hospital

The inpatient survey involved 169 acute and specialist NHS Trusts in England and responses were received from more than 88 000 patients (for questions reading from top to bottom: n=60 831; 51 975; 64 644). The young patient survey involved 150 acute and specialist NHS Trusts and responses were received from more than 62 000 young people or their parents (for questions reading from top to bottom: n = 49 798; 35 173; 41 358).

Chart 4.17

See note for Chart 4.15.

Chart 5.1 Extent of change required: international comparison
Chart 5.2 Extent of change required: UK time series
Chart 5.8 Choice in physicians: international comparison
Chart 5.11 Interactions with GP: international comparison
Chart 5.12 Doctor–patient communication (GP)
Chart 5.13 Patient access to medical record: desired and achieved

The 2004 Commonwealth Fund International Health Policy Survey focused on primary care and ambulatory care experiences. It consisted of telephone interviews with random, representative samples of people aged 18 and older: in 1400 in Australia, 1410 in Canada, 1400 in New Zealand, 3061 in the United Kingdom and 1401 in the United States. The Commonwealth Fund provided support for random samples of 1400 in each country. The Health Foundation partnered with the fund to expand the UK and enable future analysis by UK country. For the intra-UK survey, sample numbers were England 1561; Scotland 503; Wales 500; Northern Ireland 500.

Chart 5.3 Getting better or worse: perceptions in Scotland
Chart 5.6 Ratings of care in Scotland
Chart 5.9 Choice in referrals
Chart 5.14 Extent of public influence on NHS in Scotland

In 2000, Fieldwork was carried out by using Computer Assisted Telephone Interviewing (CATI). A sample of telephone numbers was generated by Random Digit Dialling and interviewers then worked to quotas, which were based on the results of the Scottish Household Survey and designed to reflect the characteristics of the population in terms of age, sex, working status and tenure. In total, 3052 interviews were conducted with adults (aged 16 and over) in September to October.

In 2004, 2600 telephone interviews were conducted in March and April with a representative sample of adults aged 16 and over, from all parts of Scotland. The sample frame consisted of randomly generated numbers in proportion to the population distribution across Scotland. The sample profile was quota-controlled by sex, age, working status and region.

For information, the expectation results in 2000 were much better 14%; a bit better 30%; unchanged 27%; a bit worse 22%; much worse 8%.
www.scotland.gov.uk/cru/kd01/purple/panhs-00.asp
www.scotland.gov.uk/library5/government/panhss-00.asp

Chart 5.4 Patient ratings at hospital and mental healthcare in England
Chart 5.9 Choice in referrals
Chart 5.10 Involvement in decision-making
Chart 5.15 Patient perceptions: treated with respect and dignity
Chart 5.16 Patient perceptions: confidence and trust
Chart 5.18: Cleanliness
Chart 5.19 Mixed-sex wards

The inpatient survey involved 169 acute and specialist NHS Trusts, and responses were received from more than 88 000 patients.

The young patient survey involved 150 acute and specialist NHS Trusts, and responses were received from more than 62 000 young people, or their parents.

The mental health survey involved 81 NHS Trusts that are responsible for providing secondary mental health services (including combined mental health and social care trusts, and primary care trusts). Responses were received from more than 27 000 service users.

The primary care trust (PCT) survey involved 303 primary care NHS Trusts, and responses were received from more than 122 000 registered patients.
www.nhssurveys.org

Chart 5.5 Public ratings of healthcare services in Northern Ireland
Chart 5.17 Fair treatment: Northern Ireland

Telephone interviews were conducted with 1500 adults in April–May 2004. In the first instance the Northern Ireland Electoral Register was used as the sampling frame for the survey with a simple random sample of addresses, with telephone numbers, selected from each of the 26 Local Government Districts.
www.dhsspsni.gov.uk/publications/2004/pas/pas-report.asp

Chart 5.6 Public ratings of healthcare services in Scotland

See entry for Chart 5.3.

Chart 5.7 Choice in hospitals

YouGov/Economist survey conducted 26–29 March 2004 with 2254 respondents.

Chart 5.8 Choice in physicians: international comparison

See entry for Chart 5.1.

Chart 5.9 Choice in referrals

See entries for Chart 5.3 and Chart 5.4.

Chart 5.10 Involvement in decision-making

See entry for Chart 5.4.

Chart 5.11 Interactions with GP: international comparison

See entry for Chart 5.1.

Chart 5.12 Communicating about treatment options in primary care

See entry for Chart 5.1.

Those countries with the highest and lowest ratings (Australia and US) from the international survey were included for reference points.

Chart 5.13 Patient access to medical record: desired and achieved

See entry for Chart 5.1.

Chart 5.14 Extent of public influence on NHS in Scotland

See entry for Chart 5.3.

Chart 5.15 Patient perceptions: treated with respect and dignity

See entry for Chart 5.4.

Chart 5.16 Patient perceptions: confidence and trust

See entry for Chart 5.4.

Chart 5.17 Fair treatment: Northern Ireland

See entry for Chart 5.5.

Chart 5.18 Cleanliness and healthcare facilities

See entry for Chart 5.4.

Chart 5.19 Mixed-sex wards

See entry for Chart 5.4.

Chart 6.1: Life expectancy

6.1a ONS data. Results are rolling averages, produced by aggregating deaths and population estimates for each three-year period. Details on populations, health authority level data, and methods for the calculation and interpretation of life expectancy at birth are at www.statistics.gov.uk/statbase/Product.asp?vlnk=8841.

6.1b Healthcare Commission analysis. Uses ONS data for life expectancies for each Local Authority (LA) in England and compares with deprivation scores (Index of Multiple Deprivation or IMD 2004) for each LA (as provided by the Office of the Deputy Prime Minister www.odpm.gov.uk). A similar picture is found in Scotland, *see* www.dph.gla.ac.uk/hppu/publns/HealthInequalitiesReport.pdf.

Chart 6.2 Infant mortality by socio-economic status

ONS data, three-year rolling averages. Social class is defined by father's occupation; dataset does not include sole registrations. Categorisations of social class have been superseded by NS-SEC classification. Data from 1996–2001 uses social class groups IIIM, IV and V for routine/manual aggregation; whereas 2002 data uses socio-economic classification Groups 5, 6, and 7. Mortality data from www.statistics.gov.uk/statbase/Product.asp?vlnk=6305.
2001–03 data from www.dh.gov.uk/assetRoot/04/09/83/48/04098348.pdf.

Chart 6.3 Low birth weight by deprivation, England 2002

ONS data on percentages of low birth weight infants (< 2500 grams); Healthcare Commission analysis cross referencing deprivation (IMD 2004 quintiles) to low birth weight.

Chart 6.4 Smoking in pregnancy

Infant Feeding 2000 is the sixth national survey of infant feeding practices, surveying mothers of babies born between August and October 2000. It surveyed around 9100 mothers from the UK: 5200 from England and Wales; 2150 from Scotland; 1750 from Northern Ireland. National Statistics Socio-Economic Classification (NS-SEC) is used to stratify responses. Within NS-SEC (3 class), higher occupations include managerial and professional occupations; intermediate occupations include small employers and own-account workers; and lower occupations include lower supervisory and technical occupations as well as semi-routine and routine occupations.

Chart 6.5 Socio-economic disparities in cancer survival

2.2 million patients from England and Wales in broader study from which this data is drawn. Data was collected on patients diagnosed with 20 most common cancers 1986–2001. Patients were assigned to category of socio-economic deprivation based on their electoral ward at time of diagnosis (Carstairs deprivation index). 95% confidence intervals: Colon (M) 3.4–8.0; Colon (F) 5.1–9.4; Rectum

(M) 6.8–12.0; Rectum (F) 5.2–11.4; Breast (F) 4.8–6.7; Cervix (F) 1.7–8.4; Prostate (M) 5.5–9.0.

Chart 6.6 Avoidable admissions by deprivation

Charts a and b use Hospital Episode Statistics (HES) data and IMD 2004 deprivation quintiles.

6.6a: Data for where asthma was recorded as primary diagnosis in admission episodes, 2002–03.

6.6b: All admission episodes with diabetes in any diagnosis field. Both use indirectly age and sex standardised admission ratios, with England standardised to 100.

Chart 6.7 Diabetic control in children by deprivation

The National Paediatric Diabetes Audit is a joint initiative between Diabetes UK, the Royal College of Paediatrics and Child Health (RCPCH), the British Society for Paediatric Endocrinology and Diabetes (BSPED) and the Royal College of Nursing (RCN). The cohort for children with diabetes was 11 696, collated from 111 hospitals with paediatric diabetes services in England together with aggregated data from Northern Ireland, Wales and Jersey; of these 7.2% were from a minority ethnic group. The mean age of the cohort was 11.3 years, the mean duration of diabetes 4.0 years and the mean age at diagnosis was 7.2 years. Some 52% of the children were male and 48% were female; 97% of the children have type 1 diabetes. The overall mean HbA1c was 8.98% (target 7.5%). Where ethnicity is recorded (88% of reports) white children had statistically significantly lower HbA1c results than the combined group of non-white children. Girls generally showed poorer average HbA1c results for blood glucose control than boys and this became more apparent as they got older. Deprivation quintiles were based on the Carstairs deprivation index. 95% confidence intervals for quintile 1(Q1): 8.74–8.97; Q2: 8.80–9.01; Q3: 8.89–9.07; Q4: 8.97–9.16; Q5: 9.08–9.27.
www.diabetes.org.uk/audit/downloads/PaediatricAuditReport.pdf

Chart 6.8 Anticipated costs as a barrier to care
Chart 6.9 Cost disincentives to healthcare

The Commonwealth Fund International Health Policy Survey 2004 focused on primary care and ambulatory care experiences. It consisted of telephone interviews with random, representative samples of people age 18 and older: 1400 in Australia, 1410 in Canada, 1400 in New Zealand, 3061 in the United Kingdom, and 1401 in the United States. The authors state that the margin of sampling error is approximately ± 3 percentage points for differences between countries and ± 2 percentage points for country averages at the 95% confidence level. Poststratifica-

tion weights were applied in each country to adjust for variations between the sample demographics and known population parameters. Analysis compared responses between or within countries using t-tests and chi-square tests.
www.cmwf.org/publications/publications_show.htm?doc_id=245178

Chart 6.10 Influenza vaccinations by deprivation

Based on data collected from NHS Trusts in England for 2004 star ratings. Deprivation quintiles are based on IMD 2004.

Chart 6.11 Cancer screening rates by deprivation

6.11a Cervical cancer screening data provided by Department of Health, refers to uptake at 3.5 years for women aged 25–64.
6.11b Breast cancer screening data is provided by Department of Health, refers to uptake at three years for women aged 53–64. Both charts use IMD 2004 deprivation quintiles and primary care organisation distribution.
'Uptake' refers to the percentage of women invited for screening who attend. This figure differs from 'coverage' which is the percentage of eligible women who have been screened.

Chart 6.12 Socio-economic deprivation and heart failure: incidence, consultations and survival

This study of 53 general practices (307 741 patients) identified 2186 patients who were seen at least once for heart failure between April 1999 and March 2000. Rates shown are age and sex-standardised. Deprivation quintiles were assigned using postcodes of residence and the Carstairs deprivation index.

Chart 6.13 Gender-based disparities in revascularisation rates in patients ≥ 65 years

Data was taken from ONS in England and National Hospital Discharge Survey in the US. The study used the ratio of procedures to acute myocardial infarction (AMI) discharge rates (a proxy for disease burden).

Chart 6.14 Prescribing for older people

Data was collected from the same 62 hospitals in England in 1999 and 2000. Each hospital collected data on 100 consecutive patients aged over 65 years of age, from medical wards, but not from surgical or psychiatric wards. Data was also collected on % drugs prescribed with a generic name (83% in 1999 and 86% in 2000) and % adjusted appropriate use of anti-thrombotics in atrial fibrillation (54% in 1999 and 57% in 2000).

Appendix A: Search terms for literature search

Searches were conducted using PubMed in May 2004.

1. (Process assessment [MeSH] OR outcome assessment [MeSH]) AND quality AND NHS
2. Assess* AND health care quality, access and evaluation [MeSH] AND (Process assessment [MeSH] OR outcome assessment [MeSH])
3. Great Britain[MeSH] AND (process assessment [MeSH] OR outcome assessment [MeSH]) AND quality of care
4. Great Britain[MeSH] AND (process assessment [MeSH] OR outcome assessment [MeSH]) AND quality of health care [MeSH] AND evaluation
5. Great Britain[MeSH] AND assess* AND data AND quality of care
6. Great Britain[MeSH] AND data AND acute myocardial infarction
7. Great Britain[MeSH] AND data AND outcomes AND stroke
8. Great Britain[MeSH] AND data AND outcomes AND diabetes
9. Great Britain[MeSH] AND data AND outcomes AND coronary heart disease
10. Great Britain[MeSH] AND data AND outcomes AND depression
11. Great Britain[MeSH] AND trend AND hospital acquired infection
12. Great Britain[MeSH] AND hospital acquired infection AND (data OR surveillance)
13. Great Britain[MeSH] AND trend AND mortality
14. Great Britain[MeSH] AND trend AND morbidity
15. Great Britain[MeSH] AND data AND arthritis
16. Great Britain[MeSH] AND (Process assessment [MeSH] OR outcome assessment [MeSH]) AND quality AND surg*
17. Target* AND NHS AND data
18. Great Britain[MeSH] AND Falls AND incidence
19. Great Britain[MeSH] AND error AND incidence
20. Great Britain[MeSH] AND adverse incidents AND data
21. Great Britain[MeSH] AND medical mistakes AND data
22. Great Britain[MeSH] AND preventable adverse event AND data
23. Great Britain[MeSH] AND inappropriate treatment AND data
24. Great Britain[MeSH] AND unnecessary procedures [MeSH] AND data
25. Great Britain[MeSH] AND unmet health needs AND data
26. Great Britain[MeSH] AND ageism AND data
27. Great Britain[MeSH] AND (racism OR sexism) AND data
28. Great Britain[MeSH] AND statins AND data
29. Great Britain[MeSH] AND antibiotics AND (sore throat OR respiratory)
30. Great Britain[MeSH] AND palliative care AND data
31. Great Britain[MeSH] AND smoking cessation AND data
32. Great Britain[MeSH] AND obesity AND data
33. Great Britain[MeSH] AND caesarean section AND rates

Chartbook statistical glossary

Age standardisation is a statistical method that facilitates meaningful comparisons between two or more populations with different age structures. Age standardisation attenuates differences in mortality, incidence, or survival that reflect the fact that one population is much older and thus more likely to be diagnosed and die from a particular disease. Different datasets use different standardisation methods, e.g. European, World, Organisation for Economic Cooperation and Development (OECD). Results are not directly comparable if different standardisation populations have been used.

Avoidable mortality refers to deaths that should *not* occur in the presence of effective and timely healthcare. It tallies deaths from conditions that are *amenable* to treatment and medical care; for example, with appropriate diagnosis and treatment no deaths ought to occur from appendicitis. It also includes deaths from conditions that are *preventable*; for example, those diseases which are a result of behavioural and lifestyle choices, such as smoking-related lung cancer.

Case-mix adjustment is the process of adjusting for differences in the complexity and severity of clinical cases treated by different doctors, teams or hospitals, so that their costs or outcomes can be compared.

Confidence interval is an estimated range of values that is likely to include an unknown population parameter, the estimated range being calculated from a given set of sample data. A 95% confidence interval means that if the population were sampled many times, 19 out of 20 times the interval would contain the true result.

Deprivation quintiles separate a population into five bands according to the level of deprivation. As an illustration of the factors taken into account, the Index of Multiple Deprivation (IMD 2004) incorporates indicators from seven domains with different weights:

- income deprivation (22.5%)
- employment deprivation (22.5%)
- health deprivation and disability (13.5%)
- education, skills and training deprivation (13.5%)
- barriers to housing and services (9.3%)
- living environment deprivation (9.3%)
- crime (9.3%).

Source: www.odpm.gov.uk/stellent/groups/odpm_urbanpolicy/documents/downloadable/odpm_urbpol_029247.pdf.

Stratification into IMD deprivation quintiles is based on geographical area in which a subject lives (often local authority areas). There are alternative indexes available (e.g. Townsend or Carstairs) which use different formulae and weighting but result in similar types of stratification of the population.

Hazard ratio is the relative risk of an endpoint occurring at a given time. Using death as an example endpoint, the hazard ratio compares the risk of death in group 1 to the risk of death in group 2.

Incidence refers to new instances (or registrations) of disease that occur within a defined time period in a specified population. We include them as one measure of disease burden affecting rates of mortality.

Mean (or average) is a measure of central value for a distribution. It is calculated by taking the sum of the observations and dividing by their number (n).

Median is a measure of central tendency. It is the central value of a distribution, that is, half the points in the distribution are less than or equal to it and half are greater than or equal to it.

Mortality rates are the number of deaths occurring in a given period divided by the number of people in the population of interest. They provide an overall measure of health outcomes determined in part by the quality of healthcare along with other factors such as disease incidence and severity and socio-economic attributes and patient behaviours. Rates are not simply numbers, they are numerators and denominators.

NS-SEC The National Statistics Socio-economic Classification (NS-SEC) has been used for all official statistics and surveys from 2001 onwards. The NS-SEC is an occupationally based classification with rules to provide coverage of the whole adult population. The version of the classification, which will be used for most analyses in this chartbook, has eight classes, the first of which can be subdivided (*see* Table 1 below). For complete coverage, the three categories Students, Occupations not stated or inadequately described and Not classifiable for other reasons are added as 'Not classified'. For further details, refer to: www.statistics.gov.uk/methods_quality/ns_sec/downloads/NS-SEC-USER-VER1-2.pdf.

The **odds ratio** is a way of comparing whether the probability of a certain event or risk factor is the same for two groups. An odds ratio of 1 implies that the event is equally likely in both groups. An odds ratio greater than one implies that the event is more likely in the first group. An odds ratio less than one implies that the event is less likely in the first group.

Prevalence is the number of current cases of a disease per population at risk.

Relative risk is the ratio of the probability of developing, in a specified period of time, an outcome among those receiving the treatment of interest or exposed to a risk factor, compared with the probability of developing the outcome if the risk factor or intervention is not present.

Socio-economic classification. A classification sorts a large set of observations or entities on the basis of shared characteristics and provides a framework for the description and comparison of statistics. In the UK, the National Statistics Socio-economic Classification (NS-SEC) is one of the most widely-used standard classifications. It stratifies the population on the basis of occupational group (*see* entry for NS-SEC).

Survival rates are a measure of the effectiveness of healthcare services in early detection and treatment of disease. The time from diagnosis of cancer to death is tracked by cancer registries. The five-year **relative survival rate** is the number of patients still alive five years after their initial diagnosis and is adjusted for expected deaths from other causes.

Table 1

8 classes	5 classes	3 classes

1 Higher managerial and professional occupations
  1.1 Large employers and higher managerial occupations
  1.2 Higher professional occupations
2 Lower managerial and professional occupations
	1 Managerial and professional occupations	1 Managerial and professional occupations

3 Intermediate occupations	2 Intermediate occupations	2 Intermediate occupations
4 Small employers and own account workers	3 Small employers and own account workers	
5 Lower supervisory and technical occupations	4 Lower supervisory and technical occupations	3 Routine and manual occupations
6 Semi-routine occupations	5 Semi-routine and routine occupations	
7 Routine occupations	† – – – – – – – – – – – – – – – – – – –	† – – – – – – – – – – – – – – – – – – –
8 Never worked and long-term unemployed	Never worked and long-term unemployed	Never worked and long-term unemployed

Source: ONS.

ACC	American College of Cardiology
ADE	Adverse Drug Event
AHA	American Heart Association
AHRQ	Agency for Healthcare Research and Quality (US)
AMI	Acute Myocardial Infarction
AUS	Australia
CABG	Coronary Artery Bypass Graft
CAN	Canada
CDR	Communicable Disease Report (England & Wales)
CHD	Coronary Heart Disease
CHF	Congestive Heart Failure
CMO	Chief Medical Officer
CPO	Chief Pharmaceutical Officer
CRAG	Clinical Resource and Audit Group (Scotland)
CSBS	Clinical Standards Board for Scotland
DH	Department of Health (England)
DHSSPS	Department of Health, Social Services and Public Safety (Northern Ireland)
EARSS	European Antimicrobial Resistance Surveillance System
GP	General Practitioner (family doctor)
HAI	Healthcare-Associated Infection (*or* Hospital-Acquired Infection)
HES	Hospital Episode Statistics (England)
HPA	Health Protection Agency (England & Wales)
HPSS	Health and Personal Social Services (Northern Ireland)
HTBS	Health Technology Board of Scotland
IARC	International Agency for Research on Cancer (WHO)
ICD	International Classification of Disease
IOM	Institute of Medicine (US)
ISD	Information and Statistics Division (Scotland)

MHRA	Medicines and Healthcare Products Regulatory Agency (UK)
MINAP	Myocardial Infarction National Audit Project (Royal College of Physicians)
MRSA	Methicillin-resistant *Staphylococcus aureus*
NAO	National Audit Office (UK)
NCCMERP	National Coordinating Council for Medication Error Reporting and Prevention (US)
NCHOD	National Centre for Health Outcomes Development (England)
NHQR	National Healthcare Quality Report (US)
NHS	National Health Service (UK)
NICE	National Institute for Clinical Excellence (England & Wales)
NINSS	Nosocomial Infection National Surveillance Service (England & Wales)
NPSA	National Patient Safety Agency (England & Wales)
NSF	National Service Framework
NZ	New Zealand
OECD	Organisation for Economic Cooperation and Development
ONS	Office for National Statistics (UK)
PCI	Percutaneous Coronary Intervention
PSA	Public Service Agreement (UK)
PTCA	Percutaneous Transluminal Coronary Angioplasty
QIS	Quality Improvement Scotland
SASM	Scottish Audit of Surgical Mortality
SIGN	Scottish Intercollegiate Guidelines Network
STEMI	ST-elevated Myocardial Infarction
UK	United Kingdom
US	United States
WHO	World Health Organization
wte	Whole-time Equivalent

Index